Sudan's Nuba Mountains
People Under Siege

Sudan's Nuba Mountains People Under Siege

Accounts by Humanitarians in the Battle Zone

Edited by SAMUEL TOTTEN

Foreword by BARONESS CAROLINE COX
Afterword by ISRAEL W. CHARNY

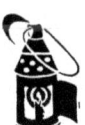

McFarland & Company, Inc., Publishers
Jefferson, North Carolina

LIBRARY OF CONGRESS CATALOGUING-IN-PUBLICATION DATA

Names: Totten, Samuel, editor of compilation.
Title: Sudan's Nuba Mountains people under siege : accounts by humanitarians in the battle zone / edited by Samuel Totten ; foreword by Baroness Caroline Cox ; afterword by Israel W. Charny.
Description: Jefferson, North Carolina : McFarland & Company, Inc., Publishers, 2017. | Includes bibliographical references and index.
Identifiers: LCCN 2016051900 | ISBN 9781476667225 (softcover : acid free paper) ∞
Subjects: LCSH: Nuba (African people)—Social conditions. | Kurdufān al-Janūbīyah (Sudan)—Social conditions. | Sudan—History—Darfur Conflict, 2003—Personal narratives. | Humanitarian assistance—Sudan—Kurdufān al-Janūbīyah. | Visitors, Foreign—Sudan—Kurdufān al-Janūbīyah—Biography. | Medical personnel—Sudan—Kurdufān al-Janūbīyah—Biography. | Missionaries—Sudan—Kurdufān al-Janūbīyah—Biography. | Philanthropists—Sudan—Kurdufān al-Janūbīyah—Biography.
Classification: LCC DT155.2.N82 S83 2017 | DDC 962.404/3—dc23
LC record available at https://lccn.loc.gov/2016051900

BRITISH LIBRARY CATALOGUING DATA ARE AVAILABLE

ISBN (print) 978-1-4766-6722-5
ISBN (ebook) 978-1-4766-2715-1

© 2017 Samuel Totten. All rights reserved

No part of this book may be reproduced or transmitted in any form or by any means, electronic or mechanical, including photocopying or recording, or by any information storage and retrieval system, without permission in writing from the publisher.

Front cover artwork: *Bombings and Extreme Hunger Force Nuba Mountains People from Their Villages and Homes*, watercolor on 140 lb cold press paper 17" × 22", © 2016 Kathleen Barta

Printed in the United States of America

*McFarland & Company, Inc., Publishers
Box 611, Jefferson, North Carolina 28640
www.mcfarlandpub.com*

First, I wish to dedicate this book to my dear wife, Kathleen Maria Barta, for her unconditional love, her remarkable and sustained support in regard to my efforts in war-torn regions of the world despite her anxieties of what may become of me, and her incredible contributions to my efforts in the refugee camps along the Chad/Darfur, Sudan border, and the Nuba Mountains in Sudan.

I also wish to dedicate this book to each of the individuals whose stories appear herein. They are a unique, caring, dedicated and intrepid group of individuals. Some are dear friends, others are acquaintances, and still others are "colleagues" of sorts whom I either know by reputation and/or only via email, but in the end they will always be an inspiration to me.

And last but certainly not least, I dedicate this book to the people of the Nuba Mountains who simply desire to live peaceful lives on their ancestral land with the opportunity to honor and practice their unique cultural ways and way of life, to enjoy their God-given rights, including the freedom to practice their religion of choice, to have a voice in their local, state and national affairs, and to be treated fairly and as equals among and along with their fellow Sudanese, no matter their "race," tribal affiliation, color, religion, or political leanings. They will always be in my heart.

Table of Contents

Glossary	ix
List of Acronyms	xvii
Foreword (Baroness Caroline Cox)	1
Introduction (Samuel Totten)	11
A Love for the Nuba People TOMO KRIŽNAR	21
Doing God's Work RYAN BOYETTE	38
On the Frontlines of Medicine TOM CATENA, M.D.	49
In the Service of Christ: My "Tours" in the Nuba Mountains SISTER DEIRDRE M. BYRNE, M.D.	64
A Son of the Nuba: From Forced Exile to My Return as a Humanitarian GEORGE TUTU	75
Confronting War Crimes in the Nuba Mountains of Sudan MATT CHANCEY	101
A Moral Imperative: From Conducting Research in the Nuba Mountains to Hauling Food to Those in Most Critical Need SAMUEL TOTTEN	114
Sojourns Through Worlds of Suffering JOHN C. JEFFERSON	160
Doctoring in the Nuba Mountains During Wartime JOHN P. SUTTER, M.D.	189
Medical Missions to the Nuba War Zone CORRY CHAPMAN, M.D.	204

Sowing Seeds of Peace: My Life at Mother of Mercy Hospital
　MARGARET CAMARCA   210

A Small Town Doctor Responds to the Needs of the Nuba
　C. LOUIS PERRINJAQUET, M.D.   225

Afterword (Israel W. Charny)   246

Annotated Bibliography   251

About the Contributors   259

Index   261

Glossary

Abdel Aziz Adam Al-Hilu (commonly referred to as simply Abdel Aziz): Aziz was a SPLM commander in the south's fight against the north (1983–2005). Subsequently, he became deputy governor of South Kordofan, Sudan. In 2011, he ran for the governor of South Kordofan against Ahmed Haroun and lost. The SPLM–North decried the election as rigged. Shortly thereafter, war broke between the SPLM–N and the Government of Sudan, with Aziz serving as the commander of SPLM–N.

Abid: "Slave" in Arabic.

African Union (AU): Formerly the Organization of African Unity (OAU), the AU is a union of 54 African States concerned broadly with African solidarity, development, security, sovereignty, politics, and economics. According to the AU's vision statement, the AU strives for "an integrated, prosperous and peaceful Africa, driven by its own citizens and representing a dynamic force in the global arena."

Antonovs: The Government of Sudan planes that carried out attacks on the black African villages in Darfur in the early 2000s and that have carried out (and continue to do so through today) (June 2011–present or January 2017) attacks against the civilian population of the Nuba Mountains. Purchased by Sudan from Russia, Antonovs are Russian cargo planes retrofitted to serve as bombers.

Arabization: A phenomenon involving ever-increasing cultural influence on a non–Arab area, gradually resulting in one that becomes Arabic in speech, worship, social and political practice, education and often legally (e.g., Shari'a, Islamic law). A key goal of Arabization, then, is the complete transformation of an area/society.

Ban Ki-moon: Secretary General of the United Nations from 2007 through 2016.

Bashir, Omar al-: The president of Sudan (1989–present). Al-Bashir became president of Sudan in 1989 following a coup d'état that he and his fellow military officers carried out. He is wanted by the International Criminal Court on charges of crimes against humanity, war crimes and genocide for alleged atrocities perpetrated in Darfur between 2003 and 2008.

Black Africans: The Arab people of Sudan refer to non–Arabs as "black Africans," and the so-called black Africans refer to themselves as black Africans in order to distinguish themselves from the Arabs.

Blue Nile State: A state in Sudan. Since August 2011, primarily resulting from serious differences concerning the implementation of the Comprehensive Peace Agreement in the region, a faction in the Blue Nile State rebelled. Subsequently, the Government of Sudan (GoS) have carried out wholesale attacks on the populace of the region. As a result of the attacks by the GoS, massive numbers of civilians have fled their villages.

Comprehensive Peace Agreement (CPA): Following the catastrophic Second Sudanese Civil War (1983–2005), in which an estimated two million people died and another four million were forced from their villages and homes, a peace agreement (The Comprehensive Peace Agreement) was signed in 2005.

Under the mediation of the Intergovernmental Authority on Development (IGAD), the Government of the Sudan and the SPLM/A signed a series of six agreements:

x Glossary

- The Protocol of Machakos: Signed in Machakos, Kenya, on July 20, 2002, in which the parties agreed on a broad framework, setting forth the principles of governance, the transitional process and the structures of government as well as on the right to self-determination for the people of South Sudan, and on state and religion
- The Protocol on security arrangements: Signed in Naivasha, Kenya, on September 25, 2003
- The Protocol on wealth-sharing: Signed in Naivasha, Kenya, on January 7, 2004
- The Protocol on power-sharing: Signed in Naivasha, Kenya, on May 26, 2004
- The Protocol on the resolution of conflict in southern Kordofan/Nuba Mountains and the Blue Nile States: Signed in Naivasha, Kenya, on May 26, 2004
- The Protocol on the resolution of conflict in Abyei: Signed in Naivasha, Kenya, on May 26, 2004.

The last series of talks were held between the First Vice-President Ali Osman Taha and the Chairman of the SPLM/A, John Garang.

Crimes against humanity: Widespread systematic violence against a civilian population, which includes: murder; extermination; enslavement; deportation or forcible transfer of population; imprisonment; torture; rape, sexual slavery, enforced prostitution, forced pregnancy, enforced sterilization, or any other form of sexual violence of comparable gravity; persecution against an identifiable group on political, racial, national, ethnic, cultural, religious or gender grounds; enforced disappearances of persons; the crime of apartheid; and other inhumane acts of a similar character intentionally causing great suffering and serious bodily or mental injury. Since 1948, crimes against humanity have fallen under the jurisdiction of the United Nations Security Council, which now refers cases to the International Criminal Court for prosecution.

Darfur: A region in West Sudan comprised of five states: North Darfur, South Darfur, East Darfur, West Darfur, and Central Darfur. From 2003 to 2008, Darfur was the site of a brutal counter-insurgency against the JEM and SLM/A that targeted black African civilians from the Fur, Zaghawa, and Masalit tribal groups. The United Nations Commission of Inquiry (January 2005) defined these atrocities as crimes against humanity (January 2005), while the United States defined them as genocide (September 2004), and the International Criminal Court defined them as crimes against humanity and war crimes (2009) and genocide (2010).

Ethnic cleansing: The term ethnic cleansing has been used in various ways by different scholars, human rights organizations, attorneys, and victims of human rights violations. In its simplest and easiest to understand definition, it is the systematic and forced removal of an ethnic group from a city/town, region or society via deportation. Generally, the threat of violence, if not actual violence, is used to carry out the deportation. In some cases, scholars and others have used the term as a synonym for genocide, which is incorrect. While ethnic cleansing could certainly take place as genocide is being perpetrated, they are not one and the same.

Garang, John: Garang was the leader of the People's Liberation Movement in southern Sudan during the Second Sudanese Civil War (1983–2005) between the north and the south. Following the signing of the Comprehensive Peace Agreement (CPA), which brought the war to a close, Garang became the Vice President of Sudan.

A Dinka who was raised by a Christian family, Garang attended Grinnell College in Iowa, and later earned a graduate degree in economics at Iowa State University. Upon his graduation from Grinnell, Garang returned to Sudan where he joined the Anya Nya rebel group, which was based in a region of the south that was largely populated by Christians and animists. Following the signing of the Addis Ababa Agreement (1972), Garang, along with many other rebels, was absorbed into the Sudanese military. As a colonel in the Government of Sudan military, he underwent additional training at Fort Benning, Georgia. But then, in the 1980s, as the Government of Sudan became increasingly Islamist, Garang was tasked with putting down an uprising in the south in May 1983. Balking, he left his post and joined up with the rebels, out of which he organized and led the Sudan People's Liberation Army.

In late July 2005, shortly after he had become the Vice President of Sudan, Garang died when the helicopter he was flying in crashed.

General Union of the Nuba (GUN): The GUN emerged in the aftermath of the 1964 forced resignation of General Ibrahim Abboud as president of Sudan. It is considered a key turning point for the Nuba people, who emerged as a major political force in opposition to the ruling elite in Khartoum. The GUN spoke on the behalf of the Nuba, both clearly spelling out how the Nuba had been under the thumb of Khartoum, and calling for basic rights. The GUN was a key player in the establishment of a rural alliance in which leaders of the south, the east and Darfur came together to speak on their peoples' behalf. Many see it as a precursor to the New Sudan ideology that was to be conceived and formalized later in time.

Genocide: According to the 1948 United Nations Convention on the Prevention and Punishment of Genocide, genocide is defined as: "any of the following acts committed with intent to destroy, in whole or in part, a national, ethnical, racial or religious group, as such: killing members of the group; causing serious bodily or mental harm to members of the group; deliberately inflicting on the group conditions of life calculated to bring about its physical destruction in whole or in part; imposing measures intended to prevent births within the group; [and] forcibly transferring children of the group to another group."

Genocide by attrition: "Genocide by attrition occurs when a group is stripped of its human rights, political, civil and economic. This leads to deprivation of conditions essential for maintaining health, thereby producing mass death. Genocide by attrition is epitomized by the Warsaw Ghetto (1939–43), Democratic Kampuchea (1975–79), and Sudan (1983–93)" (Fein, 1997, p. 9).

Government of Sudan (GoS): The government of Sudan is essentially run by the National Congress Party (NCP), which came to power following a military coup d'état in 1989. Black African refugees frequently refer to Government of Sudan troops by simply saying "the GoS." Still others often refer to it simply as Khartoum, which is where the seat of the federal government is located. It is also referred to simply as "the North."

Haroun, Ahmed: Under Sudanese President Omar al-Bashir, Haroun has served in many different positions within the Sudanese government. During the Darfur crisis in the early 2000s, Haroun served as the Minister of State for Interior Affairs, and from April 2004 to September 2005 he oversaw the Darfur Security Desk, which coordinated various government agencies involved in the counterinsurgency campaign in Darfur, including the infamous Janjaweed. From 2006 to 2009, he served as Sudan's State Minister for Humanitarian Affairs during which he was responsible for overseeing the two million internally displaced persons in Darfur. Various humanitarian aid organizations decried what appeared to be Haroun's interference in their operations. Accusations by others asserted that Haroun was responsible for tasking the Janjaweed with policing various IDP camps. In September 2007, the GoS assigned Haroun to conduct an investigation in order to ascertain whether any human rights violations had been perpetrated in Darfur. The GoS also appointed him to serve on its committee responsible for overseeing the United Nations African Union Mission In Darfur (UNAMID).

As a result of his alleged decisions, directives and actions in relation to Darfur, on April 27, 2007, the International Criminal Court (ICC) issued a warrant for Haroun's arrest on charges of twenty counts of crimes against of humanity and twenty-two counts of war crimes. ICC prosecutor Luis Moreno-Ocampo accused Haroun of recruiting and arming *Janjaweed* militias for the express purpose of squelching the black African rebel attacks against the Sudanese government. Moreno-Ocampo asserted that Haroun was "present as arms were distributed to fighters, had full knowledge of atrocities including rape and murder happening on the ground, and incited militias to slaughter civilians in speeches." The operative term is "civilians."

In May 2009, Haroun was appointed governor of South Kordofan, the home of the Nuba Mountains. The people of the Nuba Mountains did not want anything to do with Haroun, because of (1) the purported atrocities he had overseen in Darfur, (2) the fact they did not like having one of al-Bashir's cronies foisted about them as governor, and (3) their preference for governor was one of their own, Abdel Aziz. Some Nuba may have also been cognizant of the fact that in the 1990s Haroun had taken part in mobilizing the Muraleen militia for the express purpose of carrying out attacks in Kordofan.

In May 2011, a gubernatorial election was held in which Haroun ran against Abdel Aziz. On

May 16, 2011, Haroun was named the winner, but the Sudan People's Liberation Movement/Army decried the results, claiming that the election had been rigged. In June 2011, warfare broke out between the Government of Sudan and the Sudan People's Liberation Movement/Army–North, and has continued unabated ever since.

In July 2013, the GoS reinstated West Kordofan as a state. Ultimately, Haroun was appointed acting government of North Kordofan, with Adam al-faki Mohamed al-Tayeb taking on the position of acting governor of South Kordofan.

Internally displaced persons (IDPs): Those individuals who, for whatever reason (massive human rights violations, armed conflict, ethnic cleansing, etc.), are forced from their villages, towns, cities and homes and thus compelled to seek sanctuary somewhere else in the country.

International Criminal Court (ICC): The International Criminal Court (ICC), governed by the Rome Statute, is the first permanent, treaty based, international criminal court established to help end impunity for the perpetrators of the most serious crimes of concern to the international community, including crimes against humanity and genocide. The ICC is an independent international organization, and is not part of the United Nations system. Its seat is at The Hague in the Netherlands. It was on July 17, 1998, that the international community reached a historic milestone when 120 States adopted the Rome Statute, the legal basis for establishing the permanent International Criminal Court. Following its ratification by 60 countries, the Rome Statute entered into force on July 1, 2002.

Janjaweed: Arab militia groups used by Khartoum during the counter-insurgency in Darfur. Reportedly, the Janjaweed are now active in South Kordofan, fighting with Government of Sudan troops against the people of the Nuba Mountains.

Justice and Equality Movement (JEM): The Justice and Equality Movement (JEM) was one of the first two rebel groups to engage in battle with the Government of Sudan (GoS) in Darfur in the early part of the first decade of the 21st century. It is Islamist based with most of its supporters, at least early on, coming from the Kobe Zagahawa group in Northeastern Darfur. Over the years, it has split many times over.

More recently (2013/2014), JEM has joined the Sudan Revolutionary Front and has become active in South Kordofan, fighting with the SPLM/A–N against the GoS. In various cases, JEM members have acted irresponsibly and failed to heed the commands of the SPLM/A–N and have had to be reigned in by the latter.

Kadugli: The capital of the State of South Kordofan, Sudan.

Kalashnikov: An automatic assault rifle. It was first developed in the Soviet Union by Mikhail Kalashnikov in the 1940s.

Kauda: A relatively large town in the heart of the Nuba Mountains.

Khartoum: The capital of Sudan. It is located at the confluence of the Blue and White Nile Rivers. The Government of Sudan is often referred to as "Khartoum."

Kuwa Mekki, Yousif (August 1945–March 31, 2001): A renowned and highly revered SPLA governor-commander in the Nuba Mountains. Kuwa was a member of the Miri tribe. He was raised a Muslim, actually believing he was an Arab, when his family was actually considered to be "black." In 1975, as s a young university student and political science major, he was instrumental in co-founding Komolo, the first political organization comprised of Nuba youth. The express purpose of Komolo was to raise cultural and political awareness among the Nuba. Following a career as a teacher both in Darfur (Sudan) and the Nuba Mountains, Kuwa was elected to the Kordofan regional assembly in 1981. However, discovering that his position in the assembly was not conducive to helping the Nuba Mountains people gain their basic civil and human rights, he joined the Sudan People's Liberation Movement/Army in 1984. Under his leadership, the Nuba Mountains people resisted the war carried out against them by the government. Not only was Kuwa a commander but he was also considered a visionary. In that regard, he strove to help his people help themselves; and in doing so, he founded a teachers' training college and a nursing school.

For sixteen years he served as a commander of the SPLA in a fight to gain basic human rights for the people of the Nuba Mountains. Ultimately, Kuwa became the SPLA–appointed governor of the Nuba Mountains. During his period as governor he implemented a form of self-government in which the Nuba Mountains people elected their own village leaders, district representatives and county administrators. In 1994, Kuwa organized and headed up the National Liberation Council of the SPLM movement, which in turn helped to establish civil administrations, along the line he had implemented in the Nuba Mountains, in all of the areas under the control of the SPLA. Subsequently, Kuwa helped to create the Nuba Relief, Rehabilitation and Development Organization (NRRDO) in order to provide the people of the Nuba Mountains people with food, cooking oil, and clothing.

Lyman, Princeton N.: Served as the United States special envoy for Sudan and South Sudan from March 2011 to March 2013.

National Congress Party (NCP): The NCP is the major the political party of Sudan. Prior to the secession of the South (South Sudan) in 2011, the NCP's base was primarily in the north.

National Islamic Front (NIF): The National Islamic Front is the political organization that has controlled Sudan for decades under Sudanese President Omar al-Bashir. The NIF was a direct offshoot of the Muslim Brotherhood. It was under the auspices of the NIF that al-Bashir carried out the 1989 coup d'état in Sudan, which brought him to power. The NIF is now known as the National Congress Party.

Nimeiri, Jaffar: President of Sudan from 1969 to 1985. Nimeri rose to power in 1969 when he and a group of young fellow army officers carried out a coup d'état. The coup dispatched a group of civilian rulers who had been in power for five years and had gained a notorious reputation for being corrupt and inept, especially when it came to handling the economy. Nimeiri was a devout Moslem and imposed Shari'a law in 1983, which many claim was the major catalyst for the 20-plus year-long war between the Government of Sudan and southern Sudan. To throw his rivals off kilter in an ongoing attempt to remain in power he made a number of radical shifts in policy. Over the years, his style of rule became increasingly authoritarian. He lost his own presidency in 1985 as the result of a coup d'état. After he was overthrown, he was granted political asylum in Egypt. He died on May 30, 2009, at the age of 79.

Nongovernmental organizations (NGOs): Civil society organizations that are independent of governments and are not for profit corporations. Frequently created by citizens, the focus of NGOs is rather eclectic: human rights, the environment, health, education, development, and self-help. NGOs can have a local, regional, national or international focus. They are funded in various ways, from foundations to businesses to grants from governments.

"The North": The way in which many people in the Nuba Mountains refer to the Government of Sudan, which is based in Khartoum.

Nuba: For the people of the Nuba Mountains, the term "Nuba" refers "to the myriad cultures and traditions of the more than fifty different tribal groups in the Nuba Mountains" (African Rights, 1995, p. 5). On the other hand, "for the dominant class in Sudan, and in particular the ruling National Islamic Front [NIF], 'Nuba' refers to second class citizens—'primitive' black people, servants and labourers" (African Rights, 1995, p. 5).

Nuba Mountains: A region located in the Sudanese state of South Kordofan, home to a religiously and ethnically diverse population consisting of more than 50 different tribal groups adhering to Christian, Muslim, and/or animist beliefs.

Nuba Mountains Cease-Fire Agreement: A cease-fire agreement signed by the Government of Sudan and the SPLM/Nuba on January 19, 2002, at the Bürgenstock (NW), Swiss Confederation.

Nuba Relief, Rehabilitation, and Development Organization (NRRDO): An indigenous aid organization that works with both donors and NGOs "to improve the livelihoods of poor communities and to promote and defend the human rights and interests of Southern Kordofan State/Nuba Mountains."

Nuba Reports: Eyes and Ears of the Nuba: A group of Nuba citizen journalists, founded by American Ryan Boyette, who have assiduously documented Khartoum's violence against civilians in the Nuba Mountains since 2011. The team relies on a network of members based in South Kordofan. Once an incident is reported, a citizen journalist is dispatched to document and verify the event, establish GPS coordinates, and upload the report online where they are frequently picked up by the international media and available to the general public to read on the Internet. The posts are in English. A key source for anyone who wishes to keep abreast of the latest attacks by the GoS in the Nuba Mountains.

Operation Lifeline Sudan (OLS): Operation Lifeline Sudan was a consortium of UN agencies—including the World Food Program and UNICEF, and some 35 nongovernmental organizations—that provided humanitarian assistance throughout southern Sudan during the years of war and famine from 1989 through the late 1990s. OLS was established following negotiations between the UN, the Government of Sudan (GoS), and the Sudan People's Liberation Movement/Army "to deliver humanitarian assistance to all civilians in need, regardless of their location or political affiliation." Due to a blockade by the GoS, Operation Lifeline Sudan was not able to reach the Nuba Mountains, which was one of the major factors contributing to the genocide by attrition of the Nuba people between late 1980s and the mid 1990s.

"Peace camps": As they attacked village after village in the early to mid–1990s, Government of Sudan troops rounded up and forced tens of thousands of civilians from the Nuba Mountains into so-called "peace camps" or "peace villages," which were essentially concentration camps. These camps were armed camps controlled by the GoS army and government-created militia, the Popular Defence Force (PDF). In the camps many girls and women were forced to "marry" their captors, while many others were simply used as "concubines." In many cases, the captives virtually became slave labor. Children were often taken from their parents and forced to attend fundamental Islamic schools, where they were inculcated with beliefs antithetical to their parents. While the GoS brazenly asserted that the Nuba were placed in the camps to remove them from the war zone for purposes of safety, some scholars have characterized it as a form of ethnic cleansing driven by economic motives to remove the people from their land for the government's own use. Some also argue that in order to prevent the general populace from harboring or assisting members of the SPLA and to punish people for purportedly helping the SPLA, the GoS formed the camps.

Popular Defense Force (PDF): The paramilitary militia force deployed by the Government of Sudan in Darfur, the Nuba Mountains, and other regions of Sudan.

Refugees: People who have fled their home country due to war, persecution, ethnic cleansing, famine or natural disaster, etc.

Republic of South Sudan: On July 9, 2011, the Republic of South Sudan became the newest country in the community of nations. Following a referendum (a requirement spelled out in the 2005 Comprehensive Peace Agreement, the latter of which brought to an end 20 years of civil war that resulted in some two million deaths) in which 98.83 percent of the population of the south voted, the southerners chose to secede from Sudan.

Satellite Sentinel Project (SSP): Conducts satellite surveillance in Sudan's major areas of conflict, including Darfur and South Kordofan (Nuba Mountains). According to its website, SSP "launched on December 29, 2010, with the goals of deterring a return to full-scale civil war between northern and southern Sudan and deterring and documenting threats to civilians along both sides of the border [i.e., dividing Sudan and the Republic of South Sudan]. SSP focuses world attention on mass atrocities in Sudan and uses its imagery and analysis to generate rapid responses on human rights and human security concerns…. DigitalGlobe satellites passing over Sudan and South Sudan capture imagery of possible threats to civilians, detect bombed and razed villages, or note other evidence of pending mass violence. Experts at DigitalGlobe work with the Enough Project to analyze imagery and information from sources on the ground to produce reports. The Enough Project then distributes releases to the press and policymakers and sounds the alarm by notifying major news organizations and a mobile network of activists."

Sharia Law: In Arabic, "sharia" means "path." Sharia law is essentially a religious code that impacts all aspects of Muslim life (e.g., religious obligations, familial obligations, financial affairs, daily routines). While there are different forms of sharia, it is primarily derived from the *Koran* (the Muslim holy book) and the Sunna (Islamic custom or practice)—the teachings, sayings, and practices of the Prophet Mohammed.

Sheik: A traditional leader of a village.

South Kordofan: A state in Sudan that shares a border with the Republic of South Sudan. It is an oil rich area that was the site of significant battles during the 20-year civil war between north and south Sudan. The Nuba Mountains are located in the heart of South Kordofan.

Sudan Armed Forces (SAF): The official army of the Government of Sudan. Khartoum's regular military force.

The Sudan People's Liberation Movement (SPLM): A political party in Southern Sudan which began as a rebel movement, and led the twenty plus year fight against the north (the Government of Sudan) during the course of the Second Sudanese Civil War. Its military wing is known as the Sudan People's Liberation Army (SPLA).

In 1983, Lieutenant Colonel John Garang formed the SPLA. Initially, Garang was tasked with quelling a mutiny in Bor, where some 500 southern troops refused to be rotated to the north. However, instead of squelching the mutiny, Garang encouraged other garrisons to mutiny and established himself as the leader of the rebellion against the Government of Sudan.

The SPLA grew from a small group of disenchanted soldiers into a force of tens of thousands that ultimately pressured the Government of Sudan to sign the Comprehensive Peace Agreement, which resulted in the termination of hostilities between the north and south in 2005 and a vote on a resolution in January 2011 to decide if the south would secede from the north or remain as part of Sudan.

Today, the Sudan People's Liberation Movement–North (SPLM–N) is active in South Kordofan and the Blue Nile state as it engages in battle with the Government of Sudan.

Sudan People's Liberation Movement–North (SPLM–N): The SPLM–N was crafted from the remnants of the Sudan People's Liberation Movement/Amy that remained in the south following the South's vote for independence in 2011. It was formed in view of what it perceived to be threats by Sudanese President Omar al-Bashir (including the establishment of sharia law throughout Sudan), and out of fear that the Government of Sudan would continue to treat the people of the region as second class citizens or worse. It was also feared that the GoS might seek to retaliate against those who fought with the south during the Second Sudanese Civil War and continued to live in South Kordofan, which remained part and parcel of the north. The aim of the SPLM–N is to take the fight this time around all the way to Khartoum.

The SPLM–N asserts that it is "a Sudanese national movement that seeks to change the policies of the centre in Khartoum and to build a new centre for the benefit of all Sudanese people regardless of their religion, gender or ethnicity background." For the past six years (June 2011–January 2017), the SPLA–N has been engaged in an all-out battle with the GoS.

Suq: Open air market that is common in many African and Middle Eastern countries.

Tukul: The traditional abodes of the people of the Nuba Mountains. The foundation is generally made of natural rock with large poles, made from the branches of trees, forming a frame to which woven dried sorghum stalks are attached in order to form a broad, conical-shaped roof.

Umda: A traditional leader, head of all the sheiks in the region/area.

United Nations High Commission for Refugees (UNHCR): Established by the United Nations General Assembly in 1950, the UNHCR "is mandated to lead and co-ordinate international action to protect refugees and resolve refugee problems worldwide." It provides assistance for stateless people, and protects their rights and safety.

Unity State: The oil-rich border state in South Sudan; many refugees from the Nuba Mountains have flooded across the border into Unity State. The Yida Refugee camp is located in Unity State, along the Republic of South Sudan and Sudan border.

U.S. Agency for International Development (USAID): USAID is considered the principal U.S. agency for extending "assistance to countries and peoples recovering from disaster, trying to escape poverty, and engaging in democratic reforms. USAID supports long-term and equitable economic growth and advances U.S. foreign policy objectives by supporting: economic growth, agriculture and trade; global health; and, democracy, conflict prevention and humanitarian assistance."

Wadi: A valley, gully, or streambed located in northern Africa and parts of the Middle East that remains dry except during the rainy season when they often swell up with torrents of water.

War crimes: War crimes constitute a violation of international humanitarian law. Examples of war crimes include deliberate attacks on non-combatants; deliberate attacks on hospitals; the use of chemical or biological weapons; the murder or ill-treatment of prisoners of war; the murder of hostages; and the destruction of cities, towns, and villages "not justified by military necessity."

World Food Program (WFP): Under the auspices of the United Nations, The World Food Program (WFP) provides emergency food aid for refugees and internally displaced persons (IDPs) in dire straits all across the globe. It also supports economic development and social development.

Yida Refugee Camp: A refugee camp in The Republic of South Sudan, along the South Sudan-Sudan border. Refugees from the Nuba Mountains have flooded into the camp since June 2011, when the SPLM/A–N and the Government of Sudan took up arms against one another.

REFERENCES

African Rights (1995). *Facing Genocide: The Nuba of Sudan*. London: African Rights.
Fein, Helen (1997). "Genocide by Attrition in Sudan and Elsewhere." http://www.crimesofwar.org/sudan-mag, Spring 2002, p. 9.

List of Acronyms

AU	African Union
CPA	The Comprehensive Peace Agreement
GoS	Government of Sudan
GUN	General Union of the Nuba
ICC	International Criminal Court
IDP	internally displaced person
JEM	Justice and Equality Movement
NCP	National Congress Party
NGO	Nongovernmental organization
NIF	National Islamic Front
NRRDO	Nuba Relief, Rehabilitation, and Development Organization
OLS	Operation Lifeline Sudan
PDF	Popular Defence Force
RPG	Rocket-propelled grenade
SAF	Sudan Armed Forces
SPLM	The Sudan People's Liberation Movement
SPLM/A	The Sudan People's Liberation Movement/Army
SPLM-N	The Sudan People's Liberation Movement–North
SSP	Satellite Sentinel Project
UN	United Nations
UNDP	United Nations Development Program
UNHCR	United Nations High Commission for Refugees
USAID	United States Agency for International Development
WFP	World Food Program

Foreword

Baroness Caroline Cox

The Nuba Mountains rise like a rugged green spine traversing the heart of Sudan. The people who have lived there from time immemorial are renowned for their distinctive culture, including formidable wrestling, dynamic dancing and music with traditional instruments. The Nuba people enjoy harmonious relations transcending diverse religious beliefs: Christians, Muslims and adherents to traditional beliefs all happily participate in each other's joyful ceremonies such as weddings and share the grief of funerals.

I am delighted that this book will be a timeless record of these dignified, courageous and hospitable people and a tribute to their unique culture, traditions and resilience. I am also grateful that the book records the sustained and barbaric suffering inflicted on the people of the Nuba Mountains by Islamist governments in Khartoum. I therefore pay tribute to Samuel Totten for his vision of the book—and to all the authors who have contributed in their own distinctive ways. All the contributors explain their deep concern for the Nuba people and describe personal experiences of being alongside them as they endure, with courage and fortitude, the genocidal tribulations to which they are being subjected by the regime of Sudanese President Omar al-Bashir.

It is a great privilege to be invited to write this foreword. In doing so, I wish briefly to put on record a few memories of my own visits as my personal tribute to the Nuba people and as a context for my appreciation of the contribution of the authors of the essays in this book.

My journeys to the Nuba Mountains have spanned three phases of their recent history. First, I made a number of visits during the 1990s and the early years of the new millennium, during an era of massive suffering inflicted by the Islamist National Islamic Front (NIF) regime during its self-declared military *jihad*. This war raged from the NIF's military coup in 1989 until the so-called Comprehensive Peace Agreement (CPA) was signed in 2005.

Second, I visited the Nuba people several times during the years between the signing of the CPA and the attainment of the independence of the southerners in 2011. During these years, with the absence of military offensives inflicted by the Government of Sudan (GoS), we witnessed valiant attempts by the Nuba people—who were forced to remain under the fist of Khartoum—to return to normality. But we also heard the people's concerns about their future once the people of the Republic of South Sudan achieved their independence. People throughout the Nuba Mountains expressed the very real fear that the Islamist regime in Khartoum would impose its avowed agenda of Islamization and

Arabization on them. This threat posed by the Islamist regime's determination to impose its hard-line ideology boded ill for the traditionally African peoples of the Nuba Mountains.

In those years we supported programmes by NRRDO (Nuba Relief, Rehabilitation and Development Organization) to help war widows establish co-operatives to generate mutual support, income and economic independence. Whenever we visited we were always deeply impressed by the women's courage, creativity and resilience—and we loved to celebrate their achievements.

Third, I have returned several times during the current situation in which the people are suffering the fate they dreaded: entrapment within the confines of the Republic of Sudan, still ruled by President Omar al-Bashir and the same regime responsible for the previous war. He is now perpetrating at least war crimes and perhaps crimes against humanity against the people of the Nuba Mountains, using sustained aerial bombardment of civilian targets: schools, clinics, places of worship and markets. The bombers also target civilians trying to plant or harvest crops in order to prevent them from growing food—thereby inflicting what could lead to a case of genocide by attrition through starvation and death from hunger-related illnesses. What makes this particularly likely is that al-Bashir absolutely refuses to allow any international humanitarian organizations from entering the region in order to provide food and medicine to the civilians who are in desperate need of both. In fact, he has threatened to slice the throats of anyone crossing into Sudan without direct permission from the GoS. And, the GoS has also virtually established a no-fly zone over South Kordofan State (which is the home of the Nuba), thus ensuring that humanitarian airlifts are not feasible.

Most recently, in January 2016, we were again with some of the thousands of women and children forced to flee aerial bombardment and seek sanctuary in horrendous conditions in caves infested with deadly snakes. They told us: "We would never usually even enter these caves, *but we are more afraid of the bombs than the snakes.*"

The ongoing onslaught against the people of the Nuba Mountains is the context for this important book. It is an honour to introduce the authors whose contributions provide compelling, authoritative and powerful accounts of these valiant people and their heartbreaking predicament.

As you read the book, you will experience a kaleidoscope of emotions.

Each evocative essay provides unique insights into the horror of the suffering deliberately inflicted by the GoS on innocent civilians. Some essays are especially painful to read, with heart-wrenching descriptions of excruciating injuries and illnesses and the painful stress of valiant doctors and nurses trying to treat patients in terrible need, too often with inadequate medical supplies.

But I believe that you, like me, will experience other emotions: profound admiration for the poignant resilience of the Nuba people, as well as their graciousness, hospitality and courage.

And I think you will also feel profoundly humbled by the detailed accounts of the experiences of those who risk life and limb to be with the Nuba people in this time of desperate need. You will feel you are actually travelling with them, experiencing their bone-shattering journeys over rocky roads, their fear at the sound of the dreaded Antonov bombers and their greater fear of the Sukhoi jets which come so fast it is impossible to take cover. You will be deeply impressed by their determination to take life-saving medical and food supplies to communities facing death from starvation and hunger-related illnesses—and, in many essays, their overt testimony to their Christian faith which motivates and sustains them.

Finally, I think you will feel, like me, intense anger at the international community's refusal to designate this manifest, systematic killing of civilians and destruction of the means of survival as the international crime it undoubtedly is. The GoS's sustained military offensives—especially the deliberate destruction of the Nuba's food sources as the genocide by attrition it certainly is—are criminal acts that the world does not want to acknowledge. The words "Never Again" ring very hollow in the hills and caves of the Nuba Mountains when they are echoing with thundering explosions of bombs dropped from the Antonovs, the Sukhoi fighter jets and long-range missiles fired from GoS bases.

From here forward, I offer a brief "introduction" to each essay in order to provide you, the reader, with an overview of this book's vitally important message as well as to encourage you to read each of the author's personal stories—of their fascinating experiences in the Nuba Mountains, their love for the people, their passionate commitment to provide life-saving help, and their continuing endeavours to seek long overdue justice.

Tomo Križnar describes his yearning to tell the story of the people of the Nuba Mountains in order to generate the recognition, protection and support they need and deserve—a yearning which has led him to encourage many famous people over the years to report their experiences.

They include Leni Riefenstahl (1902–2003), a renowned German screenwriter, film director, producer, photographer, and Nazi propagandist, who was equally famous for her extensive travels in the 1970s in the Nuba Mountains and her two books, rich with remarkable photographs, *The Last of the Nuba*, and *The Nuba People of Kau*. Tomo desperately encouraged her to revisit the Nuba people as they faced an onslaught of terror at the hands of the GoS. His account of her problematic visit is riveting reading.

But the most riveting stories are Tomo's detailed descriptions of his own many visits to the Nuba Mountains with formidable logistical challenges and at great personal danger. The passion for the truth to be told and to goad the international community to help and protect the peoples subjected to al-Bashir's genocidal policies which motivated Tomo Križnar to risk his life in so many ways over the years, still continues today. As he notes, The Tomo Križnar Foundation and the humanitarian organization Hope, established by Klemen Mihelič in 2009, are trying to help these innocent and endangered indigenous people by equipping them with information technology. Tomo concludes his essay with these words in regard to the latter efforts: *"We are at the beginning. We are looking for support and like-minded people."* I passionately hope this book will help to elicit that support.

Ryan Boyette, born in the United States and brought up a Christian, felt "called" to go to Sudan to help people in need, and thus he approached Samaritan's Purse, an evangelical organization with projects across the globe. Despite many anxieties, he landed in the Nuba Mountains on April 27, 2003, and has been living there ever since. In 2007, he met the beautiful Jazira, a local Nuba woman. They married in February 2011, in a local church. Astonishingly, some 6,000 people attended their wedding.

In June 2011, when the fighting began again between the GoS and the Sudan People's Liberation/Army–North (SPLA-N), most of the non–Sudanese people working for international nongovernmental organizations pulled out of the area within two days due to the danger of the situation. Ryan and Jazira remained, committed to telling the world the truth about what was happening.

Deciding he had to do something beyond merely witness the tragedy unfolding around him, Boyette came up with the idea of creating a group of "citizen journalists" to cover the war and report on it. Thus, *Nuba Reports* was born. Risking their lives, Boyette and his team, equipped with cameras, travel to the hot spots in the Nuba in order to objectively document the events. After writing up their reports, they disseminate the facts to the international media, international human rights organizations, and even foreign policy makers. *Nuba Reports* also helps to bridge divisions fuelled by the Sudan Government's propaganda over three decades by bringing together staff who are Arabs and Africans, Muslims and Christians.

Ryan and Jazira live in great danger. On May 11, 2012, at 9:50 a.m., the Sudan government targeted their home. An Antonov airplane flew over the house and dropped six bombs which fell within 30–50 meters of the building. However, Ryan is keen to emphasize that the real heroes who take the greatest risks are the Sudanese reporters and editors with *Nuba Reports*. They are building an archive of life in the Nuba Mountains—a living, evolving memory of the war. Also, they are providing information which calls the international community to account—no one can claim they "do not know" what is happening.

Tom Catena, M.D., has been providing life-saving medical care for the people of the Nuba Mountains since March 25, 2008—only leaving briefly on two occasions. The Catholic-sponsored Mother of Mercy Hospital where he works was established to serve a huge catchment area, the size of Georgia in the U.S. Busy before the war flared up again, Mother of Mercy is now inundated with the often horrendous casualties of war as well as patients suffering from the inevitable range of illnesses such as malaria, severe malnutrition to starvation, and serious gynaecological/obstetric problems.

One example of Dr. Tom's way of life is indicative of the stress, courage, pain and commitment which are required for him to maintain his ministry: on the night of June 8, 2011, Dr. Tom got his first taste of being a war surgeon as several casualties from the fighting in Heiban arrived around 10:00 p.m. "The soldiers lay in their blood soaked uniforms, many crying out in pain," he writes. "*Any notions I ever had of war being anything but a gruesome exercise of man killing man quickly vanished.* As the only referral hospital and only one offering surgical care in the Nuba Mountains, we quickly became inundated with war wounded."

Dr. Tom describes many similar scenes of horrendous suffering inflicted by the Government of Sudan's ruthless bombardment of innocent civilians. He also describes his own personal feelings and commitment: trying to maintain some sort of perspective is a challenge, particularly with such prolonged periods of isolation in the remote Nuba Mountains. But he says he wouldn't want to have it any other way. As a medical missionary, he adheres to the teaching attributed to St. Francis of Assisi: "Preach always and sometimes use words." And he prays for strength to keep helping people even though he sometimes feels the life force "being sucked out of me."

Sister Deidre M. Byrne, M.D., grew up in a devout Catholic family in Washington, D.C., and felt called to serve Jesus by serving the poor. Since January 2000, she has been a fully professed member of the Little Workers of the Sacred Heart, committed to overseas medical missionary work providing free medical care for the poor and uninsured.

She joined the Active Reserve of the U.S. Army Medical Corps, attaining the rank of colonel and was posted abroad, including in Afghanistan. At the request of the Order, she retired from the military in 2009 after 29 years of service and professed final vows with the Little Workers in 2011. Sister DeDe has visited the Nuba Mountains three times, serving at the Mother of Mercy Hospital. She describes her "tour of duty" in 2010 as "almost romantic." The hospital was fairly new, the rainy season had ended, and the peanut plants were in full growth.

Her second "tour" began in October 2011. South and North Sudan had recently split into two countries and the atmosphere in the Nuba had changed to one of fear that the Nuba and the GoS might find themselves back at war against one another. That fear came to fruition in June 2011, and on her third visit the situation had changed drastically: now there were serious injuries resulting from the constant daily bombings of civilian areas. Also, the journey to reach the hospital was hazardous because Khartoum's bombers targeted vehicles. With a wry sense of humour, Sister DeDe writes, "Thank God they had lousy aim."

Sister DeDe makes numerous tributes to the faith, courage, resilience and love which characterize the people of the Nuba Mountains. She also testifies to her own faith and the inspiration she finds in the words of St. Therese of Lisieux: "We can do no great things; only small things with great love." Her account is, in fact, an inspirational testimony to her love and admiration of the Nuba people and to the way in which she puts her faith and love into practice in situations of extreme danger and the constant challenge of trying to treat patients with horrific injuries.

George Tutu's vivid accounts of his youth provide many first-hand insights into the plight of the people living in the Nuba Mountains under the GoS and the latter's attempts to force the Nuba to leave their ancestral culture and to adopt the Arabic-Islamic culture. He also addresses the GoS' jihad, which resulted in the death of his father and many other relatives. In part, George's response was to work with other Nuba friends to found the Nuba Christian Family Mission (NCFM). After moving from Egypt to the United States, George immediately began raising money to help meet the many needs of his people back home, including the construction of water wells and pumps and the establishment of schools (including the first Teacher Training Institute in the Nuba Mountains). He returned to the Nuba Mountains in 2007 and again in 2013 and 2014. His graphic account of the suffering of the people echoes in every horrible detail the reports of other writers who feature in this book—as does his passionate commitment to try to deliver whatever help he can to his people who are in such desperate need (and have been left bereft thanks to the actions of the GoS and the inactions of the United Nations, the African Union and virtually every other intergovernmental organization comprising the international community).

The personal account by Matt Chancey describes how Matt's engagement with Sudan developed slowly, initially through his friendship with an individual named Brad Phillips whom he met when Brad was working as a "Hill Rat" (legislative assistant) in Washington. Phillips' passion was foreign policy, especially as it related to Africa. While on Capitol Hill, he met Sudanese NBA (National Basketball Association) star Manute Bol, who told Brad his personal story and how he had fled persecution by the National Islamic Front (NIF) government in Sudan.

In 1997, Phillips launched a campaign called the Persecution Project. Initially, it was his attempt to use his background in government and advocacy to raise awareness about the incidence of religious and racial persecution in Africa. In 1998, one of Phillips' friends, Hedd Thomas, who worked for Christian Aid, invited Phillips to meet Philip Neroun, then Director of the NRRDO. Neroun shared his own experiences regarding the targeting and persecution of Christians in Sudan's Nuba Mountains by the GoS with Phillips, and also arranged for Phillips to meet the now late Yousef Kuwa, one of the most renowned leaders of the Nuba people.

Phillips was so moved and motivated that he established the Persecution Project Foundation (PPF). PPF subsequently became aware of the GoS policy of declaring areas of Sudan as "Red No-Go" zones, where aid could not be delivered. Often, these areas were selected because of security problems. But more often they were "off limits" because of the NIF's political agenda. PPF therefore decided to focus on delivering aid specifically to Red No-Go areas.

In 2005, shortly after the Comprehensive Peace Agreement was signed, Matt accompanied Phillips on a relief trip. Subsequently, Matt decided to quit his desk job and devote most of his energy to the day-to-day work of PPF. In January 2011, he moved his family to East Africa. It was an increasingly turbulent time in the Nuba Mountains, and in June 2011 fighting broke out when al-Bashir's army tried to forcefully disarm Nuba fighters who had sided with South Sudan during the previous war. When they resisted, Bashir's army sacked the capital city of Kadugli and massacred many hundreds of Nubans.

Matt interviewed dozens of survivors only weeks after the attack, and they all said that GoS troops went from house-to-house killing people according to three criteria: ethnic Nubans, members of the Sudan People's Liberation Movement–North, and Christians. That was when PPF went in. On July 4th, 2011, Matt flew with Phillips and a small team on one of the last flights into the Nuba Mountains—the first of several missions they conducted as they carried in urgently needed medicines.

This moving essay highlights the poignant situation of children: the heart-breaking reality that during times of war—especially wars of terror—children endure most of the suffering—"Most of the sickness. Most of the wounds. Most of the death," as Matt puts it.

For Matt, the children's courage and suffering arouse deep anger and challenging questions: "In witnessing all these events, I know I am looking into the very heart of evil. These children are not 'collateral damage.' They are the targets of a sadistic regime hellbent on wiping them out. And for what? Uncontested political dominance? A pure Arab state? Money?'"

The account concludes with a condemnation of Western policy and a request—which I hope will generate positive responses from the readers of this book:

> Many policy-makers around the world have been silent about this blatant policy of ethnic cleansing in Sudan. All the while, Bashir's [public relation's] machine works overtime to excuse and deny. He discovered a long time ago that he can curry favor with both the U.S. government and the international community by sharing intelligence on jihadist activities (as though Bashir's behavior doesn't qualify!) with Western countries in great need of more Arab allies in the "War on Terror." As for me and my organization, our money is on the children, not their abusers. We can only hope the rest of the world wakes up and follows suit. But we're not waiting for the rest of the world. We're working now. And we invite others to join in the cause of "active compassion for the persecuted."

Samuel Totten's essay is a truly masterly, comprehensive overview of this complex, tragic, challenging situation covering the historical, political, military and cultural characteristics and experiences of the Nuba people.

In part, he describes, in graphic detail, his various gruelling journeys transporting food to people suffering from severe malnutrition and dying from starvation and hunger-related illnesses. As you read his essay, you "travel with him" and experience, vicariously, the challenges confronting him and his colleagues as they try to obtain scarce food and fuel and as they encounter the raw suffering following Antonov bombing raids.

You will also begin to understand why Sam has become so passionately committed in his endeavours to convey to the world the al-Bashir regime's ongoing, serial perpetration of crimes against humanity and genocide against the people of Sudan. His various initiatives in bringing the truth into the public domain, along with other authors in this book, means there is no excuse for anyone, anywhere, to claim ignorance of what has and is transpiring in the Nuba Mountain. Indeed, there is abundant evidence on the record to call the international community to account for failure to intervene.

The title of Sam's essay "A Moral Imperative: From Conducting Research in the Nuba Mountains to Hauling Food to Those in Most Critical Need" encapsulates the essential message found in this book. That is, there *is a moral imperative* to stand beside these victims of genocidal policies and to challenge the GoS's refusal to allow aid to reach its victims and the international community's unconscionable capitulation in the face of human tragedy.

In June 2012 he wrote a guest commentary, "Obama's Empty Promises to Halt Genocide Leave It to Us to Act," (*South Sudan News*, June 28, 2012) that spells out his position. The conclusion read as follows:

> One has to really wonder what lessons the world—leaders and ordinary citizens alike—has learned from [past genocides]. Even those who espouse such heartfelt sentiments/words/phrases such as "Never Again!" are among those who look away when new tragedies break out —and here I include former survivors of genocide, scholars, and educators at all levels. And if they don't look away, then far too often they stand slack jawed and silent. Neither is admirable; and, in fact, both reactions are unconscionable.
>
> Not one to suggest that others should pursue an avenue I am not willing to undertake, I shall place my name at the top of the list to take part in any of the above suggestions [which included hauling food up to the Nuba Mountains people] that gain traction. *Those willing to step up and be counted and thus avoid the tag of being a bystander in the face of certain crimes against humanity and potential genocide by attrition can contact me at samstertotten@gmail.com* [Totten, 2011, n.p.].

A week or so after the article was published Sam received a call from a fellow named John Jefferson, a businessman and evangelical Christian from California. Jefferson told Sam that an acquaintance of his, Billy White, an old Sudan hand, now based in South Sudan, had sent him a copy of Sam's article and challenged him to act upon it. His introduction was followed by, "Were you really serious about the challenge and about being ready, willing and able to act?"

"Without a doubt," Sam replied.

John C. Jefferson takes the reader on several visits to the Nuba Mountains with gripping and graphic accounts of challenging—and at times dangerous—journeys to some of the most remote locations in the region. One of these is Kao Nyaro, which has been *totally* "off the radar screen" of aid organisations. As his words powerfully express, the destitute people—including the 6- or 7-year-old boy, with dried snot under his nose, whom he describes as possessing as much charisma as Martin Luther King, Jr., delivering one of his famous speeches—made a profound impression on him.

The passion to provide help for the Nuba people led John to first co-initiate, with Samuel Totten, the End Nuba Genocide (ENG) coalition and, subsequently, the Greater Nuba Action Coalition (GNAC).

As the onslaught by al-Bashir's regime continues unabated, John concludes: "Where my sojourns in the land of the suffering strong will take me next only God knows. What

I do know is that I remain dedicated to helping the Nuba, both to grow in Christ and to help ease their physical and emotional suffering as the current war takes its daily toll on so many innocents."

John P. Sutter, M.D.'s fascinating and detailed account of volunteering his medical expertise at the Mission of Mercy Hospital alongside Dr. Tom Catena takes the reader through the daily hospital routine, introducing the patients with their challenging range of illnesses and injuries and their suffering and their courage. John also describes personal challenges, such as the decision every night whether to sleep on a bed or, given the bombing raids inflicting death and injury by night as well as by day, to sleep on the floor among the scorpions and the fat, hairy spiders.

Addressing why he volunteered in such a dangerous, challenging place as the active war zone of the Nuba Mountains, John says: "The short and totally honest answer is: The longing for adventure, to see the world, and to challenge myself.... At Mother of Mercy Hospital, all resources are limited and nothing is wasted. All decisions and actions are necessary and important, and the actions save lives. That is a very satisfying way to practice medicine."

But he pays especial tribute to the people with whom he worked and the reminder that his "small adventure and small contribution pale in comparison to those that are up in the Nuba working day-in and day-out, month after month for years on end. What is an adventure—and now a story for me—is daily life for those such as the drivers that dodge the Antonovs to bring supplies to the hospital as well as for Dr. Tom, the sisters and the Nuba staff, *who risk everything, every day*, to serve the victims of war and disease."

John concludes with a final tribute—to the Nuba people: "The Nuba are good people, and it is odd how their plight is, for the most part, ignored, especially by the West. It is a shame that no one has stepped up to stop the bombers from carrying out their daily bombing missions. The Nuba I met have values and traits that mirror what we strive for in the West—tolerance (Muslims and Christians living together without issue in the Nuba), a fair rule of law, respect for women and children, an appreciation for education, and an emphasis on the preservation of the family unit. I'm lucky to have been able to work with them, and once again, I'm inspired."

Corry Chapman, M.D., a physician based in Washington, D.C., has traveled to the Nuba Mountains on three different occasions, each time serving as a visiting doctor at Mother of Mercy Hospital in the Nuba Mountains. The last time he was in the Nuba, in 2014, was when the SPLA-N was at war with the Government of Sudan. Of that last trip, he writes:

> That was a new development. I understood it to be more dangerous than it had been in the past, but I didn't realize how bad it was until I got there. The upshot is, after that last trip, with the bombing and death, I don't think I can go back any time soon. I can't get myself killed. That wouldn't be fair to my kids. Plus, I'm scared now. The bombing and death I saw up there scared me.

Dr. Chapman is extremely modest in regard to that which he brought to Mother of Mercy, meaning his medical expertise and gracious assistance in a hospital that he describes as essentially a MASH unit. Of his time in the hospital, Dr. Chapman says:

> I had seen injury and death before, but never in such a catastrophic way. It's grotesque what exploding metal does to the body. Arms and legs ripped off, faces destroyed, intestines hanging out, blood, pain and death. The minute I saw it, I was afraid and wanted to go home. I realized there was no law,

no safety, no civilization [when it came to the actions of the Government of Sudan]. And that there was no reason I wouldn't be shredded by the next bomber. My sense of myself as a special person, a doctor working hard to help people, was gone. The banality of the chaos and violence terrified me. I wanted to get out.

Margaret Camarca originally qualified as a nurse, but on arrival at the Mother of Mercy Hospital, worked as a pharmacist. As she noted, "The position, nonetheless, was a perfect fit for me. I was able to support the employees, care for and visit with patients, organize the pharmacy and most importantly be touched by the villagers' stories. I feel privileged to share some of these stories with you." Continuing, she says:

> Not a few ask why I remained in the Nuba and at Mother of Mercy after the war broke out. My reasoning was simple: I was completely confident that I was living the life God had prepared for me. This instilled in me an overwhelming sense of peace. From the beginning I understood that the region was not safe. In 2003 I visited the memorial site of fourteen children and one teacher from Holy Cross Primary School in Kauda who had died during a bombing in 2000. During this visit, I met a school girl who had been maimed in the attack. I understood that President al-Bashir wanted to eradicate the region of the Nuba people and I was aware that all of us caring for the sick were considered criminals by the Khartoum government. Ultimately, I understood that my life was in the hands of God, so nothing else mattered. I witnessed firsthand the dedication of others in the region making exceedingly greater and more dangerous sacrifices than mine and I wanted to continue supporting them and the villagers.

Margaret also pays tribute to lessons she learnt from the local people: "The villagers taught me much about courage and trust in God. I was inspired by their strength, humility and tenaciousness. I clearly experienced how very little we actually need in life to get by. A case in point: I enjoyed learning that the local blacksmiths collect pieces of metal from exploded bombs and fashion them into hoes and other household items to sell in the market. Nuba resourcefulness is truly unrivalled."

In conclusion, Margaret says: "Upon my departure I knew I was going to miss Nuba hope and joy. Despite living for decades under a brutal regime, the Nuba are quick to celebrate life. The villagers know they've been long abandoned by the international community, but are confident that God is with them. Although the distance between my life among the Nuba and my U.S. home is great, they will live eternally in my heart. Mother Teresa once said works of mercy are works of peace. Together, let us continue to sew these seeds of mercy throughout the world confident that they will eventually bear an enduring peace."

C. Louis "PJ" Perrinjaquet, M.D., humbly refers to himself as "a small town doctor," but as one reads his story it is obvious that he has a big heart and an adventurous soul. For the past twenty plus years he has travelled to out of the way places in order to volunteer medical services to those in need, including, for example: Honduras, Nepal, Darfur, Sudan, and most recently, the Nuba Mountains.

His descriptions of working alongside Dr. Tom Catena at Mother of Mercy Hospital provide the reader with a vivid and upsetting picture of the suffering experienced by innocent civilians at the hands of the Government of Sudan. Those same descriptions also speak volumes about the incredible heart Dr. PJ has for the people of Darfur and the Nuba Mountains. Speaking of his efforts in El Geneina in Darfur, he writes:

> I spent some time at the Therapeutic Feeding Center. It had actually been built by Save the Children many years before the outbreak of the Darfur crisis, in response to previous food shortages before the conflict in Darfur. The mothers themselves were malnourished and could provide no breast milk. On arrival the more severe patients were mere skeletons draped with loose brown skin that once covered

muscle and fat. Too weak to even drink from a bottle, a feeding tube had to be inserted in their nose and on down to their stomachs in order to give precision formulas to save their lives.

Later in the Nuba Mountains, while working alongside Dr. Tom Catena, Dr. PJ relates the following in tersely written notes:

> Two children die during morning rounds today. Less than 1-year-old child in feeding program for the past week, fever, not doing well, gave few agonal breaths [agonal breaths of a person in agony are slow dying gasps] as we entered ward, his mother sobbing and holding scarf over her face as the father rocked the baby.
>
> As soon as I left this part of the children's ward, a nurse summoned me to help adjust the dose of IV Quinine for a six-year-old boy who had been admitted in a coma the night before with cerebral malaria. He had a seizure as we approached his bed. There was little to do but wait and see if the medicine would work or not. Later that morning I knew he had died when I heard the wailing of a crowd of women gathered outside the main walls of the hospital and then noticed that the boy's bed was now empty.

If only the world had more Dr. Tom Catenas and Dr. PJs. Then again, if only the world didn't need the services of Dr. Tom Catenas and Dr. PJs. But since it does, the world, in general, and the Nuba, in particular, are lucky that such good souls exist.

~ * ~

Knowledge of the truth may not yet be sufficient to bring the Khartoum government to account or to bring peace, justice and "a happy issue out of all their [the Nuba people's] affliction." But as the Bible teaches, "It is only the Truth which can make us free." Without the light of truth, the deeds of darkness can continue unchallenged. This book will be an invaluable resource for all who are striving to bring the plight of the Nuba people to the awareness of the international community with the hope that the moral imperative will eventually prevail.

Baroness Caroline Cox is a cross-bench member of the British House of Lords and founder and CEO of Humanitarian Aid Relief Trust (HART).

Introduction

Samuel Totten

Do unto others as you would have them do unto you?

Imagine, if you will, that you are a member of a group of civilians whose basic human and civil rights have been trammeled for decades by your nation's government. Imagine, as well, that the particular region in which you reside is largely bereft of schools, hospitals, roads, bridges, etc., while the region around the capital of your country is rich in all of these. Years of calling on the government to recognize and honor the fundamental rights of your group, as delineated in the UN Declaration of Human Rights, has come to naught. Upon holding peaceful rallies to decry the intransigence of the government, your group is threatened with punitive action by leaders at the highest level of the government. Ultimately, in abject frustration, a sector of the population within your group forms a rebel band for the express purpose of going head-to-head with the government. The vast majority of your group continues on as they always have—putting in long, arduous hours of work in order to eke out an existence for yourself and your family. As the rebels and government troops engage in warfare, the government makes the calculated decision to carry out daily aerial bombings of those areas where civilians congregate (marketplaces, places of worship, schools, etc.) The bombings are so deadly that many in your group flee in fear, thus leaving behind their homes, their jobs, and their way of life. Those who remain face the daily fear of being maimed or killed. Many, in fact, suffer horrific injuries, including the loss of arms and legs or worse. The daily aerial attacks go on for months on end. Months turn into years. Years turn into a half a decade and more. Despite your desperate calls for help, none is forthcoming from the international community. Talks among government officials, the rebel group, and outsiders ensue, but all the talk about creating a peaceful resolution continues to be nothing but talk, talk, and more talk. Daily life becomes more tenuous by the year, hunger sets in and slowly becomes the norm, as does malnutrition. More and more of your group flee from the region. Intent on winning at all costs, the government decides to ramp up the costs to the rebels and their purported supporters (the members of your group, the public, civilians all), and begin to use even more deadly and accurate weapons. Fear among your members increases exponentially. Children are so fearful that they will be killed as a result of aerial attacks on their school they refuse to attend school, and thus all schools have closed down. And yet nothing concrete is done by the international community to either bring the killing to an end or to ameliorate the abject hunger that has now become so serious that people in the region begin to suffer the entire gamut of hunger: malnutrition, severe malnutrition, and, ultimately, starvation. Finally, when talk among members of the international community begins to focus on the possibility of providing humanitarian aid (food and medicine), the leaders of your government issue a warning in no uncertain terms: anyone crossing the border into our sovereign territory without first seeking permission will be dealt with swiftly and mercilessly. Suddenly, all the talk by outsiders about providing humanitarian aid evaporates like the steam rising from a hot cup of coffee. The one thing, though, that does not end, are the daily aerial attacks against you and your fellow citizens.

What do you do? Who do you look to for help? What options are left on the table? *What do you hope will be done?*

The above scenario is essentially what the people of the Nuba Mountains in Sudan faced in the 1990s, during a period that scholars now refer to as a case of "genocide by attrition" (African Rights, 1995; Totten, 2015b), and it is what they face today as war (which broke out in June 2011) has engulfed South Kordofan State, and in particular, the people of the Nuba Mountains.

"Nuba Mountains?" one might ask.

A fair question. It is, in fact, a safe bet that most people across the globe (outside of Africa) have never heard of the Nuba Mountains.

Sudan.

While most have certainly heard of Sudan, it is probably an equally safe bet that most people across the globe would be hard-pressed to, first, state exactly where Sudan is located in Africa, and second, name those nations with which it shares a border—let alone provide any information at all about the government or its policies.

This is not to be critical, but rather to acknowledge that the crises that have haunted the people of the Nuba Mountains over the past two and a half decades under the regime of Sudanese President Omar al-Bashir are not on the radar of most people across the globe. And that, in and of itself, is just one of the many aspects of this book that make it so unique. We shall return to this a bit later. First, though, a little background is called for.

The Nuba

As for the Nuba people, it is important to note that "the Nuba" does not refer to a single group of people, but rather 50 different tribal groups roughly numbering an estimated 1.07 million people who reside in the Nuba Mountains in South Kordofan State. The vast majority are farmers and/or herders of cattle and goats. While most speak Arabic, the official language of Sudan, some 100 languages *in toto* are spoken by those who reside in the Nuba Mountains. The Nuba practice a variety of religions, including: Islam; Christianity; animism; plus, a mixture of Islam and animism, and a mixture of Christianity and animism. Many of the Muslims are moderate, as opposed to fundamentalist, in their beliefs. Tellingly, for the most part, no matter what one's religion is, the people of the Nuba get along extremely well. For example, within the same family one finds both Christians and Muslims. A Muslim man may have two wives, one being Muslim and one being Christian. There are not a few cases where children brought up as Muslims have, in their later teens to their early to mid-twenties, converted to Christianity and are readily welcomed by the family, still loved and still respected.

Since June 2011, war has raged in the Nuba Mountains (Sudan) between the Sudan People's Liberation Army–North (SPLA-N) and the Government of Sudan (GoS). Typical of its modus operandi in its battles with different groups within Sudan (i.e., in Darfur, in Blue Nile State, etc.), the GoS has not limited its attacks solely against the Sudan People's Liberation Army–North (SPLA-N or the Nuba rebel forces), but has carried out almost daily aerial bombings against the civilians of the Nuba Mountains *and* used food as a weapon of war against them as well.

Exacerbating matters is the fact that the GoS continues to refuse foreign aid groups (be they international nongovernmental organizations such as the United Nations or nongovernmental groups such as Doctors without Borders) from entering the Nuba Mountains. To a large extent, it appears as if the international community has rolled over and acceded to the demands of the GoS in this regard.

Exactly how many combatants there are on each side is impossible to state with any certainty. That said, the GoS certainly has tens of thousands of soldiers in the region. In one battle alone in January 2015, some 1,500 GoS soldiers took part in the attack against the main SPLA-N stronghold, the town of Kauda, in the Nuba Mountains (*Totten*, 2015a, n.p.).

The roots of the war are many, but the most significant are as follows:

(a) As a result of being marginalized and disenfranchised politically, socially, and economically by the GoS, the Nuba Mountains people joined the south in battling the north (Khartoum) during the Second Sudanese Civil War (1983–2005);

(b) In 2005, the international community, including the United States, helped to broker a peace that brought an end to the Second Sudanese Civil War (1983–2005), which claimed an estimated two million deaths. With the signing of the Comprehensive Peace Agreement (CPA) between the Sudan People's Liberation Movement/Army (SPLM/A or the southerners) and the GoS (or Khartoum, the northerners), those in the south were accorded the right to hold a referendum to decide whether they would remain part of Sudan (a "New Sudan," or a united and secular Sudan) or to secede and establish their own nation. Despite the fact that the people of the Nuba Mountains fought on the side of the south during the civil war, they were not allowed to vote on the referendum, which was largely due to various compromises and side agreements made by the international community and the GoS. Held between January 9 and January 15, 2011, an astonishing 98.83 percent voted in favor of independence. On July 9, 2011, the Republic of South Sudan officially became the newest nation in the community of nations;

(c) Ultimately, the Nuba were not allowed to secede from Sudan with the rest of the southerners. Thus, even though they fought with the south against Khartoum, the Nuba people remained under the dictatorial rule of Omar al-Bashir[1];

(d) Initially, al-Bashir named Ahmed Haroun, who is wanted by the International Criminal Court (ICC) on 43 charges of crimes against humanity he allegedly perpetrated in Darfur during the early part of the century, governor of South Kordofan, which understandably incensed the Nuba people;

(e) Later, in May 2011, following an election between Haroun and Abdel Aziz, Haroun was elected governor of South Kordofan, but the Nuba asserted that the election was rigged;

(f) As a result of a series of vociferous protests by the Nuba in late 2010 and early

2011 over (1) being left out of the CPA, (2) the election of Haroun as governor, and (3) their ongoing political, social and economic disenfranchisement by the GoS, al-Bashir ordered the protesters to cease and desist immediately. If they didn't, he threatened, he would see to it that the Nuba faced the same fate that they did during the 1990s (which essentially meant that they would face relentless attacks by the Sudanese Armed Forces (i.e., Khartoum) and potential starvation as they did during the genocide by attrition); and,

(g) At one and the same time, al-Bashir threatened to establish *sharia* (or Islamic) law as the law of the land, which the Nuba recoiled at, particularly in light of the fact that they are comprised of Christians, moderate Muslims, and animists.

Furious at the fact that they were forced to remain under the fist of the dictatorial regime of al-Bashir, the Nuba not only voiced their displeasure but asserted that they would rearm themselves if they were not treated fairly and justly. Following increasingly heated exchanges, accusations, counter-accusations, and threats, the Nuba and the GoS went to war in June 2011. The continuous threats by al-Bashir essentially constituted the trigger that ignited the war in June 2011, at which point the SPLA–N carried out its initial attacks against the GoS.

By early July, the UN peacekeeping observers based in Kauda and Kadugli in the state of South Kordofan were essentially "paralyzed," and it was not long before they pulled out of the region altogether. In July and August one humanitarian aid group after another also pulled out of South Kordofan due to the danger posed by the fighting in the region.

The GoS' Aerial Bombings of Civilians

If attacked, any government anywhere will retaliate, either arresting and/or killing those who have carried out the attacks. When the SPLA–N attacked GoS facilities in June 2011, the GoS not only struck back at the rebel group, but immediately began carrying out ground and aerial attacks (using both Antonov bombers and attack jets) against the civilian population of the Nuba Mountains. Attacking civilians is against international law.

The initial attacks by the GoS against the civilian population ranged from aerial attacks that came in low and pinpointed civilians, leaving many dead bodies looking as if they had been rendered in a slaughterhouse, to door-to-door searches in Kadugli (the capital of South Kordofan State) by GoS' operatives who killed suspected SPLA–N supporters by slitting their throats and letting them bleed out where they dropped.

Ever since 2011, GoS' Antonov bombers have carried out daily attacks on Nuba civilians, primarily targeting large groups congregated in such places as *suqs* (open marketplaces), schools, churches and mosques, and villages. While most villagers and shop owners have dug deep holes (seven to eight feet deep) that serve as bomb shelters (thus providing them with a relatively safe place to wait out the aerial attacks), many who have been caught out in the open have either been killed or had limbs (legs and arms) sheared off. Furthermore, since many aerial attacks have been carried out against the Nuba's farms, many fear the results of continuing "to cultivate," which has resulted in the production of fewer crops and ever-increasing hunger.

The Use of Food as a Weapon of War

Just as it did during the genocide by attrition in the Nuba Mountains between 1989 and the mid–1990s, the GoS is once again using food as a weapon of war against the civilians of the Nuba Mountains. During the genocide by attrition, tens of thousands of Nubans were forced off their farms as a result of SAF ground and aerial attacks. The civilians fled up into the mountains by the tens of thousands seeking relative safety in the caves that honeycomb the mountains in the region. Without access to their farms and granaries, many Nuba resorted to eating wild grasses, leaves, and roots. When the latter had been consumed, many had no recourse but to begin eating leaves and roots that they knew were poisonous. The Nuba would cook and strain the roots three times, allow them to dry in the sun, beat the roots into granules and add the granules to any sorghum they might have. Because their systems could not process the latter, it was not unusual for both infants and the elderly to perish from eating such "food."

Today, daily hunger in the Nuba Mountains is a fact of life and death again as no one has enough food to eat. In fact, many, if not most, are down to eating a single meal a day. Those, however, who reside in the most remote parts of the Nuba Mountains and/or are the most impoverished continue to face, as they have over the past six years, the entire gamut of hunger, from malnutrition to severe malnutrition to starvation.

Some Nuba who fled their villages and farms and attempted to cross the border into The Republic of South Sudan where refugee camps are located have perished along the way as a result of starvation. Undoubtedly, more are likely to do so as the GoS continues its attacks on Nuba farms and villages and refuses to allow international humanitarian aid agencies from entering the region. (For a detailed discussion of the genocide by attrition, see *Genocide by Attrition: Nuba Mountains Sudan* by Samuel Totten, and *Conflict in the Nuba Mountains: From Genocide by Attrition to the Contemporary Crisis* co-edited by Samuel Totten and Amanda Grzyb.)

As alluded to above, in January 2012, rumors were afloat that both the United Nations and the United States were considering the possibility of establishing a humanitarian corridor in order to distribute food and medical aid to those Nuba civilians in dire straits. The rumors continued apace until May, when they abruptly and virtually disappeared.

Risking Life and Limb to Help the Nuba

Those whose stories are related in this book are a fairly eclectic group with diverse backgrounds and interests. Two are female, ten are male. Their ages range from their early 30s to their early 70s. Most are ardent Christians. A few do not comment on their faith. Nine are Caucasian, and three are black (one is Nuban and two are African-American). Amongst them are physicians, nurses, journalists, a university researcher in the field of human rights and genocide studies, a business executive, and charity workers. One individual is a Catholic sister. *The one thing they all have in common is the fact that they have risked life and limb to help the people of the Nuba Mountains at a time when war rages all across the Nuba Mountains.*

Individually and collectively, the stories in *Sudan's Nuba Mountains People Under Siege* constitute a countervalence to the way the international community has reacted to the ongoing crisis in the Nuba Mountains. More specifically, while the international community has largely acceded to al-Bashir's demand to cease and desist from providing humanitarian aid of any kind into the Nuba Mountains, a small number of private individuals have stepped up of their own accord and volunteered to do all they can within their power to help the Nuba.

Obviously, different people have different reasons, different motivations and different aims for helping others. Some are inclined to reach out and help those who share the same origins (i.e., ethnicity or nationality), the same religion, the same race, etc. Others are motivated by principles and commandments inherent in their faith (i.e., The Golden Rule and the Good Samaritan in the Christian faith; *tzedakah* or charity in the Jewish tradition; or *zakat* or support of the needy in Islamic faith). Still others may be motivated by their fierce belief that each and every person across the globe is inherently entitled to inalienable fundamental rights based on the dignity and worth of the human person—or, putting it in even simpler terms, simply because she or he is a human. And, of course, others are inclined to help those who are friends or, on the most basic of terms, simply because fellow humans are in need. All of these motivations and more are at the heart of what motivates the people (contributors) whose stories are related in this book.[2]

In a day and age when the term "hero" is tossed around rather loosely, most, if not all, of these individuals have actively resisted the appellation of hero being applied to them. Almost to a person, the contributors are incredibly modest in regard to their efforts. They are also astonishingly modest in regard to what they may have accomplished (or the good they've done). Ultimately, all have gone about their work in the Nuba in a matter of fact way. It is what they do. Granted, it is conducted in a region of the world that is extremely remote and where warfare rages, but it is what it is.[3]

While the personal story of each contributor is remarkable in its own way, one thing that each of them has in common is *their tremendous commitment to help those in dire need when no one else on the face of the planet is willing to do so* (including such organizations as the United Nations, the World Food Program, and all of the other entities whose missions are purportedly to assist those who are facing crises that impact their very existence). While they may not perceive themselves as particularly special and do not seek the limelight or special recognition for their humanitarian efforts, their stories are well worth relating due to the fact that unlike the vast majority of humanity they have refused to allow themselves to become bystanders when their fellow members of humanity are facing life-threatening actions at the hands of murderous perpetrators.[4] *Put another way, they stand in stark contrast to the mainstream of indifference that far too often is the rule versus the exception when innocents are in extremis.* And, unlike most, they are willing to put their own lives on the line in an attempt to help those who otherwise would be forsaken, and they seemingly do so due to their belief that all human life is precious and that all people everywhere are part and parcel of their universe of obligation.

Conclusion

Not a few of the contributors to this book were somewhat tentative about writing pieces about themselves and their efforts. Ultimately, they were convinced to do so when they came to appreciate the fact that their stories were yet one more way to get the story out about the trials and tribulations of the Nuba Mountains people—a people, who like most others across the globe, simply want to live their lives in peace with their loved ones and friends and enjoy those fundamental rights all people across the globe are entitled to as a result of being members of the human family. No less, and no more.

In light of that, it is hoped that the inspiring stories that comprise this book help to shine a bright light on the plight of the Nuba Mountains people at this particular juncture in time—that is, how the Nuba and their very culture face an existential threat as a result of the policies, stances and actions of the Government of Sudan.

It is also hoped that readers will be moved to contribute in their own way(s) to help focus ever greater attention on the plight of the Nuba so as to push, prod and cajole the international community to act—and act effectively—sooner rather than later, to protect the Nuba culture, the Nuba people's basic human rights, and the Nubas' very existence.

Finally, it is hoped that the stories of the individuals herein will spark deep thought and reflection in readers about what it means *to not be a bystander* in the face of cruelty, injustice, and oppression no matter who the victims are or what they believe or where they reside. It almost goes without saying that innocents caught up in the maelstrom of violent conflict—where fear and dread are constants, where the potential to lose loved ones is never far away, and where the potential for grievous injury and death are stark realities—frequently feel all alone in the world and that no one cares about their plight, let alone their fate. One can only attempt to imagine what that feels like in the deepest chambers of their hearts and minds.[5]

All human beings have aspirations, hopes, dreams, desires, and wants. All human beings cry when they are sad, are desperate when confronted with overwhelming odds, and suffer in the face of profound loss. All human beings facing desperate straits hope against hope that someone, somewhere will help them, that they and their loved ones will not be subjected to horrific atrocities and made to suffer for nothing they have done but simply because of who they are (i.e., this or that race, ethnicity, gender, nationality, etc.) or because it was their fate to live in a particular region of the world at a particular point in time under a particular set of circumstances. Indeed, all hope they will not be (or haven't already been) forgotten.

In the end, it is my hope that readers will truly and deeply consider what it means to "do unto others as you would have them do unto you" in relation to those who are caught up in nightmarish situations where dictators, rogue governments, so-called intelligence agencies (no matter which country they "work" for), and extremists of any stripe (i.e., Nazis, Stalinists, Boko Haram, ISIS, etc.) run roughshod over innocents and terrify and kill at will.

Notes

1. In regard to the eventual establishment of the new nation of the Republic of South Sudan, see the following articles by Samuel Totten that have appeared in *Social Education*: "The Birth of a New Nation: The Republic of South Sudan," and "The Birth of a Nation Is Only the Beginning: The Travails of South Sudan."

2. A good number of the individuals whose stories are featured in this book were actively involved in helping the Nuba in various ways *prior to* the start of the war in June 2011. Two individuals, for example, lived and worked in the Nuba Mountains for many years prior to 2011: Ryan Boyette and Dr. Tom Catena. Others, while not residing in the Nuba Mountains year around, have served the Nuba in various and significant ways for many years prior to 2011. George Tutu was born and raised in the Nuba Mountains, but due to his efforts to gain basic rights for his people he was forced into exile by the al-Bashir regime. Ever since making it to the United States in 1998, George has continued to return periodically to the Nuba for the express purpose of delivering food and medication

to those of his people in most need. He has also served as a strong voice for the Nuba in the United States, and has put in long hours working with various groups who are keen to help the Nuba. Additionally, he has taken on the responsibility of guiding many humanitarians into the Nuba, thus risking his own life over and over again.

Tomo Križnar first traveled to the Nuba back in the 1990s. In the subsequent years he has spent months on end crisscrossing the Nuba, befriending the people, producing remarkable books and documentaries about the Nuba, and speaking on their behalf in Europe and beyond. Notably, Tomo has also crisscrossed Darfur and the Blue Nile State, when each region raged with warfare. In a word, Tomo is "indefatigable" in his dedication to the Nuba people.

Still others had traveled to the Nuba for short spans of time for various purposes prior to the outbreak of war in 2011: Sister Deirdre M. Byrne (to volunteer and apply her medical expertise at Mother of Mercy Hospital), and Samuel Totten (to conduct research), and only later to deliver food to those communities facing the greatest "food insecurity").

3. It is also true, of course, that travel in the region is anything but easy. During the dry season temperatures often reach well over 100 degrees Fahrenheit. The "roads" are rutted and rock strewn and result in head rattling and body battering rides. Swirling dust is also a constant. And the distances between various points are often long and result in hours of rough travel. Even if one carries one's own liquids, it is not unusual for the temperature of water, for example, to quickly rise to 70 degrees Fahrenheit or higher, which is far from thirst quenching.

Furthermore, those who enter the Nuba Mountains today do so illegally. Since the GoS does not want witnesses to the crimes committed every single day against civilians and do not want outsiders to provide the Nuba with humanitarian aid, it does not grant visas to travel in the region. As a result, one must cross illegally and then travel illegally in the country.

Anyone who remains in and/or enters a new a war zone takes an enormous amount of risk. While it may be a calculated risk, it is still a risk. It is, obviously, not a decision to be made lightly.

4. It is a simple fact that relatively few people are willing to purposely remain in and/or head into a war zone if they don't have to do so. It is also a sorrowful fact that far too few people in the world care enough about the plight and fate of others, particularly in far away places, to speak up on their behalf, let alone to act on their behalf.

At one and the same time, though, it is also true that more people today than ever before do contribute time, thought, effort and, yes, money, to help those who are less fortunate and/or in dire straits. Even a short list of the many international human rights organizations that are comprised of members from around the globe is telling in regard to the desire and commitment of many to speak out on the behalf of the beleaguered, the threatened, the unfairly imprisoned, the tortured: Amnesty International, Amnesty International USA, PEN, and Women's International League for Peace and Freedom. Then there are such remarkable nongovernmental organizations that do the most fantastic work on the behalf of the oppressed and downtrodden in some of the toughest, most violent places on the globe: *Médecins Sans Frontières* (MSF) or Doctors without Borders; Oxfam International; Catholic Relief Services; Mercy Corps; American Refugee Committee; CARE (Cooperative for Assistance and Relief Everywhere); Norwegian Relief Council; and the United Nations Office for the Coordination of Humanitarian Affairs, among many others. All of these organizations individuals can support through donations. Many also have opportunities for volunteer work, both in the U.S. and/or overseas. The same is true of the following organizations that address violations of international human rights across the globe: Human Rights Watch, Refugees International, Protection International, and the International Committee of the Red Cross.

There is, of course, a medium ground between (a) individuals risking their lives in conflict zones and (b) solely supporting an organization by donating money. And it is there, in that medium ground, where individuals who really care deeply about the plight of others, who deeply desire to help others, and who are willing to commit themselves to a sustained effort versus a one-off action (the latter of which is more of a feel good approach versus a serious commitment to address the problem) can make a real and significant difference.

5. Sadly, the Nuba Mountains is hardly the only place in the world today where innocent civilians face such fears and concerns. Among some of the many others, for example, are: the Democratic of the Republic (DRC), the Central African Republic, Libya, Burundi, Nigeria (where the Boko Haram run wild), Somalia, Yemen, Afghanistan, Syria, Iraq, Mynamar (Burma), North Korea, China, Darfur, Sudan, and the Blue Nile State, Sudan.

REFERENCES

African Rights (1995). *Facing Genocide. The Nuba of Sudan*. London: Author.

Totten, Samuel (2015a). "Bombs Rain Down: Attacks to Intensify Against Nuba." *Arkansas Democrat Gazette*. November 6. Accessed at: http://www.arkansasonline.com/news/2015/nov/06/bombs-rain-down-20151106/?f=opinion.

Totten, Samuel (2015b). *Genocide by Attrition: Nuba Mountains, Sudan*. New Brunswick, NJ: Transaction Publishers.

Totten, Samuel, and Grzyb, Amanda (Eds.) (2015). *Conflict in the Nuba Mountains: From Genocide by Attrition to the Contemporary Crisis*. New York: Routledge, 2015.

United Nations (1948). The Universal Declaration of Human Rights. New York: Author. Accessed at: www.un.org/en/universal-declaration-human-rights/

A Love for the Nuba People

Tomo Križnar

For the past twenty plus years I have dedicated my life's work to helping to prevent the extermination of the Nuba people, "the last natives" in Central Sudan. In doing so, I've traveled what feels like every single inch of the Nuba Mountains. And I've done so in every which way possible: cargo planes, motorcycles, bicycles and on foot. I love the region and I love the people. And that, simply, is why I have done what I've done (much of which will be addressed herein).

Back in 2003, when my adventures in the Nuba Mountains were coming to an end, just when I was beginning to feel good again (meaning, it appeared the Nuba were going to be OK), a new rebellion broke out in Sudan, this time in Darfur. Abruptly, I moved from writing articles and books to producing documentaries (i.e., *Voices from the Other Side*, and *Dar Fur—War for Water*). Documentaries, I figured, would reach many more people in much less time than articles and books.

My express purpose in producing a documentary about Darfur was to attempt to create the critical mass needed to awaken the world, the international community, to the slaughter that was underway in Darfur: the onslaught of destruction against the so-called Black Africans of Darfur by the Government of Sudan (and, in particular, the government of Sudanese President Omar al-Bashir, the army colonel who had carried out a coup d'etat in Sudan in 1989 and had ruled ever since). That disaster is still ongoing, though one would never know it from the lack of attention given to it by the leaders of the world, the United Nations, and, yes, even activists.

In June 2011, war broke out again in the Nuba Mountains.

Herein, I shall highlight my efforts on the behalf of the Nuba people. In doing so, I shall reach back to the 1990s, when I first traveled to the Nuba. I shall touch on the different periods I've been in the Nuba Mountains—when, why, where and what I was doing, as well as how the Nuba were/are doing. Chapters in books are, of course, limited in how long they can be, and in light of that readers will appreciate that what I delineate herein is, by necessity, a very truncated story of my time, experiences and efforts in the Nuba Mountains.

My Meeting with Leni Riefenstahl, October 1999

Leni Riefensthal. For many, at least those who are conversant with the history of World War II and Nazi Germany, the name Leni Riefensthal calls to mind a young female photographer's friendship with Adolf Hitler and the propaganda film she produced, *Triumph of the Will*. What many are unlikely to know, though, is that she is equally famous among professional photographers and Africanists as the one who photographed the Nuba people in all their glory.[1]

I decided I needed to meet her, because of her work about the Nuba. During my visit with her at her home in Pökingen, a village about fifty kilometers south of Munich, she appeared, for all the world, like a "star." Seated on an expansive white sofa, below which spread a beautiful white carpet, her legs crossed, she rubbed one thigh against the other in an incredibly flirtatious manner. And she was 99 years old!

"What is happening to my Nubas?" she asked me, sadly. "What happened to my Gabik? Where is my Massala now? What is Kaka doing?"

She began crying.

Oddly (I say "oddly," because I never knew this about her and had never noticed it in any photos of her), I noticed that she was cross-eyed. Each eye looked in a different direction.

I had gotten her phone number from a friend of mine, Vito Babic, who had gotten it from an acquaintance at the Neue Slowenische Kunst (a controversial art collective in Slovenia), who had been tirelessly attempting to reach her as he was very keen to interview her. I called her at least ten times. All to no avail. It finally dawned on me that I needed to provide her with a good reason to meet with me. And so, during my next call to her, I informed her that I had news for her from Kau, Niar and Fungor, each of which are the names of three locations in the Nuba Mountains that she photographed in her now famous pictures of the Nuba back in the 1960s and 1970s, and had published in her books, *The Last of the Nuba* and *People of Kau*. Long story short, my ploy worked. In fact, I was informed by her secretary that "Madam, was very anxious to meet me." I was then told, immediately, that "Madam will get up and ready herself for your visit."

Upon my arrival at her home, I was greeted by Horst Kettner, who had been Riefenstahl's companion since he was 20 years old and she approximately 60 years old. He escorted me into the living room where Riefenstahl was seated, and then stood next to her in order to serve as her interpreter.

Immediately, they both claimed that Riefenstahl was not fluent in English, which I knew was not true.

"They are dying!" I more or less spat out. "They are finished! If you do not respond at once and do something, they will be exterminated!"

Her hand, shaking, covered her mouth as she acted as if she could not believe what she had just been told.

Not holding back, I hit her with something a lot more personal: "One of the survivors in Kauniar, a local man, told me that the main pogrom started with your *El Kitab* [an Arabic wedding]. As you know, in your books you included photos of the indigenous animists bare naked, which the Muslims in northern Sudan see as a national shame. When President Nimeiry honored you with Sudanese citizenship and a Sudanese passport for your merits in promoting Sudan, he also sent a death squad to the Nuba Mountains, executioners with a sword in one *hand and the Koran in the other. Those who would not accept the Koran were systematically exterminated.* All naked, all natural, all primal, all pagan, all that co-existed symbiotically with Mother Nature, all had to die."

She flinched, either at my words or the truth of the matter or due to the fact that she was embarrassed that the truth had been spoken.

"In your book you wrote that in no other place or time had you been happier than amongst the Nuba; not even when you were one of the most powerful women in the world. If you truly love them, then for the love of God, help them now!"

I shared with her that my initial interest in the Nuba began around 1980 when I first saw a photograph of the ash-covered winner of the famous Nuba arm wrestling competition sitting on the shoulders of his fellow men. The photograph had been taken by a British colonial officer, George Rodger, immediately following World War II. It was, interestingly, the very same photograph, as she stated in her memoir, that spurred Riefenstahl to travel to Sudan in the first place—after she had failed to locate any "extras" in all of East Africa to use in a documentary on contemporary slaves that she was filming.

I placed ten videotapes on the table in the living room. They contained information about the extermination of Nuba farmers in Kau, Niaro, and Fungor, among others. I had personally recorded them illegally the summer before in an area that had been off limits—a no go zone—and a place where no reporter had made it to ever since the beginning of the Second Sudanese Civil War in 1983. I told her how the GoS's military troops, along with various Arabic nomadic militia groups hired by the GoS, were systematically forcing more then fifty Nuba tribes from their homes in the mountains to the deserts in the north. I also informed her about how many of the people who were forced from their homes were dying from a lack of food. Furthermore, I told her about how those Nuba who refused to acquiesce with the demands of the GoS and would not leave their land were being attacked, bombarded, in order to force them out. I shared with her that many Nuba were being taken and used as slaves: girls and women for sexual purposes, and boys as janissaries. Many of the most elderly were being murdered since they were not perceived as useful. I decried the fact that no powers that be (neither individual nations nor the United Nations) seemed to care anything at all about the plight and fate of the Nuba.

But, I pointed out, there are a handful of scholars, journalists and activists who are attempting to doing something to draw the world's attention to their plight, but few seem to be listening to them. For example, I said, Alex de Waal, who conducted research in the Nuba Mountain for his doctoral dissertation at Oxford, co-founded a group called African Rights, which is based in England, and had been ardently working on a number of different fronts in an effort to wake the world up about what the Nuba are facing. African Rights, for example, I told her, had published a highly informative book entitled *Facing Genocide: Nuba of Sudan*. I also told her that a journalist named Julie Flint, along with de Waal, had produced a BBC documentary entitled *Sudan's Secret War*.

I also told her about an activist named Arthur Howgh, who secretly produced an important documentary about life in Sudan under the regime of Sudanese President Omar al-Bashir, *The Kafi Story*. But, I said, not a single television channel agreed to air it.

Continuing, I said, "We are all trying to support Suleiman Rahhal, a doctor in London, born to a notable Nuba family. He has established a self-help organization called *Nuba Survival*. But all the European governments, even the Scandinavians and Washington, D.C., are apparently under the influence of oil lobbies that cooperate with the Islamic fundamentalist authorities in Khartoum.

"So we really need you! Someone who knows the Nuba, someone who is famous, someone who the world might listen to! If your love for the Nuba is as true as you say it is, then you must go to Sudan immediately!"

"Leni is too old and too sick to undertake such a journey,'" Horst spoke up, obviously not pleased with my suggestion.

Not saying a word, I pulled a copy of my most recent book, *Nuba, the Pure People*, from my bag, and I jotted a dedication to her and signed it.

I then made a point of showing her the photographs I had taken and explained how easy it had been to get into the illegal zone with a plane, which had been hired by the German Emergency Doctors (*Kap Anamur*), the only foreign organization that, at the time, was attempting to help the Nuba people.

I went on to tell her about Father Kizito, an Italian missionary in Kenya, who personally made at least one trip to the Nuba with stocks of salt, medicines, and school supplies.

Finally, I told her that she could, without a doubt, get a flight to the region from NRRDO—(the Nuba Rehabilitation Relief Development Organization), a Nuba organization secretly supported by other small western donors, which operated charter flights at least once a month.

I found myself musing: "And if the trip proved to be the last she ever took? Hadn't she, back in the seventies, chosen to be buried among 'the noble savages'"? If the rival of Eva Braun should die in the Nuba Mountains, the whole world would hear about the genocide of the innocent that very same day!"

But then I actually said, "Go back to the mountains, Leni, and we will do everything we can so that history remembers you as a shining example to all humanitarians worldwide."

Three hours later Riefenstahl and I were caught up in reminiscing about many of the rituals the Nuba perform in gratitude of the first raindrops that announce the coming of the rainy season and the ritual calling for fertility. Riefenstahl also spoke movingly of how deeply touched she was by the unity, cooperation, care and modesty amongst the Nuba and how they all seemed to deeply care for every person in the tribe—a quality that enabled the Nuba people to survive thousands of years in one of the most inhospitable environments on the planet.

"I am a living witness to how traditional conflicts over access to land and water between native African farmers and Arabic nomadic immigrants are used," I said, "by the Arabic government in Khartoum to force the natives, the Nuba, off their farms, out of their villages, and how they do so by supporting the *mujahedeen*, the Arab nomads, as they attack one Nuba village after another. I witnessed the establishment of massive, mechanized farms that Khartoum established on Nuba land, which it had virtually stolen from the Nuba."

Riefenstahl listened to me in silence, but with obvious interest.

"But when the American company Chevron found oil south of the demarcation line that divides northern and southern Sudan, war over land and water morphed into war for oil. The cowboys are co-responsible for the civil war in Sudan."

"*Nein! Nein!* The Jews are to blame!" Riefenstahl exclaimed and instantly straightened her eyes. "*Die Juden! Die Juden!*"

"It is not enough for them to control all the world's gold, they want to control all the oil too!" Horst interjected. "All over eastern Europe, in Slovakia, Ukraine and in some of the countries carved from out from the former Yugoslavia, Jews are buying used weapons and shipping them in containers to black rebels in the southern Sudan. By supporting the rebels in the SPLA they are provoking the Arabs and destabilizing the Sudan."

"Then hit back at them and return to the mountains and show the whole world who is driving black tribes away from the oil fields and water sources," I begged. "Please, return to the Nuba Mountains, film everything, take photographs, show the famous Jew Susan Sontag that you're not only concerned with Nazi aesthetics."

"Susan Sontag? How can someone so intelligent say such foolish things about me?" Riefenstahl asked, indignantly. "I am interested solely in art and beauty, only in what is wonderful. Politics I do not care about. I have nothing to do with politics. Look, you can see it here!"

She proceeded to hold up a copy of her book *Mein Afrika*.

Then, on the first page, she wrote: "To Tomo Križnar, who came to tell me about Nuba."

A week later Riefenstahl called me on the phone. "I am going! Our German ambassador is on very good terms with the Arabs in the Omar Bashir government. Our ambassador in Khartoum has promised me that he would personally organize a visit to the Nuba Mountains."

Two weeks later, Riefenstahl called me again: "Sixteen thousand Mesakin Nubas in the Rekha village will dance in my welcome! Filmmaker Ray Muller is also coming with us. He will make a new documentary about me." That was Riefenstahl!

When Julie Flint heard about Riefenstahl's plan, she immediately responded in protest. "Big mistake! Big mistake! The Arabs in the Sudan government will create a perfect show for Leni, who will then try to convince the whole world how happy the Arab-occupied Nuba families are. The Arabs will use Leni as propaganda, how very well the Nubas who have let themselves be Arabised by Islamic fundamentalists are doing."

Still, Riefenstahl continued apace with her plan, which was to travel to various areas controlled by the Nuba rebels, purportedly so she could compare and contrast what life was like for the Nuba under Khartoum versus life under the Nuba rebels, thus enabling her to attempt to ascertain which side the natives would more likely have a real chance of saving their indigenous coexistence with. It was my hope that once she saw the reality on the ground, then perhaps she would choose to work on the behalf of the Nuba.

But a wrench was thrown in the works. More specifically, I discovered that legendary commandant of the Nuba rebels, Yousif Kuwa Makki, who would have undoubtedly won Riefenstahl over and convinced her to side with those who were fighting for righteousness, for the right to be Nuba, was in London being treated for prostate cancer. Long story short, Riefenstahl's plans were, for the moment, nixed.

But then, the first week of January 2000, Leni, Horst and Ray Muller made it to Khartoum, where they awaited their official permit from the Sudanese Ministry of Interior to travel south.

"This is not going to be good," I thought. "More like a disaster, without Kuwa there."

I called every day from a free phone in the editing room in the basement of the TV Slovenia building (the Slovenian national broadcasting company), where we were working on my documentary, *Nuba, the Pure People*. I called Julia and Kuwa in London and Leni and her team in Khartoum trying to work something out.

"She will be cautioned once more, maybe twice—if she does not desist, she will have only herself to blame!" Yousif's voice warned over the phone.

On January 29th, Riefenstahl's team took off from Khartoum in a rickety helicopter heading towards Kadugli, the capital of South Kordofan State, which is the state where the Nuba reside. The landing was far from perfect and resulted in the puncture of one of the helicopter's tires. That, in turn, forced the team to travel by jeep as it headed on towards the Rekha "peace camp."

Upon reaching their destination, they were, as Riefenstahl said they would, greeted by Mesakin Nuba. But it was far from the sixteen thousand she had predicted, but it was still quite a welcome. Everyone wanted to shake her hand and then, as they traditionally do, danced to welcome her. Many invited her to their *tukuls*. She said she only recognized a few old friends from her earlier visits.

She also said, though, that something was not quite right. The Nuba, she noticed, were tense, with some visibly frightened. Gradually, it dawned on Riefenstahl that what she and the others were seeing was staged. Everything! Everything from the people, the village, the animals. Essentially, Riefenstahl and her team witnessed a parallel to, though much less extravagant in its set-up, what the Nazis had created in its phony makeover of the Theresienstadt concentration camp.[2]

They had been taken to a so-called "peace camp." A concentration camp, actually. Such camps had been established all over the region; it was where those Nuba, mainly women and children and the elderly, who had been captured by GoS troops and their militia, were incarcerated

Riefenstahl was then informed by one of the Nuba that one of her oldest Nuba friends had just been killed. And as she was told that, the crowd started to get agitated, panicky. And with that, the GoS officials told Riefenstahl and her team that the visit was over, and they had to return to Khartoum immediately.

A half an hour or after their takeoff, the rickety aircraft they were in crashed to the ground. Riefenstahl and Ray Muller were both injured. She suffered two broken ribs, while he suffered a cracked pelvis bone.

Rupert Neudeck: Lokichogio, Turkana Land, Kenya, April 2001

I was resting in the shade in the pub garden of the Norwegian People Aid camp located in a place called Lokichogio, close to the Kenya and Sudan border, when a man who looked extremely familiar crossed what served as the dance floor. My neck was aching badly and I was massaging it. It hurt so badly I had even contemplated the possibility of returning home. Thin, even bony, the man had a grey beard. It was Rupert Neudeck, who I last saw in a German national television documentary.

"Herr Rupert Neudeck, I suppose," I said as I rose from my chair.

"From Slovenia?" he asked with a smile. "That new little country that fell blessed on its knees because it was on its soil that Bush and Putin met for the very first time? Did you really clear out the whole city in their honor last week?"

I started defending myself saying that the presidents met there by mistake since they had confused Slovenia for Slovakia. I then immediately boasted that Slovenia used that opportunity to show itself as a world scale humanitarian super power. Twenty-one eminent Slovenians had signed a petition calling on the two leaders of two of the world's powers to focus attention on the suffering of the people of the Nuba Mountains, who had recently suffered what was being referred to as "genocide by attrition." The petition was signed by a real who's who of Slovenia: the most prominent of statesmen, heads of parliament, the Slovenian archbishop, noted academics, highly respected journalists and artists.

"Is that why no media mentioned the country or the city of their meeting?" he asked sarcastically, as he pushed the latest issues of *Time Magazine* and *Newsweek* towards me.

I perused the articles in each magazine and saw that he was right: neither Ljubljana nor Slovenia had been mentioned.

"People who own the media collaborate with people who own oil lobbies and they immediately sabotage any initiative that would allow for the great shame to come out," he said, with contempt in his voice. "They are all in it together. They are organized. Birds of a feather flock together. Look around you. The truth lies bare naked here in Africa."

Three years before, in 1998, when I first visited the rebels in the Nuba Mountains, the German Emergency Doctors was the only foreign organization I came across that was helping the besieged families in the Nuba Mountains. Of all that are bound by their statute to help the most threatened, the young Germans were the only ones risking their lives to help the victims.

The name Rupert Neudeck first rang in my ears when it was shouted through a radio connection by one of four team members of the German Emergency Doctors responsible for logistics, Roberto Vilone. He wanted Rupert to send, posthaste, twenty five thousand square meters of plastic sheets so he could cover the only landing strip that was not occupied by government forces, and thus attempt to keep it dry in the rainy season that had just started.

That was two months after I had done everything I could to "smuggle" myself into the Nuba Mountains by bicycle through the war zone that had been declared by the Sudanese government military, and which no observer, reporter or humanitarian organization was allowed to cross. By the time I arrived in the Nuba, Sudanese Arabs had already been carrying out ethnic and cultural cleansing of the natives for a full decade. The naked people in the Nuba Mountains were, like those in the south of Sudan, a remnant of the past and were considered such an awful disgrace that they had to be approached with the *Koran* in one hand and a Kalashnikov in the other and then forcibly dressed, Arabized and Islamized. During my four months of illegal cycling in the region, I was arrested five times, but released each time after a maximum of four days. I was not allowed to continue on my way, though, until the military intelligence agents tried to infuse me with their propaganda that the extermination of the "naked savages" in the mountains was an absolute necessity if Sudan was to develop into a modern, prosperous country like United Arab Emirates and the United States of America or those in Europe.

The longer I rode my bicycle in this region and the more I spoke to different GoS officials and officers, the clearer it became that the Second Sudanese Civil War was neither so much about ethnic, cultural and religious conflict between the Muslim Arabs in the north and Christian Africans in the south, as the media was reporting to its followers in Europe and the United States, nor so much about freeing the south from traditional slave hunters from the north. It wasn't about any of that anymore. It was, I came to believe, mostly about oil.

The reason why I wanted to manage to reach the Sudanese rebels in the Nuba Mountains was because I wanted to see for myself what had happened to my friends in the Mesakin Quisar tribe, whom I first met as a student in 1980. I wanted to see if it was true that the UN (UNICEF and the World Food Program) was involved in the extermination of "the last naked pagans" in the Nuba Mountains, together with the Sudanese government, like Alex de Waal from the African Rights organization, stated in his book. But what worried me the most was what Peter Werney stated in the book *Oil and Conflict in*

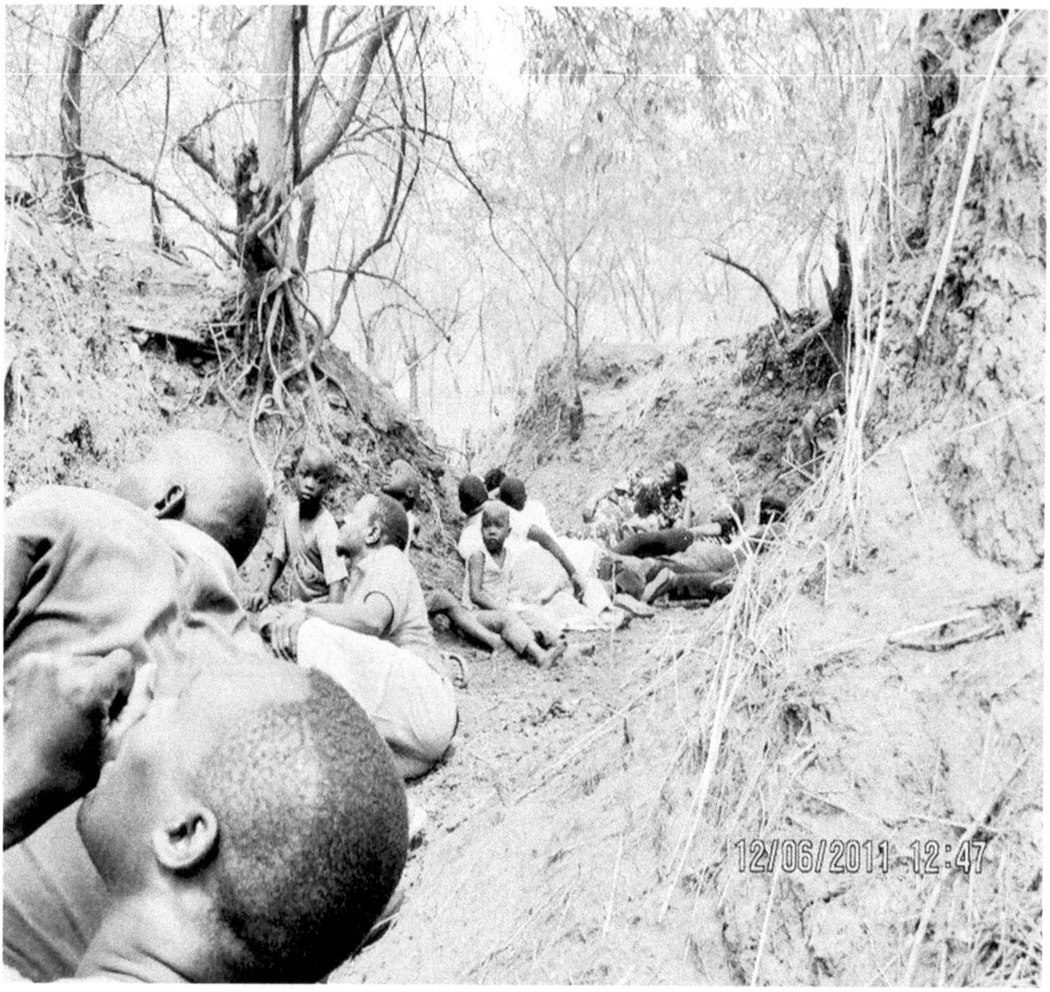

Nuba civilians seeking safety from an Antonov bomber overhead (Tomo Križnar).

Sudan: essentially, the Sudanese government was making use of certain weapons purportedly in place to protect the workers of western companies on their oil drilling/pumping sites—that is, they were said to be using them to systematically gun down the natives. Not only the U.S. companies, but also European multinational corporations, were allegedly involved in such actions, including such Scandinavian countries as Denmark, Finland, Norway, and Sweden.

Roberto died a week later of a viral lung disease he supposedly caught while rummaging around cluster bomb oddments. The plastic sheets never arrived because the entire team left the mountains in a light aircraft together with Roberto's body. I was the only one who remained. Russian Antonovs were dropping cluster bombs on villages throughout the Nuba Mountains in August and September 1998 while I was there. Government spies were about, funneling information to government garrison posts.

I was interviewing the representative of the Nuba self-help organization NRRDO one afternoon when we heard an Antonov, and that ominous whistling sound of falling death that changed my life forever. That was the day I was bombed for the first time.

Afterwards, we proceeded to pick up the pieces of explosion-torn children with our bare hands. We ended up burying a few small heaps of torn remains of four children and two women.

Rupert and I crossed paths again, and this time we found ourselves talking about Leni Riefenstahl. We condemned her because in all her life not once did she ever—in all her interviews in prestigious cosmopolitan magazines—not once commented about her return to the Nuba people and what they were facing. She bragged about her life force, bragged about *Triumph of the Will*, wondered how nothing could destroy her, and even speculated about whether Adolf Hitler had left her the secret of the elixir of life, but not once had she ever, in any way whatsoever, disclosed that "her Nuba" (as she often referred to them) were victims of genocide.

"*Die Juden! Die Juden!*" I see Riefenstahl with a raised index finger. "Jewish conspiracies are to blame for everything!"

Leni had never accused the Arabs in Sudan of exterminating the Nuba people because she believed until her last breath that the Jews are at the root of every single problem on this planet. She sided with the Arabs to her dying day because in her view the Arabs were also victims of the Jews. It is most likely not a coincidence that Sudanese president/dictator Nimeiri presented her with honorary citizenship and a Sudanese passport.

We also talked about William Gaisler, the influential German statesmen in Helmut Kohl's political party, who after the passing of Leni Riefenstahl, accompanied by Rupert, without a Sudanese-issued visa, illegally visited the Nuba Mountains and saw with his own eyes in what circumstances our friend Roberto Vilone died. When he returned home he did what we forever expected Riefenstahl to do. On the most-watched ZDF's television talk show ever produced, he phoned in front of the German audience the president's palace in Khartoum and told them that he had just been in the Nuba Mountains and saw the whole thing and then threatened the Sudanese government with diplomatic excommunication and abolishment of German aid if they did not immediately stop exterminating the innocent African children and women.

We also talked about Franco Jurij, the state secretary with the Slovenian Ministry of Foreign Affairs, who managed to convince the UN Commission on Human Rights to finally start dealing with the genocide of the Nuba people. A Slovenian initiative to send international observers to the Nuba was first backed by Scandinavian countries and later by the European Union.

We talked about the head chief of Ljubljana's Caritas, Stane Kerin, who, the year before, along with an Italian missionary based in Kenya, Kizit, and an American Comboni missionary, Paul, visited the Nuba Mountains and inserted humanitarian aid for the Nuba civilians. In doing so, they reassured the Nuba that they were not outcasts and that they were, despite the overwhelming silence in the face of all of the horrors, cared about and supported by fellow human beings in Europe and beyond.

Finally, we talked about the Slovenian director Maja Weiss, and her sister, producer Ida Weiss, and Zvone Judež of TV Slovenia, and the documentary *Nuba, the Pure People*, which earned us the honorable prize for best documentary at the film festival in Telluride, Colorado, and drew the attention of *National Geographic*, which immediately offered to produce a new documentary on the subject. Their team wanted to join me in the Nuba, which I kindly refused as I could not vouch for their safety. I did commit myself, however, to getting everything I could get on film so that a new documentary could be produced.

A Very Ordinary Trip to the Other Side, May 2011

One evening a young Turkana fellow on the street who offered me some chewing khat told me that there was a compatriot of mine staying at Kate Camp (a Hotel in Lokichoggio), a UN aircraft maintenance guy from Slovenia. On impulse, I went to see who it was, and thus I met Milan, a.k.a. Monkey, a chubby-legged, fat-bellied Serb, still in his prime. We sat down by the pool, ordered a beer with an elephant on the label, turning away child prostitutes.

One of those fellows who was drawn to war zones, he bragged about having worked all over Africa. As we continued to toss down the beers, a Ukrainian colleague of Milan's joined us. As we talked, he mentioned that he had just flown into the Nuba a week before for the SPLA. The upshot was that Rupert and I ended up hiring the plane that the Ukrainian flew. The plane, which was small, carried a small load of German medicine that was being donated to the Nuba. In an effort to get around registering at the Operation Lifeline Sudan (OLS) office, which was mandatory, we flew out before daylight. OLS was a coalition of nongovernmental organization (NGOs)—many of them among the most powerful NGOs in the world—whose express purpose was to transport food and medicine to those civilians residing in those areas under the control of the SPLA in the southern part of Sudan. OLS' mandate prevented it from entering the Nuba Mountains, as Omar al-Bashir asserted that the Nuba Mountains was off limits.

The pilot purposely flew as low as he could in an effort to evade GoS' radar. As I stared out at the passing terrain, I found myself wondering: "What happened to the nomad shepherds who tended their flocks?" "Where are those tall naked Dinkas who waved so enthusiastically at me in greeting during the rainy season in 1983, when I pushed my 49cc motorcycle on my way to the Congo and onward, following the trails of slave hunters across Rwanda and Burundi, all the way to Bagamoyo in Tanzania at the Indian Ocean coast?" They were covered in ash to protect themselves from mosquitoes, appearing to my eye like otherworldly ghosts. "But where are they?" I asked myself again.

Upon landing on an open field, which served as a makeshift airstrip, I noticed both the new green military uniforms of the SPLA and the new weapons they had. I also noticed that the number of rebels had increased greatly since I had been there last, a year ago, when the rebels were still under the command of the legendary Nuba commander, the late Yousif Kuwa Maki.

A week into my stay, an estimated seven thousand GoS troops, along with approximately 1,000 Arab mujahideen, attacked the villages of Um Durdu in the east and Como in the west. Abdel Aziz al Hilu, the new commander of the SPLA, and his men, some three thousand strong, fought the larger force to the point where the GoS troops and their allies retreated. But it was a battle that took a great toll: move than 300 Nuba civilians were killed, approximately 3,000 *tukuls* were burned to the ground, along with the churches and mosques in the region, as well as a small German medical clinic. The GoS troops and their militia also ripped off all of the recently harvested sorghum and all of the Nuba's animals. And worst of all, thousands of boys and girls were kidnapped.

I filmed interviews of the survivors, made my way out of the Sudan, and left straight for the U.S. Holocaust Memorial Museum in Washington, D.C.

Nuba Mountains, 2002–2011

There were not many of us working on the behalf of the Nuba back at the start of the new millennium. Beside Father Kizito, Stane Kerin and Bishop Makram, I recall Alex de Waal, Jamira Ron, Julie Flint, Peter Moszynski, Nana Ende, and several others whose names I cannot recall. We lobbied politicians, wrote articles, ranted on radio shows, published books, and produced documentaries about the plight of the Nuba. Some of us became famous, some of us landed jobs, and some simply gave up. When my film "Nuba, Pure People" received an award at the film festival in Telluride, it attracted the interest of both the National Geographic and a fellow named Daniel Lupinsky. The latter sent hundreds of copies of the documentary out to some of the most influential and powerful people in the United States, including key officials at U.S. State Department and John Danforth, George W. Bush's Special Envoy to Sudan.

In January 2002, a cease-fire between the SPLA and the GoS was signed with the help of "Friends of Nuba." The peace did not last long. In 2003, a new rebellion erupted in Sudan, this time in the western province of Darfur. The so-called black Africans of Darfur (mainly members of three tribal groups: The Fur, the Massaliet and the Zagahwa) were so distraught over their ongoing disenfranchisement and mistreatment at the hands of the Government of Sudan that they finally rebelled.

Many of us who had been working on the behalf of the Nuba hastily headed to Darfur, and started all over again. This time we succeeded, with the help of many others around the world, to gain enormous attention from all across the globe. Essentially, the crisis in Darfur became a cause *célèbre*, if you will.

On a personal level, I succeeded in getting the president of Slovenia, Dr. Janez Drovšek, involved. Ultimately, he sent me to Darfur as his special envoy.

Following six months of work among both the internally displaced persons in Darfur and Darfurian refugees in Chad, I was scheduled to leave the region. A peace agreement had just been signed in Abuya between the GoS and the SLA led by Minni Minnawi (the only rebel leader who signed the agreement). The war, though, continued apace. Instead of helping me to exit Darfur into Chad as negotiated with the United Nations by my president, I found myself stuck. The exit by land to Chad was cut off. So, for some unknown reason the UN handed me over to Sudan Military Intelligence. Long story short, I ended up in Shalah prison in El Fasher, where I was sentenced to two years on charges of espionage and false reporting on Sudan. Two months later, as a result of a special request of my president, al-Bashir granted me presidential amnesty. Subsequently, I was expelled from Sudan, but not before my cameras were confiscated.

When the Comprehensive Peace Agreement was signed by al-Bashir and SPLA commander John Garang, Suleiman Rahal with Nuba Survival in London immediately got word out to a lot of us, saying: "Nuba got nothing of what they had fought for in the previous war with the SPLA. The people of Nuba Mountains in Blue Nile did not get the right of self determination. The war will start again."

Six years later, just prior to the outset of the new war between the Nuba and the GoS, al-Bashir threatened to impose Sharia Law all across Sudan, cavalierly dismissing the rights of ethnic and religious minorities. That was a direct threat aimed at the Nuba, but not only the Nuba.

After an interim period of six years, on January 9, 2011, the people of the south who had fought against Khartoum finally voted in a referendum: to either remain with a reformed Sudan or to secede and establish a new nation. (The Nuba, however, were prevented from voting in the referendum.) The result was overwhelmingly in favor of seceding from the North and establishing their own nation. There was great jubilation upon the announcement of the outcome of the referendum. I, however, was not as sanguine as many others; indeed, I did not believe peace would now, once and for all, prevail, as so many of my colleagues did. This is exactly why I returned to the Nuba Mountains and Blue Nile a week before the referendum was held with my first load of digital cameras. There had been absolutely no public consultations in the Nuba Mountains as there was supposed to be under the CPA. People in the Nuba Mountains were also furious that Ahmed Haroun (who was and is wanted by the ICC for alleged atrocities perpetrated in Darfur earlier in this century) had been named governor of South Kordofan by al-Bashir and was now running for that office again. There were angry demonstrations in Kauda and other main towns. "We do not want war, we want peace!" screamed young and old. But there was no international media present except Agence France Presse. No representatives of the CPA. No activists except Julie Flint, who said, "Expect the worst!"

The first mini spy camera inserted into the Nuba Mountains I entrusted to the vice governor and SPLA commander Abdel Aziz el Hilu. The second went to Jacob Williams, who was in charge of SPLA media and public relations. Others were given to those who understood that photographs of what was taking place in the Nuba Mountains could help make a difference, as they had in the case of Darfur, where I had been training local reporters since 2008.

Five days after the war actually started again in June 2011, I returned to the Nuba Mountains with 80 cameras, computers and satellite modems. Together with Ryan Boyette (who had, by that time, lived in the Nuba for about ten years), who selected the volunteers to be trained as citizen journalists, we started a project we called Eyes and Ears of God—video surveillance of Sudan. This was our first report:

> Kauda: 21, June 2011: The system to photo and video to provide ground monitoring in the SPLA rebel areas of the Nuba Mountains has started this morning. Eleven highly motivated men divided into five teams hastily left the NRRDO compound in Kauda en route to the front lines in Kadugli, Kurchi, Talodi, Western Jebels, Heiban and Delami, equipped with ten spy mini video cameras, ten common "tourist" cameras, four lap tops and two mobile internet satellite modems, all organized [provided] by the Slovenian humanitarian organization, HOPE.
>
> They are competing to see who will end up taking and submitting the most professional photographs and footage of the new war, which started on June 6, to the outside world from the sealed off and besieged South Kordofan. The aim of the project, which the founding members named The Eyes and Ears of God ("because God hears and sees everything"), is to enable the international community to see what is going on here, and to provide proof that Omar Bashir, president of Sudan and Mohammad Haroun, governor of the province, both accused by the International Criminal Court in the Hague of having committed atrocities in Darfur, are laying claim to this province, populated mostly by indigenous Africans, who are to remain, following the secession of the South from the North on July 9th, with their traditional enemy, Khartoum, although they [the Nuba] fought in the previous war side-by-side with the southerners (the SPLA).
>
> In the last several weeks, more then 50 villages have been bombed. SPLA commander Abdel Aziz has said that a half million people have been displaced. Nobody knows yet how many civilians have been killed. All international humanitarian agencies have pulled out of the area.
>
> The main battle between Sudan army forces and SPLA rebels is being fought in Kadugli, the capital of South Kordofan. Nuba intellectuals who escaped from Kaudugli have claimed to have been hunted house by house, where, when caught, many were killed. Some people were even killed in front of the nearby UN compound near Kauda's makeshift airstrip. Breathing is unbearable due to rotting corpses lying everywhere.

Then another sort of a struggle began: an effort to get the photos, footage and reportage of our Nuba citizen journalists picked up by the global media.

"We cannot trust this footage," a director of a TV program with high international visibility said. "The footage could easily have been falsified. We need professional cameraman."

"O.K. Let them [professional cameramen and/or journalists] join me. I will show them around," I said.

"No, it would be illegal, and too dangerous!"

That was a sentence that I heard over and over again. So many times. Too many times.

Frustrated but not defeated—far from it—together with my co-director, Maja Weiss, and Television Slovenia, we produced a feature length documentary film titled "Eyes and Ears of God—Video Surveillance of Sudan." Kudos and film awards at international film festivals came in left and right, as did kudos for our lobbying politicians. But in the end, nothing changed.

I didn't know what to do. I *knew* more needed to be done, but just what it was I was not sure.

Ever since I've returned every year at least twice to Nuba Mountains and Blue Nile State with cameras, computers and satellite connections. I continue to do everything I possibly can to get word out to the wider world about the plight of the Nuba: articles, radio shows, short video reports, interviews with the international media, etc.

But this time things have not gone as before—as in the first war in the Nuba Mountains or even as in the case of Darfur. Not at all. And the question, of course, is WHY?

Four Years Later, March 2015

The bumpy and dusty and seemingly endless ride with a SPLA–N convoy lasted three days. We headed out from the Nuba Mountains south to the "border" separating Sudan from the new nation of The Republic of South Sudan, and then east to the Nile River onwards to Fashoda and then Kodok. As the saying goes, Fashoda and Kodok are like night and day. While what one sees in Fashoda are cows lumbering down the street amidst healthy looking people, not a few of large girth, sartorially dressed in bright-colored traditional garments, whereas in Kodok, it's makeshift houses jury rigged of bricks and boards and roofed with metal sheets along trash strewn, muddy streets. It seems like nearly every single sign sporting the official insignia of the new Republic of South Sudan is either riddled with bullet holes, twisted out of shape and/or crusty with rust. Electrical wires hang idly from broken concrete posts. The only place that feels more than half alive is the *suq*, where rickety stalls variously have this or that for sale: onions, spices, bananas, salt, soap, matches, cigarettes, cheap flashlights, cheap sun glasses, jellabiyas, etc. People mill about, but they look worn out, strikingly thin, at a loss. There is no evidence of what had been touted for the new state of South Sudan: no peace, no prosperity, no real happiness or satisfaction.

But that is not all one sees. There are others: groups of guys who look healthy and strong in military uniforms, flip-flops on their feet, cradling Kalashnikovs. When they ask me what I am doing there, I say, "I am here just to get to some other place," which is the explanation I use most often in conversations with those who look at me with bewilderment. But from here you cannot go any further. The border with Sudan is closed. It was almost impossible to get to Upper Nile in the first place.

At the office of UNHCR in Juba, the capital of the new nation of South Sudan, I was told in January that the government of President Salva Kiir doesn't like reporters. The authorities of South Sudan are probably most leery of journalists because they fear they will publish reports about the endless perpetration of horrific atrocities committed by both the Dinka and the Nuer in the civil war that has riven the new nation.

Because of all the skirmishes between these two tribes and the bandits that operate independently, there is no way to get to Upper Nile by land. There are also no commercial flights into Kodok, therefore I asked the Red Cross to help me out. They turned me down, despite the letter of reference I received from the Slovenian Red Cross. The regional director, Franz Rauchenstein, told me he could not let me onto one of their planes because they promised the South Sudanese government they would only use the planes to transport their own staff. I got a similar response from World Vision. They said their hands were tied, due to the fact that they receive almost 60 percent of their funds from the UN. The UN doesn't like independent reporters because we criticize their inefficiency and expose corruption in their ranks. If word got out that they smuggled me into Kodok that could endanger the cash flow from the UN to the Red Cross.

In the end, it took me two months of negotiations with my friends among the rebels in the Nuba Mountains to finally get to Kodok. I eventually traveled there with a commander of the SPLA North, Salih Atlan, in military lorries loaded with bags of sorghum seeds, some medicine and certain unconventional items. Kauniaro is an area under the control of the SPLA North. It is in Sudan, approximately 150 kilometers northwest of Kodok. It cannot be reached directly from the main SPLA North-controlled area because the Sudanese army and the Janjaweed have been guarding the savannahs between the mountains since the start of the war in June 2011. Traveling there from Kodok is generally not safe either because of the proximity of Nuer forces, which get their weapons and equipment directly from Khartoum to fight the Dinka. I had to wait for Salih to organize more than 100 soldiers and two Mercedes Unimog lorries and the requisite petrol before we could make the journey.

Three mountains—Kau, Niaro and Fungor—in the eastern most part of the Nuba Mountains are some of the most glorious and fantastic red granite formations imaginable. In any other place such a landscape would be deemed a national park. In order to reach the region where the formations exist, one has to cross wetlands west of the Nile and thick acacia forests.

The people there are incredibly resilient. Miraculously, they even survived pogroms by Islamic fundamentalists in the aftermath of Riefenstahl's documentation of their lives in her book, *The People of Kau*. The photographs of the naked, tattooed and scarred bodies of the people caught the unwanted attention of Islamic fundamentalists, who perceived the Kau as not only backward and embarrassing but as infidels.

No one was supposed to know of our passage through the Republic of South Sudan, because the new country isn't allowed to help the rebels in Sudan, even though they were part of the same SPLA army until South Sudan gained its independence. Patrons of South Sudan in Washington and Brussels demand that. So does the UN Security Council.

Rebels that form the SRF (Sudan Revolutionary Front) are fighting the central Sudanese government all along the border from Darfur to the Nuba Mountains and Blue Nile State. Civilians who reside in the region the rebels control are largely on their own.

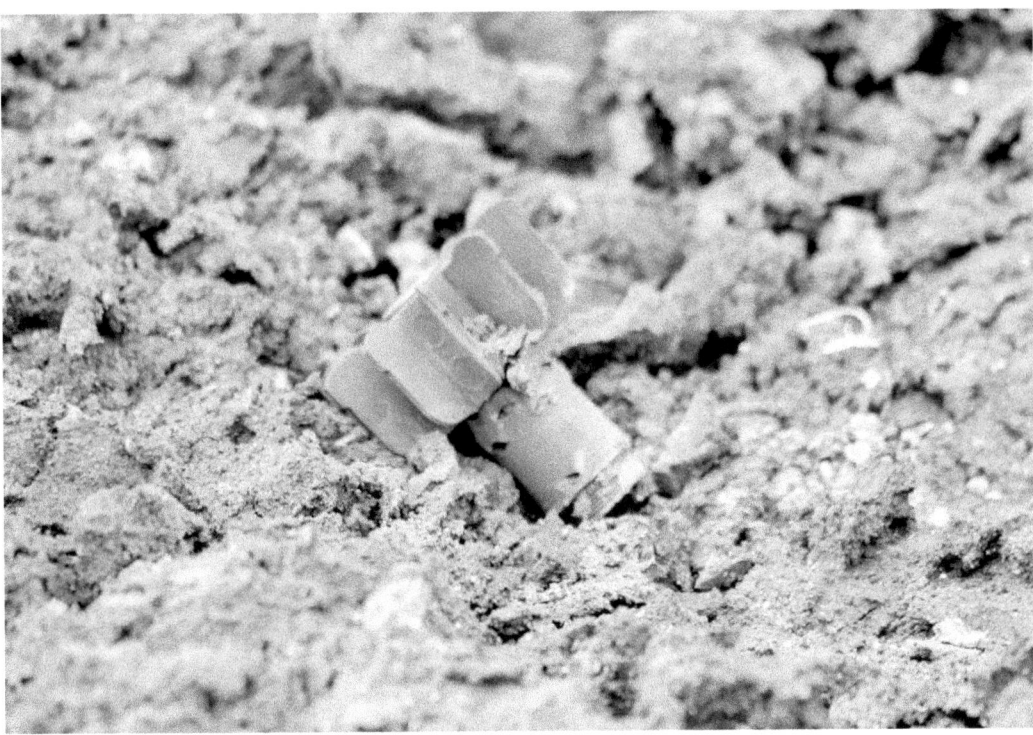

The remnants of a shell fired by the Sudanese Armed Forces in an attack against the Nuba people (Tomo Križnar).

Few journalists venture into the Nuba Mountains or Blue Nile State, and thus what the Nuba civilian populations are facing there is largely unknown by most in the world.

This spring I witnessed several air strikes by GoS Antonov bombers and MiG fighter jets in the Nuba Mountains and the Blue Nile State. My assistants and I, with sick hearts, witnessed the dismembered bodies of children, women, and the elderly. We sent out photos and reports but western politicians were seemingly uninterested in the cries for help. Stopping the genocide in Darfur used to be one of their priorities, but no longer. The military junta of Omar Bashir understands the ignorance of the general global public as a silent agreement to finish its work.

Where this will all lead, no one knows.

Postscript

And so the effort to draw international attention to the plight of the Nuba and the Blue Nile continues apace. With The Tomo Križnar Foundation and the humanitarian organization Hope, which was established by Klemen Mihelič in 2009, we are trying to help the most innocent and most endangered indigenous people in the middle of this incredible mess on both sides of the border between the two Sudans by equipping them with information technology. Since January 2013 we've been testing drones with video cameras in order to document, monitor and, hopefully, prevent total extermination. And even more: right in the eye of this great storm, in the eastern part of the Nuba Mountains,

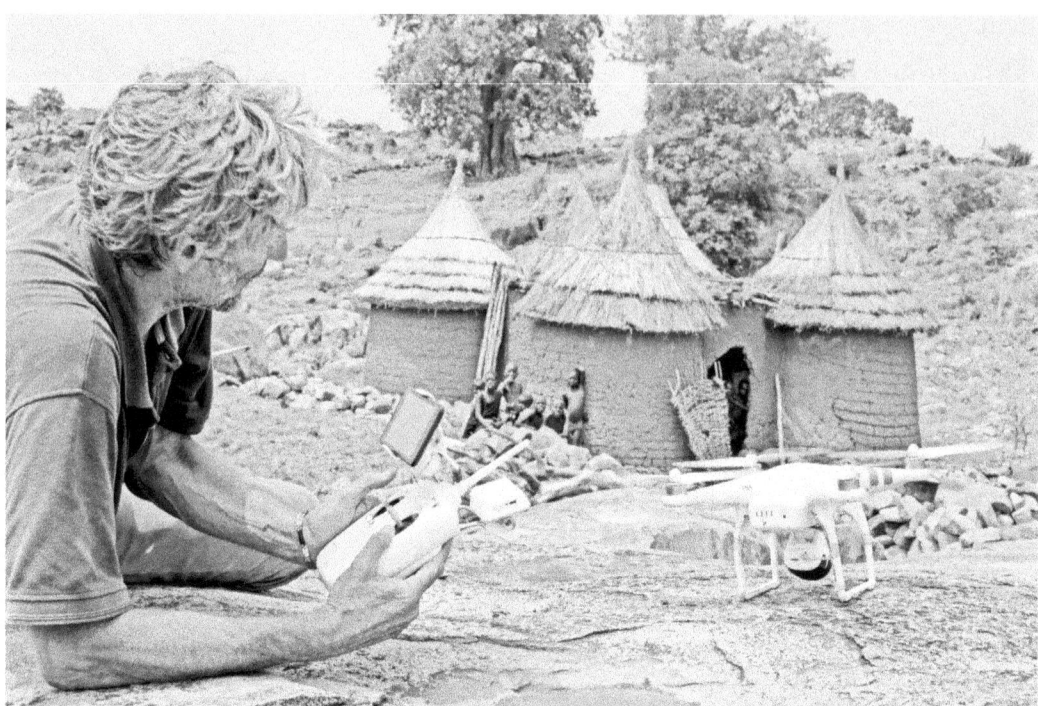

The author and a drone, which he used to film attacks by the Government of Sudan on villages in the Nuba Mountains (Tomo Križnar).

we are trying to establish a "supranational park"—a natural park that would be protected by flying robots instead of "heroes" of the UN, which cleared out its minuscule mission in the region as soon as the fighting began in 2011. The landscape of Kauniaro is as impressive as that of Yellowstone National Park, if not moreso.

In Kauniaro, as in Todoro and other villages of Mesaquin tribe country, where Leni Riefenstahl photographed and filmed her famous images of "noble savages," the most natural, the most noble, the most innocent of indigenous peoples across the globe—the Nuba—are most at danger. I can honestly say that since I have systematically visited most of the indigenous communities residing on every continent across the globe.

We are editing a new documentary titled "Drones Over Roots of Humanity" in which we try to explain the idea behind a supranatural park in the Nuba in the hope that we shall be able to convince the sensitive part of humanity that the Nuba and other indigenous people on Earth need at least such protection as enjoyed now by gorillas in Virunga National Park in the Congo.

We are at the beginning. We are looking for support and like-minded people. We need advice. We need support.

NOTES

1. Leni Riefenstahl (1902–2003) was a German screenwriter, film director, producer, photographer, and Nazi propagandist. While she is most well known for her film *Triumph of the Will*, another of Riefenstahl's films, *Olympia*, about the 1935 Olympics, is, along with *Triumph of the Will*, considered to be one of the two most powerful propaganda films ever produced. In the aftermath of World II, Riefenstahl claimed, time and again, that she had not been cognizant of the Holocaust. Many, if not most, did not believe her. She, however, won close to 50 libel cases.

In 1932, Riefenstahl heard Hitler speak at a rally, and said that she was almost literally mesmerized by his speaking ability. Describing the latter experience in her memoir, she claimed: "I had an almost apocalyptic vision that I was never able to forget. It seemed as if the Earth's surface were spreading out in front of me, like a hemisphere that suddenly splits apart in the middle, spewing out an enormous jet of water, so powerful that it touched the sky and shook the earth."

Hitler, who found Riefenstahl's work impressive, asked her to film what came to be called *Triumph of the Will*, a piece of propaganda about the 1934 Nazi party rally in Nuremberg at which more than one million Germans purportedly attended.

In the early 1970s, Riefenthal traveled extensively in the Nuba Mountains. Ultimately, she published two books rich with remarkable photographs of the Nuba tribes. They were published in 1974 and republished in 1976 as *The Last of the Nuba* and *The Nuba People of Kau*.

2. As explained in the United States Holocaust Memorial Museum:

One of the most notorious Nazi efforts at deception was the establishment in November 1941 of a concentration camp for Jews in Terezín, in the Czech province of Bohemia. Known by its German name Theresienstadt, this facility functioned both as a ghetto for elderly and prominent Jews from Germany, Austria, and the Czech lands, and as a transit camp for the Czech Jews residing in the German-controlled Protectorate of Bohemia and Moravia.

Anticipating that some Germans might discover the truth that the Jews were being sent to the East to perform slave labor and/or to be slaughtered in a Nazi death camp, the Nazi regime cynically publicized the existence of Theresienstadt as a residential community, where elderly or disabled German and Austrian Jews could "retire" and live out their lives in peace and safety. Purportedly, the inhabitants were not only treated well, with plenty of food, but happily engaged in artistic and musical activities. This fiction was invented for domestic consumption within the Greater German Reich. In reality, the ghetto served as a transit camp for deportations to ghettos and killing centers in German-occupied Poland, and killing sites in the German-occupied Baltic States and Belarussia.

In 1944, succumbing to pressure from the International Red Cross and the Danish Red Cross following the deportation of nearly 400 Danish Jews to Theresienstadt in the autumn of 1943, SS officials permitted Red Cross representatives to visit Theresienstadt. By this time, news of the mass murder of Jews had reached the world press and Germany was losing the war. As an elaborate hoax, the SS authorities accelerated deportations from the ghetto shortly before the visit, and ordered the remaining prisoners to "beautify" the ghetto: prisoners had to plant gardens, paint houses, and renovate barracks. The SS authorities staged social and cultural events for the visiting dignitaries. After the Red Cross officials left, the SS resumed deportations from Theresienstadt, which did not end until October 1944. In all, the Germans deported nearly 90,000 German, Austrian, Czech, Slovak, Dutch, and Hungarian Jews from Theresienstadt to killing sites and centers in the "East"; only a few thousand survived. More than 30,000 more prisoners died in Theresienstadt itself, mostly from disease or starvation.

Doing God's Work

RYAN BOYETTE

I grew up in Florida, a good part of it on an island, where my father was a police officer. He was always one who welcomed challenges, was adventurous, and I am much the same way.

In late 2002, when I was 21 years old, my sister read an article about Sudan. She was shocked by what she learned about the oppression of the people of Sudan and especially the persecution of Christian populations there. She shared the article with me, and I was surprised to hear about a civil war that had affected millions of people. In fact, all I knew of Sudan was that it was in Africa. I found it strange that I had never heard of this conflict. So I started to do a little research. My wonder turned into frustration as I learned how long the Sudan conflict had been going on—for twenty years at the time—and how little information existed on it.

I thought to myself, "Why is no one doing anything about what is happening there? Why is the U.S. not doing anything?" As I continued to research, though, I started to direct the question back to myself. At that time I was a recent college graduate going through the process of becoming a United States Customs special agent, but my plans for my future were beginning to shift. As a Christian I started to feel a calling to go to Sudan and help where I could.

I struggled, though, over the fear of the unknown *and* the desire to live a more comfortable life in the United States. I didn't know a single person in Sudan, the language, anything about the living conditions, what I would eat or if it was even possible for me to get there. I turned to God in prayer to help me make this decision because I knew it would shape the rest of my life.

After about a month, I decided I needed to travel to Sudan in order to do what I could to help. I quickly explored different possibilities, and discovered Samaritan's Purse, an evangelical Christian aid group that has projects worldwide, including Sudan. Samaritan's Purse was founded by Franklin Graham, the son of Billy Graham, the famous evangelist. Since it was my faith that was leading me to Sudan, Samaritan's Purse was a good fit because it is a faith-based organization. I had worked construction to pay my way through college, so I was originally hired by the organization to work with people there to help construct a small hospital. I landed in the Nuba Mountains on April 27, 2003, and I have been living here ever since.

Working with Samaritan's Purse was much more than a job, it was a conviction. A mission, actually. Also, every year that I've lived in Nuba, my connection to the place and the people has grown stronger. The people of Nuba have become my friends and family. I would go visit people in their homes every day after work. We would laugh, tell stories, go to church together, celebrate at weddings, attend funerals, take people to the hospital when they were sick, and pray together for the future of Nuba and Sudan. Nuba became my life.

In 2007, I met my wife, Jazira. I fell in love with this beautiful and honorable woman who shared the same faith. I was amazed by the struggle she had endured growing up in a war zone for most of her life. I really admired her commitment to God, as well as her strong drive to get an education and to help her people. Four years after we met, we were married in February of 2011, in the local church where Jazira was raised. About 6,000 people—mainly from the region—attended the wedding.

A few months after our wedding, we started to see signs of war. Since the signing of the Comprehensive Peace in 2005, we had had about six years of peace in the Nuba. Interestingly, or maybe tellingly, year after year I had asked myself, "If war broke out again, would you leave or would you stay?" That question was *always* going through my mind. Then, in June 2011, the fighting began between the Government of Sudan and the Sudan People's Liberation Army–North (SPLA–N).

Within two days, most of the non–Sudanese people working for international non-governmental organizations pulled out of the area due to the danger of the situation. Many, if not most, had been working with the Nuban people to build a much-needed infrastructure in the long-neglected region: schools, hospitals, clean water systems, and roads. Within a couple of weeks, Samaritan's Purse also made the decision to end operations in the Nuba.

At the time, a lot of people tried to convince me to leave. But it was not that easy. My wife is from Nuba, and our family is here, plus, I had lived in Nuba for eight years. It was—and is—home for me, for us. I found it impossible to leave and fly back to the States and say to everyone under attack, "I hope to see you when this ends."

In the last war in the Nuba Mountains, in the 1990s, people were forced off their farms and up into the mountains. People literally starved to death, and those outside the region knew little about it. One of the problems was that reporters had no way of getting into the area, which is extremely isolated and even more so in wartime. And, the fact is, I sensed that the Nuba, we, could be looking at a very similar situation once again. That is, many would likely lose their lives, both due to bombings and a dearth of food (i.e., severe malnutrition, if not outright starvation).

One of the first things I thought about was, "How will the outside world even know about what's happening up here? Not only are the Nuba Mountains in a very remote region of the world, but now it's dangerous to even travel in South Kordofan due to the bombings." Then, it quickly dawned on me that there was likely to be a lack of credible information available to international policy makers, NGOs and the media about the conflict because the region is, as the saying goes, "not on a lot of people's radar," *and* because of the difficulty reaching the region. And, I perceived that as a major problem. As a result, I decided to organize some friends of mine here in Nuba to cover the war. Because my friends are locals, they know the area well and speak the languages—both Arabic and various tribal languages.

Ultimately, a Slovenian organization called Hope kindly provided us with a couple of small point-and-shoot cameras. Initially, our guys took the cameras, headed into the field, shot photographs, wrote up reports and brought them back to me to disseminate.

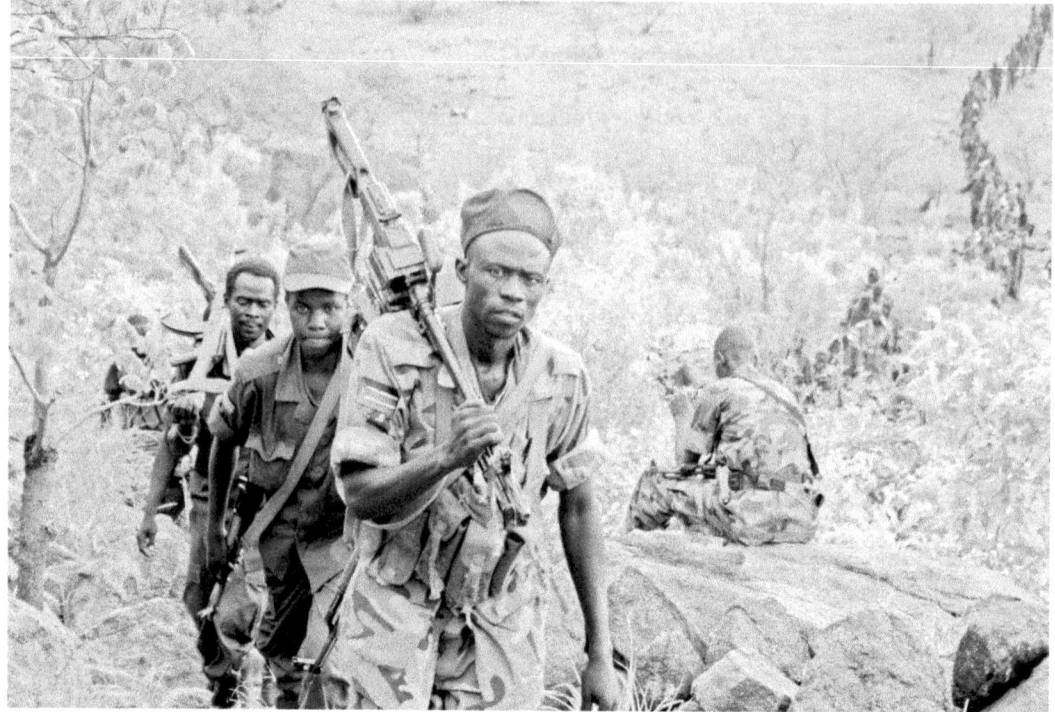

Members of the Sudan People's Liberation Army–North on the march (Ryan Boyette).

That's how *Nuba Reports* was born. Essentially, then, *Nuba Reports* was initiated in order to shed light on a complex political situation and war that would be difficult for anyone, even the largest media operations, to cover.

Tellingly, prior to joining *Nuba Reports* not a single member of our Sudanese team even knew how to hold a camera, let alone use one. Likewise, they had little, if any, idea how to conduct an interview. Now, though, after having gone through various training sessions on videography and journalism, along with their experience in the field, all four of our senior journalists (Yassin Hassan, Abdu Ibrahim, Azhari Joda, and Ahmed Khatir) have become experts in telling stories via video interviews and photos. Some now are even editing videos for publication.

In the last war (during the 1990s), Nuba was completely surrounded by government-controlled regions that kept it cut off from the rest of the world. This time around, we, *Nuba Reports*, want to make sure that the plight and fate of the Nuba people will not be sucked into some black hole and thus virtually ignored.

Ultimately, we decided to focus on capturing video clips of the attacks by the Government of Sudan against Nuba civilians—the destruction and death—because I realized that verifying information in a remote war zone is not only difficult but that video documentation could prove to be invaluable to news media outlets in the verification process. And so far it has. And that is because our reporters go out to different locations all over the state of South Kordofan that are or have been under attack, take GPS-tagged photos and videos of the incidents, conduct interviews in the field, and write up their reports based on what they have witnessed and the information they have collected. It is important to note that we only report what we have witnessed ourselves and what we can confirm.

Confirmation is critical to us, and that is why we have equipped the reporters with cameras that tag GPS coordinates to every picture.

In addition to the video reports, I compile information from our journalists and send it out to different governments, numerous media outlets, and various advocacy groups.

Before any of the citizen journalists began work with *Nuba Reports*, we, of course, drew their attention to the various risks involved. Tellingly, all of the reporters have expressed that it is a risk they are willing to take for their people.

In a very real sense, our reporters are victims of this conflict. While some were forced to flee their homes with their families, others have had to delay their plans to obtain a university education or even get married. All of them have a story of how the war has affected their lives and those of their family members. That said, they're all committed and united in getting information out to the rest of the world about what is happening in the Nuba Mountains; that is, providing evidence to the world in regard to what they are witnessing day in and day out over the weeks, months and years.

At the beginning of our efforts to launch *Nuba Reports*, we didn't have a single dollar for our operations. Everyone, including myself, volunteered to work for free during the first year. As we began to disseminate our reports and video documentation, we began to garner the attention of various international media agencies. Not only that, but we helped a lot of international journalists enter the region and report on what was happening. That, of course, helped immensely in getting word out about what was taking place in the Nuba Mountains, and helped spread the word about *Nuba Reports*.

As news about the crisis in the Nuba and our work spread, we decided to undertake a crowd-funding effort. Ultimately, we raised $45,000. We used the money to purchase better equipment, and to pay for the training of our reporters, with a focus on basic journalism and basic videography.

Our journalists started out as "citizen journalists," but after a lot of training, a good amount of experience, their shadowing of international media, and their use of new state-of-the-art equipment, our guys have become full-fledged journalists. But there's always room for improvement and that is what we strive for.

As we continued our work, many different organizations contributed to our efforts. Samaritan's Purse, for example, donated a vehicle (a Land Cruiser) to enable us to carry out our work. Then an organization called Make Way Partners gave us two motorbikes for our reporters. Motorbikes are critical to our operations because fuel is extremely expensive up here, and motorbikes only use a limited amount of fuel. They are also very mobile. They can go almost anywhere, no matter how rugged the terrain. They also enable the reporters to travel with their equipment across a region with no communication infrastructure.

As I mentioned earlier, from the outset it was my firm belief that the Sudanese government would likely commit the same atrocities they committed in the last war and in Darfur, particularly if it thought international eyes would not see what was happening.

Generally speaking, journalism in Sudan is very poor and highly controlled. Most of what one receives in Sudanese news is opinion and rumor. On top of that, there is very little video being used to present the news. Sudanese TV news reports are filled with talking heads stating their opinions—primarily the opinions of the government.

Even though we started with the aim of shining a light on what was happening in South Kordofan State, the home of the Nuba Mountains, for the express purpose of keeping the international community apprised of key incidents and events during the war, it has always been our goal as well to help raise awareness among the Sudanese, themselves, about what is happening in their country, especially as it relates to the Nuba Mountains. Through our partnerships with other Sudanese media outlets, we are doing just that. And as a result, thousands, if not tens of thousands, of Sudanese are becoming better informed about their government's actions against its own citizens.

Prior to our conception and efforts, Sudanese government officials were experts at blocking information coming out of the war zones in Sudan. For example, both international and local Sudanese media are banned from reporting from Darfur, South Kordofan and Blue Nile State, all of which are engulfed in war. Furthermore, many newspapers in Khartoum have been shut down for reporting on conflict in such regions.

I believe the government of Sudan does not want the media to access the war zones in these different regions of Sudan so as to not expose the war crimes and crimes against humanity that they are perpetrating. That is particularly relevant when one realizes that several members of the current government of Sudan, including President Omar al-Bashir, have been accused of war crimes, crimes against humanity, and in certain cases, even genocide, by the International Criminal Court in regard to atrocities perpetrated in the Darfur conflict.

It is a central goal of *Nuba Reports* to contribute to a new approach of reporting the news and media in Sudan. I believe the people working with us now will be considered the founders of this new style in Sudan.

And there is also this: through our work, *Nuba Reports* is actually helping to bridge divisions fueled by government propaganda over the last three decades. What I mean is this: we have staff who are Muslims, we have staff who are Christians, we have staff who are Arabs, and we have staff from black African tribes. Prior to working with *Nuba Reports* many of them had never worked with those different from themselves; but now, they are all working together in the same organization, with the same goals in a collective effort to bring attention to what's happening in their country. This is quite revolutionary in Sudan, and we hope we will serve as a role model of sorts to prove to other organizations and people in other regions of Sudan that they can work beside one another and together.

In the beginning, I was the only U.S. citizen on our team of citizen journalists. All the others were Sudanese. A year after we started, however, a photojournalist (Trevor Snapp) who had been reporting in Sudan for about three years found himself in Nuba. We were introduced, and he ended up being intrigued with our work and had an opportunity to meet our team members. Trevor was hooked. He volunteered for a year, helping me locate funding and helping us to become more professional in our work. Following that first year, Trevor became a full-time member of the *Nuba Reports* team and went on to build a support team of international and Sudanese editors.

Our team was not only producing video and written reports on a regular basis but we were also inviting international media to the region. Essentially, we acted as fixers for different members of the international media; that is, we helped them gain access to the region, provided transport for them once they were in South Kordofan, advised them on where we thought they should head in order to capture the essence of what was taking place, etc. In turn, our reporters, including me, were able to learn from these professionals and subsequently use what we learned in our work. Among some of the many from major media outlets that we served as fixers and guides for were Ann Curry (NBC), Greta Van Susteren (Fox News) and Nicholas Kristof (*The New York Times*).

As a rule it is hard to measure the tangible results of our work—that is true for all journalists and media outlets, actually—but we have actually seen some tangible results and we believe that they are excellent indicators of our growing impact.

First, for example, since our reporters have increased their skills, and we have proven our ability to report from the region accurately and effectively, many major international news agencies have started using our reporting and video footage. In turn, this has opened doors to meet with different government and UN bodies that take an interest in the region, and thus we have been able to share our reports and data from the areas of conflict with them.

Second, we have collaborated with many organizations. One organization that gained invaluable information from our on-the-ground collaboration was the *Satellite Sentinel Project*. Our reporters passed information to me and I would in turn provide the Satellite Sentinel Project detailed information about what was happening on the ground. They then used that information to pinpoint where different events took place, using satellite imagery to provide further evidence.

Third, in addition to members of the media, among many others who make use of *Nuba Reports* are policymakers: in the U.S. Government, nongovernmental organizations based in the U.S., and scholars across the globe. Our goal is to help them be better informed about the situation on the ground, especially as it relates to humanitarian needs. That is, a key goal of ours is to draw attention to those areas where people may have been displaced and where food shortages exist. Additionally, we share our findings, photos, video reports, and character stories with several Sudanese media sources that have the ability to get it out to Sudanese audiences.

Fourth, another example of a tangible result of our work was witnessed at a UN Human Rights Council (HRC) meeting in Geneva in 2014. The HRC decided to send an independent expert to Sudan to evaluate human rights issues to ascertain whether there was any evidence they were improving or not. The Sudanese would not allow the expert to travel to the war-affected areas, and thus was only allowed to report on what the government showed him. Just two weeks ago the expert presented his findings to the HRC in Geneva, with a Sudan delegation present. Now, since the expert was not able to go to the areas affected by war, we, *Nuba Reports*, put together a video and a written report about human rights violations in Sudan's war zones. The report used our data and findings of the past three years but primarily focused on the past year. We reported on indiscriminate aerial bombardment, torture, arbitrary arrests and collective punishment. Subsequently, that video was viewed by many UN Member States, including Sudan. Several attendees notified us after the meeting that our video helped to provide valuable information that they may not have otherwise accessed.

Our video and written reports essentially come in two forms. First, and foremost, there is the breaking news. If a bombing occurs, the government attacks a town or village, or a village is burned to the ground, our reporters go directly to the site and gather as much information as possible. In every case, they shoot a short video to complement their report. Second, there are times when we may wish to develop character-based stories and reports, and when we do we put in much more time documenting and highlighting a person's experiences. Reporters will get a specific assignment to develop a story around an individual who we think has a compelling story that is worth telling.

Not surprisingly, I guess, some individuals have claimed that *Nuba Reports* constitutes nothing less than spying on Sudan. It is true that a lot of the information that we gather, the Sudan government would like to keep a secret. But I believe that is what journalism is about: keeping governments and governmental officials accountable, and providing objective information to the citizenry. Undoubtedly, the Government of Sudan would prefer that no one ever finds out about their campaign of terror against the people of Southern Kordofan, Blue Nile and Darfur, *but that is the exact reason why Nuba Reports exists*: to spotlight those actions that people in power want to keep in the darkness, hidden from everyone.

While it is imperative to remain unbiased while reporting, I must say it is difficult when your house is bombed, when your website is hacked, and when your employees are threatened. But as I said, it takes a special team to do this and to see the importance of stating the truth.

We have also discovered that in an environment where one side does not respect the media and does everything it can to limit the reach of the media, it is extremely difficult to tell both sides of the story. In a nutshell, most dictatorships perceive transparency as anathema. So, that adds to the inherent difficulty of providing various sides to the stories we cover. And, obviously, we can't approach the government for security reasons. If we did it from afar, we'd be rebuffed. And if we did it in person, we'd probably be arrested. While we've tried our best to present the government's side as well as possible, we've always been very honest about our constraints. And I should note, when other media outlets use us as a source, they often access Sudanese government officials in order to get their side of the story.

Logistics, equipment and infrastructure are our biggest practical challenges. Just getting such equipment to the region is extremely expensive. Cameras regularly break. Our motorbikes are now four years old—and in a war zone that is a long time. Four years on now, *Nuba Reports* is using state-of-the-art DSLR cameras with GPS-tagged footage and photos.

For security reasons we are always changing locations, so setting up a stable office or base of operations is time-consuming and difficult. So, that is another major challenge that we face. The good thing is, as I've noted, our team of reporters are from the region and I have lived and worked in Nuba for twelve years now. So we have learned to be creative with what we have.

We are constantly in need of new equipment to replace that which has been damaged and/or destroyed by the harsh environment. (No matter how innovative we are, if a camera breaks, then it is done!). If a motorbike breaks down and we don't have the funds to get spare parts, we can't reach the areas where the news is happening. So, we can always use help. We tell everyone we come into contact with: If you are keen to help us, we greatly appreciate any and all donations. Those who express a wish to help us we send to our website: http://nubareports.org/make-a-donation/.

Nuba Reports began its work in South Kordofan State when the war started here. South Kordofan is also where the team members resided prior to the conflict. It's also where we are most well established. And it's also where we disseminate our reports from. But, as I noted, warfare is also taking place in Blue Nile State and Darfur. Because of that, we now try to get reports out of those regions when we can, but security, extreme distances, and other challenges make it extremely difficult. Additionally, we try our utmost to cover the occasional protests against the government held in Khartoum, the capital of Sudan, as well as well as other cities in the north. Despite the logistical challenges of establishing and maintaining reporting networks in other areas of Sudan, we feel it is imperative that we expand our operations to report on other issues facing Sudan, and that's because many of the issues have the same roots as those in the Nuba, Darfur, and the Blue Nile.

On a different note, many politicians, people in the media, and activists frequently claim that this war is *only* about Arabs versus black Africans or Christians versus Muslims. In actuality, it is not like that at all. For years the government has used anything and everything it could to divide the people in Sudan. They have used ethnic, geographical, and religious issues to both divide people and justify war in order to remain in power. The conflict cannot legitimately be said to solely revolve around the issue of black Africans versus Arabs, and that is true because there are many on the government side who are also black and many on the *SPLA-N* side who are Arab, as well as other ethnicities. Similarly, those who claim it is primarily a conflict based on the animosity between Muslims and Christians are wrong as well. After all, there are Muslims fighting on both sides. From working on the ground, this has become very clear to me.

Our work is dangerous. I readily admit that. For example, our reporters get threatening emails from supporters of the Sudan government. When one knows how the GoS treats its opponents and/or perceived enemies, such threats are frightening to receive.

It is also terrifying, of course, when the GoS bombs the region. In fact, you don't feel safe at any time of day or night.

My home was actually bombed. On May 11, 2012, at 9:50 a.m., the Sudan government targeted my wife and me in our house. An Antonov airplane flew over the house and dropped a total of six bombs in a row. The first bomb landed 30 meters to the west of our house and the second about 50 meters east of our house, while the rest of the bombs landed in a line directly down from the first two bombs.

Two of our reporters, Azhari and Ahmed, were at my house when we heard the plane. I rushed outside and noticed the plane was coming directly for my house. We all ran behind the house and laid down as quickly as possible. We could hear the bombs falling through the air and within seconds there was a huge explosion less than 30 meters from where we were laying.

My wife was visiting our neighbor at the time of the bombing. She took cover behind a rock very close to where the third bomb exploded. She saw a large piece of shrapnel fly over her as she laid down. After all six bombs exploded, the plane flew back towards the north.

I rushed to find my wife and we were both relieved that neither of us was hurt. We quickly checked with other people in the area to see if anyone was wounded or killed by the bombing. Despite all six bombs landing near homes, only one 75-year-old woman named Halima had a small wound on her head. After treating the old woman's wound, we assessed the damage at our house. Some shrapnel from the first bomb hit our house, causing minor damage to the outside wall and punching a hole in our roof. My wife and I immediately sat down and prayed to thank God that we were OK.

It is important to note that *not a single soldier lives in the village that I live in*, and that *our house is far from any front line*. The point is, the Government of Sudan constantly reiterates that it is only targeting the rebels. We, *Nuba Reports* and the Nuba people, have always known that that was not true. Now, though, I have first-hand knowledge that the GoS is, in fact, targeting civilians.

I realize that I am now a target. I have experienced many bombings here in Nuba, but that day I realized someone woke up that morning and got in an airplane with the

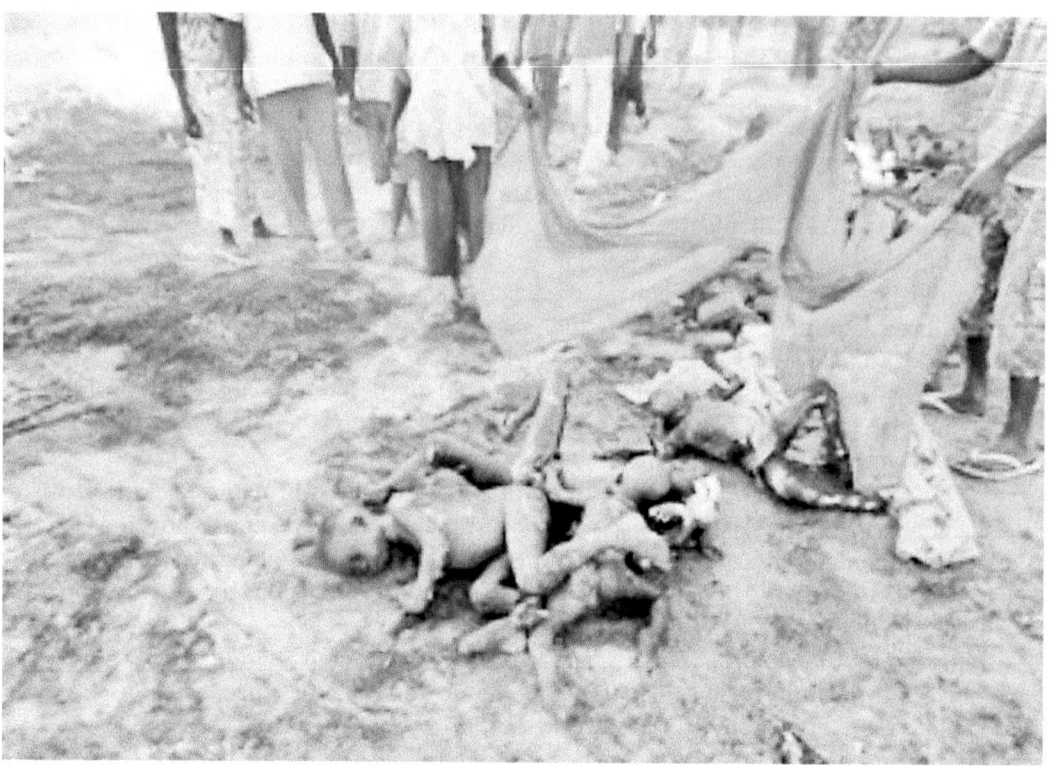

Dead babies who had been burned alive as a result of the Government of Sudan's attacks against Nuba civilians in June 2011 (Ryan Boyette).

mission to kill me. That was the closest that a bomb has exploded near me. I now fully appreciate the abject fear that men, women and children have when the bombs are falling on them.

I am not surprised that I have been targeted by the Sudan government, for, as I've said, it does not want the world to know the truth about what is happening in Sudan.

What concerns me the most about the whole situation up here is that the international community is doing nothing to halt the bombings that are affecting the lives of so many people in Nuba. Many have died, many more have been wounded and maimed, and as I write this, hundreds of thousands have been displaced from their homes due to the bombing and burning of villages. The Nuba people are hard-working farmers, but it is hard to farm with the constant threat that your government will drop bombs on you.

To say the least, it is dispiriting for everyone up here to realize that the very organizations—the Sudanese Government and its military—that are supposed to protect its citizens are actually, and purposely, destroying people's lives. Each and every year of this conflict the Nuba have known that if they are not able to plant their crops prior to the rainy season, starvation will be a major issue of concern. And the only reason they will not have planted their crops is due to the bombing and the fear of being killed in their fields. And yet the international community does nothing. And has done absolutely nothing for the past six plus years now. The international community continues to see the conflicts here—both in Sudan, in general, and South Kordofan and the Nuba Mountains, in particular—as a North/South issue, and all it can muster itself to do is repeatedly ask

Khartoum to stop its ongoing onslaught of the Nuba. Simply put, it has failed to really examine and then address the core issues as to why Sudan has no peace.

Why was there fighting for 21 years between the North and the South that led to a separation? Why has there been fighting in Darfur since 2003 up to now? Why are there protests in Khartoum? Why are there protests in the eastern part of Sudan? Why is there all-out fighting in Blue Nile and Southern Kordofan, with aerial bombardment taking place every single day? Why isn't anyone in the international community asking such questions? And if they have, how come they haven't come up with the means to address such concerns?

Nuba Reports is up against a lot. It continues to be a huge challenge to get information out about what is happening here in South Kordofan. Part of the problem, it seems, is that internationally there is what can only be deemed "Sudan fatigue." Another part of the problem is that both the United Nations and many, if not most, individual governments always seem to look for and then latch onto quick fixes. Interestingly, when I first arrived in Sudan I actually used to think about Sudan in that way. More specifically, during my first year in Sudan I used to think, "Okay, what's the most I can do this year to make the most difference, because maybe I'll go back to the U.S. at the end of year?" However, after my third year here, I knew that Sudan was going to be my home. And it was at that point that I began to think about Sudan in a completely different way—that one needs to observe what is going on, to speak to as many different people as possible, and to learn about the culture, the political issues, the economic issues, the human rights issues, and on and on. Then and only then can one begin to see why there is conflict and how it might be ameliorated.

The government of Sudan has failed its own people in Nuba, the Blue Nile, Darfur, and other parts of Sudan. The UN, the African Union and individual governments are failing the people of Sudan by allowing Sudan to bomb its own people. It astonishes me that international leaders, particularly those from other African nations, are not willing to take a stand against how the Government of Sudan treats its own people and what it is doing to its own citizens.

I firmly believe that the people of Sudan will, ultimately, be the ones to improve the situation. A first step is ensuring they have access to accurate information versus propaganda. There have been years and years of racial, ethnic, political and geographic propaganda piled up over time here in Sudan, and the Sudanese people must start peeling off these layers to the point where they can discuss their issues openly with one another. So, censorship has to go, and the fear of speaking one's mind must come to an end.

I firmly believe that by producing reports about people in the war-torn Nuba Mountains, our journalists are helping other Sudanese see the reality on the ground and to relate to their fellow citizens as people—not as this or that race or tribal group or religion but as people. If Sudanese citizens in Khartoum, for example, come to see that a farmer is unable to provide food for her family due to the daily bombings and al-Bashir is purposely blocking humanitarian aid from reaching the region or that many children have lost limbs because of the bombings, divisions between various and different groups may begin to narrow. It may help people to relate to each other, and understand the larger, underlying problems confronting the people of Sudan. The situation in Sudan is a nationwide problem and not simply isolated to the three states that are now considered war zones.

The role that I think the international community must play in all of this is to facilitate dialogue between groups that traditionally have been divided; and once that happens,

I firmly believe that the Sudanese people will begin to make collective decisions on their own on how to move forward. To me, that would constitute real success and create lasting change. My point is, no one is asking U.S. soldiers to come in and "fix" things. That's not the answer at all. I don't believe the U.S., the UN, the AU or any other body can do anything that will ultimately create stability in the region. I think local actors can and must create the type of atmosphere that lends itself to stability.

The way the international community could help to create more stability for the Sudanese people is to first stop engaging al-Bashir as if he is a man of good character. Second, it needs to actually hold him to any agreement that is made. The entire time I've lived in Sudan I've repeatedly seen the deceptiveness of the al-Bashir regime. The GoS sits down with United States and United Nations officials and as they engage in their tea-drinking political talk, al-Bashir and his cronies "work" those across from them, putting on a show pretending that the regime actually cares about the Sudanese people and is actually assisting them. It doesn't, and it's not!

What gives me hope are the Sudanese people, who have challenged their government for years, longer than I've been alive, and that they are still fighting for their basic rights. There's a song in my wife's language, in the Otoro language, that goes this way: "We're gonna fight for peace. Look at my arms. They're strong from planting my ground and building my house. Look at my legs. They're strong from climbing mountains. Look at my eyes. I've seen everything that you could possibly see." The song ends by saying, "I will continue fighting until the end of my days just so my next generation can have peace."

The people of Sudan face a great number of issues and extreme hardship even without dealing with a six-year-long violent conflict, but that they remain resilient even as the international community ignores them.

I'd like to end by returning to our, *Nuba Reports*, staff. The real heroes in this are our reporters. Those taking the real risks are the Sudanese reporters and the Sudanese editors. They're the first ones on the scene when a village is attacked and people are injured or killed and displaced. They are the ones who go inside the caves where people have sought sanctuary away from the bombs, and interview people who have fled up there with no food. They are the ones who travel great distances in order to speak with those who have fled to refugee camps. Day-by-day, week-by-week, year-by-year, they have been crisscrossing rebel territory in South Kordofan, documenting the conflict as it unfolds. As they do their work, it encourages me to work harder, to return to the U.S. to meet with NGOs, policymakers, and the media in an attempt to inform them about what is actually happening on the ground in the Nuba Mountains. During the last war in the Nuba Mountains in the 1990s, little to no information was coming out of the Nuba Mountains. Now it is, and thus no one in the international community can claim they do not know what is happening.

Our reporters are building an archive of life here—a living, evolving memory of the war. It is the only one that exists, and the only one likely to ever be produced.

When all is said and done, our efforts and experiences have taught my team and me that reporting from a remote area of conflict is not only difficult and dangerous, but it takes a special group of people to get the job done. Indeed, every member on the team must have a passion for this kind of work and must believe that fact, truth, and real life stories of the people affected by the bombings and extreme dearth of food constitute powerful sources that both the world, at large, and the society here in Sudan deserve to have access to should they so desire.

On the Frontlines of Medicine

Tom Catena, M.D.

"Doctor, we just got this patient who was hit by the Antonov, and I don't think he can survive."

Today is Sunday, February 8, 2015, and those were the first words I heard early this morning as I came to the hospital to do the usual quick Sunday rounds before going off for Sunday Mass. The patient was a 28-year-old farmer, a civilian, and father of three who had been riding in the back of a vehicle with a crowd of other people when he heard the Antonov circling overhead. He jumped out of the vehicle and began a panicked dash only to be cut down in his tracks by the large chards of jagged shrapnel. He was in a deep coma with a massive head wound consisting of an open skull fracture with gelatinous white brain matter prolapsing out of the gaping hole. His right arm was completely mangled with the fractured ends of his forearm bones sticking out. A large chunk of flesh had also been torn out of his right calf muscle. We took him to the operating room where we cleaned and closed the gaping skull wound after clearing out the brain tissue and then proceeded to amputate his right arm. He's on the ward now and we'll see if he is able to get some degree of recovery from his horrific injuries. His prognosis, though, is very poor.

This was a case of an innocent civilian maimed by his own government. Sadly, it was not isolated or unusual incident. Quite the contrary, in fact, as we've treated 29 civilians (mostly women and children) wounded by aerial bombardment or artillery fire by the Government of Sudan (GoS) over the past two and a half weeks. Many were badly wounded, with some requiring amputations and other operations. A case in point: Nine children in a single family were badly burned when an artillery shell exploded next to their "foxhole" at 4 a.m. Three children were killed on the spot and six arrived here at the hospital. The youngest, a 2-year-old girl, died from her burns three days ago.

We have a visiting journalist with us now for a couple of weeks, and he attended the operation with us. After the surgery was over, he asked me how I was feeling about this whole deal. Shock? Anger? Frustration? Sadness? I really didn't feel anything at the time, as I just wanted to get through the operation and do the best I could for the young man.

I'm trying not to become too numb to what is going on around me here in the Nuba Mountains as we enter the fourth year of war against the government. During these past four years, I've left Nuba on only two separate occasions: the first time was for a month, the second for three weeks. Otherwise I'm here at the hospital every day and rarely leave the hospital compound's immediate vicinity. Trying to maintain some sort of perspective is a challenge, particularly with such prolonged periods of isolation. But I wouldn't want to have it any other way.

Our hospital is called Mother of Mercy Hospital. It is a Catholic mission hospital located in Gidel locality and under the authority of the diocese of El Obeid. The idea for the hospital was conceived in 2001 when then SPLA Commander Abdel Aziz Adam El Hilu asked the bishop of the El Obeid diocese, Bishop Macram Gassis, to build a referral hospital in order to better serve the Nuba people. It was to be the first referral hospital of its kind in the Nuba Mountains proper, serving an area the size of the state of Georgia in the United States.

The cease-fire in the Nuba Mountains was signed in 2002, ending the decades old civil war in Sudan (1983–2005), and construction of the hospital began sometime around 2003. The work was done by local Nuba laborers, assisted by Italian architects and contractors and Kenyan builders who volunteered their time and resources in an effort to build a quality structure the likes of which had never been seen in this part of the Nuba Mountains. The walls were constructed of stones harvested from the nearby hills and secured with mud and a veneer of cement. The walls were all made two feet thick in order to withstand any potential future bombing from the Khartoum government should war break out again (as it has). The roof and trusses were brought from Italy and are of a special design that provides insulation from the intense heat. Due to the difficulties in working in such a remote region, the hospital wasn't completed until 2008.

I first heard about the hospital project in August 2002 from (now) Sister DeDe Byrne, who was a friend of Bishop Macram. DeDe and I were working together at the Kakuma Mission Hospital in the Turkana region of Kenya when she told me about the bishop's idea to build a hospital in Sudan and thought I might be interested in working there. In fact, I was very interested in working in Sudan as I saw it as an opportunity to get involved in a hospital from the ground up in an area that had a great need for the services. After leaving Kakuma, I went to work at St. Mary's Mission Hospital in Nairobi. While there, I made contact with the bishop's office in Nairobi and ended up helping with some of the planning of the hospital as it was actually being built.

I spent January and February of 2008 going around Nairobi gathering all of the supplies and medicines I could, while also interviewing and hiring Kenyan health professionals in order to be ready to open by late March. Ultimately, on March 10th, we landed with our supplies and a few staff at the Kauda airstrip and drove through the beautiful rolling hills of Nuba for 45 minutes before reaching the hospital in Gidel. We worked like crazy for the next week setting up the wards, operating room, pharmacy and laboratory in order to be ready for the official hospital blessing on March 18th. We were in full swing by March 25th and have been going strong since then.

We started off with about twenty beds, with plans to eventually have an 80-bed hospital. Due to the great demand over the years, we've now expanded to a nearly 400-bed facility.

Our initial staff consisted of fifteen local Nuba who had gone through a six week basic course in nursing a year prior to the hospital's opening, five Kenyan staff and a Ugandan matron/sister. The Kenyan staff consisted of an anesthetist, an operating room technician, a laboratory technician, a pharmacist and a general nurse. The local staff were at a very basic level, and thus had to be taught all of the procedures on the job, including everything from checking a patient's temperature and weight to inserting an IV line and administering oral drugs. At the time there wasn't a single high school graduate in the local area, and many of our staff had never finished primary school.

The first three years of running the hospital were full of great difficulties. There seemed to be a continuous series of problems. The expatriate Kenyan staff that we hired were neither prepared for the stark reality of living in the remote Nuba Mountains nor having to teach the local staff pretty much everything from scratch. The former responded to the challenges by sometimes refusing to work and demanding more pay and time off. Since there were no health professionals anywhere in the Nuba Mountains that could do their jobs, they were able to force us into giving in to their demands as we were determined to keep the hospital open and functioning. After several months of these sorts of problems, we were able to send the malcontents back to Kenya and to get some staff on board who had more of a heart for the work here.

The problems with the expat Kenyan staff were followed by problems from the Nuba staff who were threatening to strike and disrupt the work. For some strange reason even the local SPLA health officials and the local *payam* administration (local government council) were opposed to us. I got the distinct impression during our first two plus years here that the health and government officials simply did not want us here. The local people seemed more welcoming but were also wary of us. Perhaps this comes from a long history of subjugation and abuse at the hands of others. They were not going to trust us simply because we built a hospital for them. We would have to prove ourselves to them by sticking it out and persevering through some of the hardships they had endured for decades.

There was one episode that helped us immensely with the local *payam* administrator (similar to a mayor). His first wife (he had three or four) had a certain type of miscarriage, which required us to do a certain procedure in the uterus. One of the potential complications of this type of miscarriage is that the woman can bleed heavily at any time within 24 hours after the procedure. We did the procedure on a Friday late morning and everything seemed to go well; however, when I went to check on her that night, I found her lying in a pool of blood on her bed and hemorrhaging profusely from the birth canal. The only treatment in our setting here is mass blood transfusions so we immediately began searching for blood donors. Many of her relatives, including her brother-in-law, refused to donate. I ended up giving a pint of my blood, and we were able to strong arm a few others into giving their blood, eventually transfusing her with eight pints of blood and putting a stop to the hemorrhage. The *payam* administrator heard about this and finally started to warm up a bit more toward us.

~ * ~

Today is February 21st, 2015, and I just finished debriding (clearing out dead tissue) the burn wounds of a ten-year-old boy. The boy's name is Shanta and he has third degree burns over 50 percent of his body as the result of an artillery barrage fired by the Sudan army at 4 a.m. on his home village. He was sleeping with eight of his family members in a foxhole with the hope that they would be protected from the nightly artillery shelling. One of the shells struck a nearby grass hut, which caught on fire and fell into the foxhole. Three children were burned to death and six came to our hospital. The youngest of the six, a two-year-old girl, was dead within two days, but the remaining five are still hanging on to their lives. We picked out 30 or 40 maggots as we cleaned and cut away Shanta's dead skin. Can you imagine what that is like? I was reminded of a previous young female patient who was horribly burned by an incendiary bomb dropped from a Sudan air force Antonov bomber. She would scream in terror anytime she saw a fly near her as she knew it would lay maggot-producing eggs on her decaying flesh. She died after three months in agony. Did the aircrew who dropped those bombs have any idea what the result of their day's work would be? What are we doing to each other?

Although we had been busy from the opening of the hospital, the volume of work really took off in November of 2009, when we had a visiting eye surgeon conduct a two-week eye clinic, focusing primarily on doing cataract surgery. We got the word out about the clinic to the people all across the Nuba Mountains, as well into northern Sudan, and then watched as people came to our very isolated hospital from all over Sudan. It was the first time for many people to discover this new and large hospital that provided a good range of services at a minimal cost. It was fascinating to see the variety of people and dress that poured into the hospital compound. There were many Arabs in long flowing sparkling white jalabiya and turbans; Falatta, with their large Afros and mild way of speaking; and Longan people in their characteristic blue dress.

Tellingly, the crowds kept coming from far-flung places after the eye surgeon finished his work here. Patients came in rickety buses over the dirt track from Talodi, Abu Gebeha, Abu Korshola, Rahad, and Kadugli. Many even came from as far away as El Obeid and Khartoum. We even had some come to us from Darfur and Port Sudan—a bit like going from New York to Chicago for a medical or surgical consultation. Despite the many years of enmity between the Nuba and the various Arab tribes, the different groups seemed to get along rather well. It seemed people were ready to forgive and forget the injustices of the past if they could have a chance for a peaceful future. As would soon become painfully obvious, the chance for a lasting peace in Sudan seemed to fade into the sweltering summer heat.

The year 2011 started with everyone brimming with enthusiasm and a sense of optimism about the future. South Sudan had held its referendum in January and voted overwhelmingly to secede from the north, thus forming the world's newest nation (The Republic of South Sudan). The Nuba Mountains (which is located in South Kordofan State in Sudan) was not included in the South Sudan referendum, but was scheduled for gubernatorial elections in May 2011, to be followed by a poorly understood process called the "popular consultation," which most people thought would grant the Nuba some degree of self determination. The National Congress Party (the ruling party in Sudan) put up as its candidate Ahmed Haroun, who had been indicted by the International Criminal Court on 20 counts of crimes against humanity and 22 counts of war crimes as a result of his involvement in suppressing the revolt in Darfur. The opposition (SPLA-N) candidate was the well respected Abdel Aziz Adam el Hilu who was the deputy governor and former military commander of the SPLA forces in the Nuba Mountains. It seemed that everyone in our part of the Nuba Mountains was supporting Abdel Aziz and many were confident he would win the race. However, prior to the elections, the president of Sudan, Omar Hassan al-Bashir, declared that his candidate (Ahmed Haroun) would win the election "by the ballot or by the bullet." To no one's surprise, Ahmed Haroun won the election and there was a palpable tension felt throughout the Nuba Mountains. A young man in Kauda apparently committed suicide upon hearing the news of the elections. We all had a sneaking suspicion that war was on the horizon.

~ * ~

Today is February 27, 2015, and was a particularly bad day in a particularly bad week, month and year. Two children died this afternoon at 3 p.m. One was a young boy who had severe abdominal and head penetrating trauma after he pounded a (previously) unexploded artillery shell with a rock. The shrapnel ripped through his intestines, left eye and left hand and we spent a good amount of time in the operating room trying to fix his various problems. He died on the fifth post-operative day, most likely from the head injury. The other death was a young girl who had third degree burns as a result of an artillery shell fired by the Sudan army. Her burn wounds were extensive but had started to improve. Then, however, I noticed the facial rigidity of someone in the early stages of tetanus. She soon developed the agonizing back spasms and high fever typical of this dreaded complication. She died despite our best efforts at isolating and sedating her. I sought out her mother to give my condolences and found her with her other children. She was very strong and said "no problem." I was heartbroken and wandered around the hospital trying to find some solace somewhere. All I seemed to get was more patients and nurses coming after me with more crises. Losing a patient is very painful, and losing a pediatric patient is excruciatingly painful. I'll need to pull myself together so I can keep taking care of the other patients. I need to remind myself that I'm really not in charge of who lives and who dies, and that God is asking for my heart and commitment and not for perfection. How much longer can I carry on with this work? God give me the strength to persevere. I think Jesus died at 3 p.m.

The civil war in the Nuba Mountains officially started on June 6th, 2011, when fighting broke out in Amdoren. The previous day we met with the commissioner of Amdoren County who reassured us that the situation was under control and there would certainly be no fighting. During the preceding six years of peace, all of the military barracks in the Nuba Mountains were jointly occupied by soldiers of both the SPLA and SAF (Sudan Armed Forces, which constitutes the military forces of Sudan) and were known as JIU's (Joint Integrated Units). As word spread of the outbreak of fighting, these barracks erupted in an orgy of close quarters combat. At the barracks in Heiban, the SAF soldiers collected their weapons and returned to the barracks to fire on the SPLA soldiers at point blank range. That night of June 8th, 2011, I got my first taste of being a war surgeon as several casualties from the Heiban fight showed up at around 10 p.m. The wounded were all placed on gurneys in the corridor outside the operating room. There was a certain haziness in the air as the soldiers lay in their blood soaked uniforms, many crying out in pain.

One guy in particular stands out. He was shot at close range in the face and the bullet passed through his jaw into the back of his throat and out through a large blow hole at the back of his neck. His jaw was shattered and he was choking on his own blood. I can't forget the look of sheer horror on his face as we worked feverishly to try to stop the bleeding and bind up his wounds, showering me with blood as he coughed and sputtered. Any notions I ever had of war being anything but a gruesome exercise of man killing man quickly vanished. As the only referral hospital and only one offering surgical care in the Nuba Mountains, we quickly became inundated with war wounded.

Essentially, we had to change overnight from a being referral hospital primarily taking care of patients who needed elective surgery and more complex medical treatment to a trauma hospital taking care of war wounded. We had pretty much become a large MASH unit.

The sound of the Antonov and Sukhoi 25 bombers now filled the air as Kauda and other nearby villages were bombed on several occasions. I clearly remember standing on the just completed foundation of our proposed children's ward and watching a Sukhoi

25 make repeated dive bombings on the Kauda airstrip. It was all so surreal as I likened it to the many air shows I'd been to as a U.S. Navy flight surgeon with the obvious difference being that lethal munitions were never dropped on people at the air shows.

~ * ~

Today is March 6th, 2015, and we had sixteen operations in the operating room today. One case that stands out is that of a 30 some year old woman who came to the hospital last week with the complaint of constipation. An examination revealed a large, obstructing rectal cancer and we took her to the operating room hoping that we could remove the tumor and offer her a cure. Alas, the tumor was deep in the pelvis and stuck to the surrounding structures rendering it unresectable. We did a diverting colostomy to prevent a complete intestinal obstruction as a palliative procedure. Very unsatisfying case—the woman is still young and has her breast-feeding baby sleeping next to her on her bed. We tried to explain the problem to her and her husband but am not sure how much they understand. They seem to understand the word for cancer ("saratan" in Arabic), but the word doesn't seem to convey any meaning as it's outside their realm of understanding. How do we prepare them for the inevitable slow decline that will follow over the next several months? Another young, breastfeeding mother was admitted today with four months of neck swelling and nasal stuffiness and is now unable to open her right eye and unable to look medially (toward her nose) with the right eye. She had been in the clinic in the refugee camp in Yida [based in South Sudan, just over the border from Sudan, where tens of thousands of Nuba had fled to as a result of the war], and been put on multiple courses of antibiotics and TB drugs without improvement. We made the clinical diagnosis of a nasopharyngeal carcinoma as she has the typical signs and symptoms of this cancer, which is unfortunately very common here in the Nuba Mountains. Nasopharyngeal carcinoma is best treated with radiation therapy, which is only available in Khartoum, on the other side of the enemy lines, and a no go zone for anyone from the Nuba Mountains. Our staff are asking many questions—why is cancer so common now? What causes cancer? Most likely the cancers have always been here, and it's just that they are now being identified and diagnosed in a hospital. Cancer treatment is difficult, expensive and fraught with failures even in the best hospitals in the U.S., let alone here in a war zone in one of the most remote places on earth. Despite the many setbacks in our treatment of cancers, there have been some successes. Burkitt's lymphoma is a common childhood cancer here and is curable with several doses of cyclophosphamide. We've also had some success in treating Wilm's tumors (pediatric kidney cancer), and retinoblastoma (pediatric eye tumor) with a combination of surgery and chemotherapy. We've had palliative success with breast, ovarian, prostate, uterine and cervical cancers as well as Hodgkin's and non Hodgkin's lymphomas. Our goal is usually palliation of the cancer with a combination of surgery and a limited armamentarium of chemotherapeutic agents, always keeping the adage "*primum non nocere*" (first do no harm) in mind.

What I've not mentioned is that I am here in the Sudan as a lay medical missionary with the Catholic Medical Mission Board. Boiled down to its essence, a medical missionary is one who can show others the love of Jesus Christ through his or her actions and attitudes. One of my favorite quotations (rightly or wrongly attributed to St. Francis of Assisi) is "Preach always and sometimes use words." I think we'll never really know what effect our actions and behaviors will have on others. Sometimes I think my actions are having a negative effect on those I'm supposed to mentor as they observe my bad moods and fatigue. I can only pray that God keeps me humble and focused on the task at hand and gives me the strength to keep helping these people even as I sometimes feel the life force being sucked out of me.

As the fighting heated up in the first couple weeks of June 2011, the diocese of El Obeid office in Nairobi sent us messages to start thinking about evacuation of expatriate personnel. The diocese runs several schools, which employ several Kenyan teachers in the Nuba Mountains, and here at the hospital we had eight expatriate personnel. There were also several expatriate builders and field personnel. It was decided to close all of the schools and evacuate the teachers and builders. As the builders reached the Kauda airstrip to board the evacuation airplane, a Sukhoi bomber came overhead and bombed the airstrip as they all fled for cover. The expats eventually made it out on another day.

All of us here at the hospital were told that an evacuation plane was coming on the morning of June 16th, and that this would be the last chance to get out of the Nuba Mountains. We were free to stay but at our own risk, but we couldn't count on being evacuated down the road. Given this reality, all of the expatriate staff decided to evacuate. The priests, sisters and I all decided to stay and stick it out not knowing what the future held as we tried to make contingency plans based on different scenarios. One of our plans involved heading to the nearby hills and hunkering down in the caves as the people had done here in the past. One of our staff was to take us up to show us the caves but we never seemed able to find the time to go on the excursion.

The decision to stay was an easy one for me, and I believe it was also easy for the priests and sisters. It was a time of perfect moral clarity, for to leave would mean that many would die if we weren't there to offer our service. We are all missionaries, and this was our time to practice what we preach and show our solidarity with the people and stick with them in the rough times.

On the morning of June 16th, 2011, all of our expatriate staff secretly slipped out of the hospital under the cover of darkness and made it safely out of the Nuba Mountains. We had to keep all travel arrangements secret due to the fear that Khartoum had spies in the Nuba Mountains who would alert the Antonovs to come and bomb the evacuation airplane as it waited on the airstrip. The eight expats who evacuated included our administrator, anesthetist, midwife, lab technician, pharmacist and all of the nurses in charge of the wards. The only trained nurses left behind were our two Comboni sisters—the matron Sister Angelina and pediatric nurse, Sister Rocio. All of the rest of the staff had all been trained by us on the job, including all of the ward nurses, lab technicians, operating room personnel and pharmacy personnel. I'll never forget the look of shock on their faces when they realized that all of the expats were gone. We gathered them all together early in the morning of June 16th and explained that the expats were now gone and that it was now their time to pick themselves up and carry on with the work. We were very determined that we would continue on as before without any decline in our services. The staff responded by taking charge and getting the job done.

As it turned out, we had little time for self-pity as several casualties showed up just after we talked to the staff. A teenage boy and his sixteen-year-old female cousin had their arms blown off by an Antonov bomber. We amputated the boy's arm below the elbow, but had to remove the girl's arm at the shoulder due to the extensive damage. We did both cases under ketamine anesthesia as I was afraid to paralyze and intubate the patient by myself. The next case was a soldier who'd been shot through the back and out his abdomen. He had a large hole in his abdominal wall with feces spilling out of it. Now there was no choice as we'd have to give a general anesthetic in order to do the operation. After a quick consultation with an anesthesia text and drawing on my vague memories of intubating a goat during my military trauma course, I was able to intubate the patient and stabilize him, leaving a nurse to continue with the anesthesia while I scrubbed and started the operation. The surgery went well as I was able to guide the nurse on the drug doses during the case. God is good.

~ * ~

Today is March 14th, 2015. There was a series of large battles two days ago from which we received fifty casualties and have spent the better part of these two days in the operating room sorting out and operating on the wounded. The wounded just seemed to keep coming at us—the "technicals" with their mounted 50 caliber machine guns kept rolling into the hospital's courtyard and unloading their batches of wounded.

Blood, dust and the pungent smell of battle stress sweat everywhere. One man had a bullet go through his upper arm shattering the bone and into his chest. We sat him up to examine his chest and blood came pouring out of the wound in his chest as he became dizzy, fainted and started convulsing. We resuscitated him, put in a chest tube and started looking for blood donors to transfuse him. Another had his thigh ripped open by a large caliber bullet and the thigh bone was in pieces. We partially closed the wound and placed him in skeletal traction—pretty much civil war era treatment but it usually works. Amazing how the body can heal itself even after such horrific trauma.

Two of the patients were pretty much dead on arrival. I had just gotten to one of them as he was taking his last gasping breaths. Both of his legs were badly mangled, which likely led to his death by massive hemorrhage. No time to ponder this death or mourn for the loss of this young man as other wounded kept pouring in, while those who had been dropped off earlier were waiting for surgery in the operating room. The triage of casualty patients is a cold and unfeeling process as one must stay focused on trying to salvage as many as possible and not dwell on the ones who have no chance of survival.

While still working through the wounded this morning, we admitted a six-year-old boy who was confused and combative, often hitting his mother. I asked if the boy had ever been bitten by a dog and the mother revealed that a small dog had bitten the boy and two chickens two months previously. I gave the boy a cup of water to drink and his panic at seeing the water clinched the unfortunate diagnosis of rabies. Rabies affects the nerves and as a rabid patient tries to swallow, the muscles that control swallowing go into a spasm giving the patient the sensation of suffocating and thus the "hydrophobia" of rabies. His mother was in tears and quietly asked if she could just take the boy home and care for him there. Very painful to allow them to go home but think it's in the best interests of the family.

~ * ~

Today is March 29th, 2015. It's Palm Sunday and also my father's 85th birthday, and I hope to Skype with my parents later in the day. From 3 p.m. yesterday afternoon until 4 this morning, we received 61 casualties from some fighting north of here. Two were dead on arrival and the other 59 had the usual assortment of horrific injuries. One of the dead was one of the local commanders whom we all knew well. He had been one of our early detractors coming to the hospital and berating us for charging the patients the nominal one dollar fee. He said we came to Nuba Mountains just to operate a business and not serve the people. His attitude changed completely after he saw us taking good care of his many wives and children.

One young man had a gaping hole just next to his anus from a gunshot wound. Another confabulating twenty-year-old had a gunshot wound to the head with the large skull defect issuing forth parts of his brain. He had a fixed gaze to the left giving the impression that he was "looking" at his wound. Another had his scrotum shredded by a piece of shrapnel which we found embedded in one of his testicles. One young man had a very innocuous looking small wound on his right chest wall but a very tender abdomen. We opened his abdomen in the operating room to find a large laceration in his liver and a bullet from a Kalashnikov sitting in his abdominal cavity. Another young man had a gunshot wound to the area surrounding the eye, and he was unable to open it. As I was examining his wound and trying to open the eye, the lens of the eye popped out.

Most of the others had gunshot and shrapnel wounds to the extremities, producing shattered hands, legs and arms. Many of these young men will be left with permanent disabilities due to their wounds and no social services to assist them in their life out of the military. What do they do in this agricultural society when they can't farm or look after the cattle? Very painful to see so many young lives destroyed and no sign of an end to the conflict. By March 31st, the casualty count went up to 74 with another succumbing to tetanus.

I've been having some strange dreams lately. Last week I dreamt that a Sukhoi bomber jet circled overhead as we all ran to take cover in the foxholes. The Sukhoi landed in the hospital compound and some patients disembarked from the aircraft. The pilot got out and sheepishly asked if we could take care of these patients who were being referred to us from Khartoum. He then said he would fly back to Khartoum and bring us more patients if we would accept his proposal. Other dreams have been less pleasant. They usually start off with an Antonov or helicopter gunship landing in the hospital compound and us running to hide from them. Several SAF military and security personnel get out of the aircraft, track us down and start interrogating me. The interrogation centers around things they claim I have said against the government and imply that I'll be led away to one of their "ghost houses" for further questioning. I usually end up waking in a cold sweat.

Just as the nightmares were unsettling, so was the intensity of the fighting—the latter always resulting in more wounded, more surgeries, and for those whose injuries were so grievous they were past help, death.

There was no choice, but to deal with it. And so we did, giving our all. There was consistently heavy fighting throughout 2011 and into 2012. The Kauda airstrip fell out of use in June 2011 due to repeated aerial bombardments but some intrepid pilots continued to fly into clandestine airstrips in the Nuba Mountains for a few more months. The last flight into the Nuba Mountains was in November 2011, when the small plane was trailed by a Sudan air force Antonov bomber as it left the remote airfield. After that incident, no more pilots were willing to fly into Nuba.

The Antonov bombers continued to make daily passes overhead on their way to bomb any number of villages and localities. We became so accustomed to the Antonovs flying over head that I almost "missed" hearing the familiar low humming sound if the Antonov failed to pass over us. It was if the sound was somehow comforting—perhaps the brain's way to deal with the psychological stress of not knowing whether today would

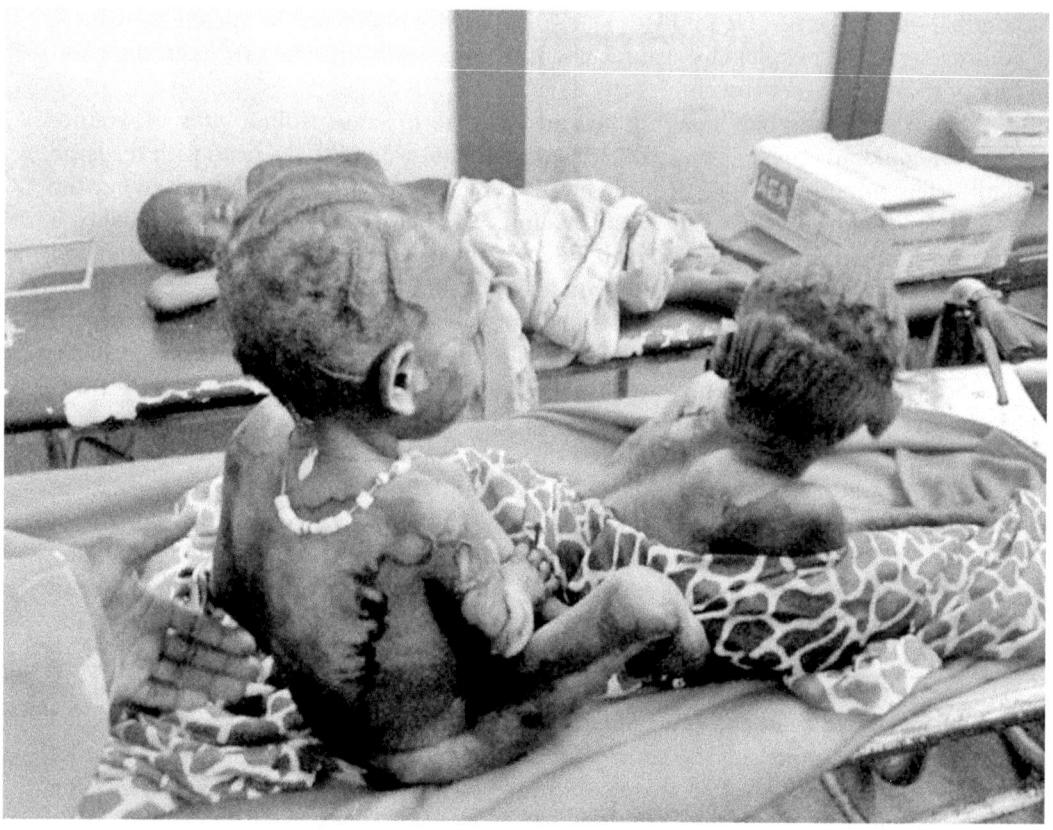

The result of stepping on a banned anti-personnel landmine (photograph by Dr. Tom Catena).

be the day they would decide to drop some barrel bombs on you.

The wounds typically produced by the Antonov bombs were particularly gruesome. Several victims had parts of their skulls torn off, exposing the soft white brain underneath. Others had been lying prone when the bomb struck and had an entire buttock taken off by the searing hot shrapnel. One six-year-old girl was hit in the neck with a large piece of shrapnel, paralyzing her from the chest down, leaving her with limited movement of her hands.

The Antonovs also dropped incendiary bombs, producing large fireballs which resulted in horrifying burns. One young boy and his 30 something year old aunt were hit by an incendiary bomb in 2012 and sustained third degree burns to 50 to 60 percent of their bodies. They both lived in agony for several months before finally succumbing to their wounds. Each time an Antonov passed over we found ourselves thinking—"I don't want to end up like Bibiana or Chalu or Mallata or Ahmed."

I remember one weekend in particular in late March 2012. It was a beautiful Friday evening and I was relaxing on our veranda with the journalist and author Jon Lee Anderson who was writing an article on the recent separation of South Sudan and on the Nuba Mountains. It had been a long day in the operating room and Jon Lee broke out a couple of cold beers. We had just started to enjoy this rare treat when one of our nurses came from the ward saying that many casualties had come from fighting in Talodi. We went down to the corridor outside the operating room and found wounded everywhere. We spent the rest of the evening and night triaging and operating on the wounded, finishing around 5 a.m. Jon Lee was able to hang with us until 2 a.m., when he signed off and went to bed. We were up at 7 a.m. to finish operating on the patients from the previous day and receive more casualties. We received over 60 individuals through Saturday evening and spent the rest of the week sorting them all out. One young man with a gunshot wound to the abdomen stands out in my mind as his wound was especially severe. We opened him up to find over twenty holes in his bowel as a result of the bullet cascading around inside his abdomen. We spent several hours closing the holes and cutting out and stitching together segments of his destroyed bowel. His postoperative course was quite rocky for the first few days and then he stabilized to the point of being able to sit up in bed, eat and talk, and I thought he was on the road to recovery. One night I was called in to see him as he had "changed condition" only to go the ward and find his now lifeless body. So frustrating to not know why someone under your care has died. Just demoralizing.

On a Sunday morning at 11 a.m. in August 2013, as we were finishing the Sunday Mass, we heard an Antonov buzzing overhead. No one got too excited as we more or less considered it a typical case of background noise, plus we had never been bombed. However, this time the usual low droning sound of the Antonov was followed by a high pitched whirring sound, which resembled the sound of a jet engine. As soon as the pitch changed, someone in the congregation yelled "get down," and we all got down in the dirt between the metal benches. This whirring sound was followed by four successive loud explosions shaking the ground under us. My overwhelming desire at that point was to make myself into a mole and burrow myself deep into the earth and escape this frightening reality. It sounded as if the bombs exploded nearby, but in fact they landed about a half kilometer away.

The next day several people were put to work digging foxholes all over the hospital compound as our sense of vulnerability increased a thousand fold. These workers were all women who came to the hospital in droves looking for work in exchange for food. The previous year's harvest was poor due to inadequate rains and people cultivating less land due to insecurity. What a pathetic reality—the only way to get enough food to survive is to go and dig foxholes to protect yourself from the bombs dropped from the government airplanes.

~ * ~

Thursday, May 1st, 2014, started out as a normal day—church, rounds, etc. It was about 9:30 a.m. and I was doing the rounds on the female ward when we heard the deafening sound of jet engines quickly followed by a loud explosion, which rocked the hospital, shaking all of the dust loose from the ceiling and blowing out windows and doors. The sound of the jet sent everyone to the floor in a hushed silence. After the explosion, everyone got up and rushed outside, yelling and screaming in panic. I headed out with the others, trying to calm them down and shepherd them into the foxholes next to the ward. I was told that the bomb had landed near the TB ward so I climbed up the small hill to investigate and found everyone pointing to a smoking hole just beyond the TB ward fence. Just then we heard the sound of the jet coming toward us so we ran to a large foxhole (actually a big hole that was to be a new pit latrine) and jumped down into it to take cover. The jet screamed low overhead, and I got a good view of the underbelly—clearly a Sukhoi-24, a supersonic jet bomber. I knew that the Khartoum government had recently purchased twelve Sukhoi-24s from Belarus, and I had been reading about their capabilities and firepower.

Just after the jet passed over, we heard a second loud explosion—this time seemingly within the hospital compound. I ran down to the compound where I found a group of people gathered just next to my room. The second bomb landed about 20 yards from where I sleep, destroying our fence and several trees. Some said they saw a rocket fired from the jet. Seems the jet was targeting my room, but the rocket sailed just over the roof and hit just beyond. The jet circled around a few more times, dropping three more bombs just outside the hospital compound. Although there were no major casualties and only minor structural damage to the buildings, we were all pretty shaken up as this was the first time we were specifically targeted. My first thought as I lay cowering in the foxhole was, "What are they doing? Don't they know that people are down here?" That night I felt more like a hunted animal than a human being.

The next day, May 2nd, we were greeted at 9 a.m. by the sound of an Antonov bomber overhead. Again, the dull droning sound of the Antonov was replaced by the high pitched whirring sound of a bomb falling through the air and then a tremendous explosion. We were being bombed for a second day in a row! Many of the staff and the patients went into a panic and fled the hospital compound. Some were just going in circles screaming about what would happen to their children. I had to take some of our staff and force them into the foxholes as they were not in their right mind. The Antonov dropped six bombs that morning all of which dropped at the periphery of the hospital and resulted in just one fairly serious casualty. We had a full list of operating room cases that day, but two of the operating room staff had reservations about continuing on with the work. After much discussion, we decided to go ahead with the schedule and were able to complete all of the cases.

The following week it was the St. Peter and Paul's primary school's turn to be targeted by an Antonov as it dropped six bombs, just missing the primary school. Several hundred children took shelter in the 200 some foxholes on the primary school grounds and none were injured. This attack was followed by a Sukhoi raid on nearby Kauda where over 50 bombs were dropped over the span of around two hours. Not a single casualty during that raid either. The message became clear that schools and hospitals were considered legitimate targets by the Khartoum government. As unsettled as we all were by these attacks, it only strengthened our resolve to stick it out and to continue to serve the people of the Nuba Mountains. No way we'd let the bullies in Khartoum win by forcing us to leave and worsening the suffering of this already beleaguered people.

In April 2014, we had started getting reports of measles cases from a place called Jemezai, which is about two hours from us. We sent one of our clinical officers there to investigate and he brought back a few of the sickest patients and a report that there were many more measles cases left behind. Over the ensuing nine months, we admitted 1,400 measles patients to our hospital alone from several villages in South Kordofan. Of this number of cases, we had 30 die from measles. There were reports of many other measles cases and deaths from other parts of the Nuba Mountains, but we'll never have any idea how many cases and deaths there were from measles as many likely stayed at home and never sought any medical care at the few functioning health facilities in the state. The time of this measles epidemic was the most difficult period of my medical career. At the peak of the epidemic, we had seven tents full of measles cases—125 children in all, and they were all deathly ill with fever, cough vomiting and diarrhea. There were two or three children to a bed and the heat and smell in the tents was overwhelming. This period coincided with our malaria season so in addition to the 125 measles cases, there were over 100 on the "regular" pediatric ward meaning we had to do daily rounds on—over 225 on the children's ward alone.

The deaths of our patients have been especially painful. We had a certain patient a couple years ago named Alawia who had lost five pregnancies at four or five months, and had no living child. She had a condition called an incompetent cervix whereby the cervix is weak and dilates on its own before the baby reaches maturity. We did a procedure on her to stitch the cervix closed, and then put her on the ward under strict bed rest for five months. When she finally reached term, we removed the stitch and she immediately delivered a healthy baby girl. Fast forward two years, and Alawia comes to the hospital with her two-year-old girl sick now with measles. The baby lasted a few days before succumbing to a combination of secondary pneumonia and diarrhea—complications from the measles infection. So much effort and care to bring a baby into the world, just to lose the baby due to lack of a single injection.

One of my favorite pediatric patients here was a one and a half year old named Kuku Azraq. He had developed a hydrocephalus (water in the brain) at three months of age, and we operated on him, inserting a tube into his brain and running the tube down under his skin into his abdomen to continuously drain off the excess cerebrospinal fluid. I saw him every month for follow up, and he was doing very well—always a cheerful and happy baby. One day I saw his sister and asked her how Kuku was doing and she told me that he had died the previous week from measles. He fell sick at night and due to the heavy rains there was no way to get him to the hospital and he was dead by the following afternoon.

I remember one Sunday morning going in the tents for rounds on the measles patients when I heard the characteristic wailing and screaming of a mother who had just lost a child. For me, it is the worst of all sounds, something I dread and feel the urge to flee from.

At the same time that we were having our measles epidemic here in the Nuba Mountains, the U.S. press was awash with reports of a large "outbreak" of measles consisting of 140 cases. To make a comparison, there were 140 cases in the U.S. out of a population of 330 million people whereas we had 1400 cases at just our hospital alone! The total population of the Nuba Mountains is perhaps 750,000 to 1 million and the total number of cases likely reached 2800. Why such an epidemic in an era when there is an effective vaccine against this virus? In the U.S. there are several parents who choose not to vaccinate their children as they believe that vaccines are linked to autism and a host of other ills. These parents are overwhelmingly upper class and highly educated—the type that would challenge the conventional wisdom of nearly every credible doctor and scientist the world over. They rely on "herd immunity" to protect their children—this is the concept that if enough children are vaccinated against a certain disease, then that disease will never make a foothold in the population and everyone will be protected. To achieve herd immunity for measles, over 90 percent of the population has to be immune from the disease.

The reasons for the measles epidemic in the Nuba Mountains are quite different. Here in Sudan, as in many other countries, a certain UN organization has the responsibility of providing vaccines free of charge to the government who then is supposed to distribute the vaccine to hospitals and clinics. This system usually works quite well in nations where the government has at least some interest in the health of its people. However, in a country like Sudan, where the government deliberately shells, starves and bombs its own people, providing their citizens with a vaccine is not a big priority. As a principle, the organization charged with providing the vaccines will not give them directly to rebel held areas without the permission of the central government as this would violate the sovereignty of the central government.

Providing the vaccines to the children in the rebel held area would constitute a "cross border" operation in UN/NGO speak, and cross border operations are anathema to the big organizations that provide humanitarian relief to most of the world's needy. These organizations fear that openly providing relief to the rebel held areas will jeopardize their work in the government controlled parts of the state.

Part and parcel of international humanitarian relief also includes drugs for tuberculosis and leprosy as these drugs are normally provided to the hospitals and clinics through the ministries of health of the central government. In fact, drugs for leprosy cannot be bought on the open market. They are only available through the government-sponsored programs. Here at Mother of Mercy we have to jump through several hoops to ensure that the leprosy patients get their drugs as we cannot access them through the central government. When you think about this scenario for a second, this entire situation approaches the theater of the absurd. What kind of a nation denies leprosy patients their drugs? Will such patients lead military campaigns against the government? What is the threat against the government of a patient suffering from the age old scourge of leprosy?

~ * ~

Today is April 13, 2015, a Monday and a fairly typical day. I finished rounds on the maternity ward and had just started rounds on the pediatric ward when a nurse from the male ward came in in a panic to tell me that one of the patients was bleeding heavily from his wound. When I got down to the patient, I found one of our patients, who had a fairly innocuous looking shrapnel wound on his lower leg, pretty much swimming in his own blood. The nurse removed the bandage and a high pressure jet of blood came pouring out of the wound as he quickly lapsed into shock. I had the nurses put his head down and hold his legs in the air as we got some blood for him and prepared for the operating room. After resuscitating him with IV fluid and blood, we rushed him to the operating room and did an above the knee amputation. As soon as we finished that operation, I went to the maternity ward to see a very short young lady trying in vain to deliver a large baby. We went back to the operating room to do a Caesarian section on her and brought out a nice three kilogram (6.6 pound) boy. Next was the drainage of abscesses on two small children, and then back to the wards to finish the rounds. By 2 p.m. I was in clinic to see a large number of patients with all manner of problems, and then back to the wards to check on some of the hospitalized patients. The evening was spent on e-mail correspondence and research.

~ * ~

Today is June 6th, 2015, the fourth year anniversary of the start of the war in the Nuba Mountains. Last week a Sukhoi bombed Kauda twice, and there are reports of the Sudan army and the Rapid Support Forces massing troops in preparation for a new offensive. Sudanese President Omar Hassan al-Bashir was just "re-elected" to another five-year term in office after a sham election. Looks like there will be no end to this conflict any time soon.

It's now the end of June and the rains thus far have been very poor and this doesn't bode well for the next year. Since 99.9 percent of people here are subsistence farmers, a poor rain means a poor harvest and no food for the next year. Seems even Mother Nature has conspired against the people this year, but we remain hopeful that the rains will pick up, peace will break out and everyone can get back to a somewhat normal life. Only time will tell.

In the Service of Christ
My "Tours" in the Nuba Mountains
Sister Deirdre M. Byrne, M.D.

Introduction

I am a general surgeon and religious sister with the congregation called the Little Workers of the Sacred Hearts.

I have ventured to Nuba three times. I love missionary work—not only because I am a religious sister who came to serve Christ in the hidden disguise of the poor, but also because I am a surgeon and the surgical cases are extremely challenging and new at times in regions of conflict overseas.[1]

I have ventured to the Nuba Mountains on three different occasions: 2010, 2011, and 2013. I have had the joy to travel to the Nuba in order to relieve Dr. Tom [Catena] so he can have a little rest and relaxation [from his duties at Mother of Mercy Hospital in the Nuba Mountains].

Formative Years

I grew up in a very devout family in McLean, Virginia, and that was the foundation, really, of my calling to religious life, which is a lifelong commitment, and began when I was a young girl. Both my mother and father attended daily Mass, which gave them the spiritual nourishment, strength, and joy to do the work they did, and that always inspired me. My mother always got all eight of my brothers and sisters up and ready for school, and then rushed off to Mass at 9:00 a.m. every morning. I think such commitment speaks for itself. My father, on the other hand, was a thoracic surgeon with a very busy schedule, but he still made attending daily mass a priority. From the faithful, loving example of my parents, my siblings and I learned what it means to have Christ within you.

Not surprisingly, as I grew up I saw and examined the events of the world through a religious lens in an attempt to find their deeper meaning. In that regard, the religious life—serving Jesus by serving the poor—always beckoned me, and ultimately led me to take vows of poverty, chastity, and obedience. I also have a private fourth vow of "free and loving medical care for the poor and uninsured throughout the world."

As an undergraduate, I attended Virginia Tech (from 1974 to 1978), which provided me with a solid foundation for both my medical career and my religious calling. I was a biology major aspiring to go to medical school, and the programs prepared me well. Because I felt the call to religious life even in college, I became involved in service-oriented activities. For example, my participation in the Newman Community (a Catholic campus ministry) at Virginia Tech provided me with a connection to the church throughout my undergraduate years.

After graduating from Tech in 1978, I attended Georgetown Medical School on a U.S. Army scholarship. In 1985 I did my residency in Family Practice at Dewitt Army Hospital at Fort Belvoir, Virginia. I then pursued a second residency program and completed my general surgery residency in 1997. I should note that knowing one's calling does not come without challenges and sacrifice. Like many women preparing to become surgeons, I spent my "dating years" working 120-hour weeks in the hospital. In my particular case, though, it was a blessing, as it strengthened my commitment to religious life. In fact, during the grueling training to become a surgeon, I was sustained by the daily reception of the Eucharist and stolen moments in the hospital chapel for quiet reflection on the scripture readings for the day. This served as spiritual sustenance for me.

It was in that very same year, 1997, that, by the hand of God, I had the wonderful opportunity to serve as Mother Teresa's doctor for five days during her visit to Washington, D.C. During that time and doing that work I took it as an affirmation that what I was doing was part of God's plan for me.

After a seven year stint in the U.S. Army Medical Corps, I spent a year working as a missionary, part of it in India. In that latter placement I worked alongside Sister Frederick, a Georgetown University trained surgeon, who spent her life serving in India. Her commitment and actions reinforced my dual vocation to religious life and work as a surgeon.

At the time I was searching for a religious order to join, and I seriously considered becoming a member of Mother Teresa's order, Missionaries of Charity. That, though, would have required that I give up my medical practice. Tellingly, I had always felt a call to the religious life but early on my passion was medicine. My mother, though, had often told me that she believed I had a vocation[2] in utero.

During a medical mission in the Sinai, which, as one can imagine, was a spiritually rich experience, I began to discern a very real call to a vocation and thus began investigating different communities. God made it very clear that He was calling me.

Fortuitously, a priest I met had served as a Catholic chaplain during the Vietnam War and he informed me about the Little Workers of the Sacred Hearts. It ended up being a perfect fit for me as work of the order included a medical component. Thus, since January of 2000, I've been a fully professed member of the Little Workers of the Sacred Heart, which performs overseas medical missionary work providing free medical care for the poor and uninsured. I began my formation in 2002 and took my first vows in 2004.

My meeting with the Catholic chaplain coincided with my helping a religious sister who was going through some medical tests in New York City. That was on September 11, 2001, when the Twin Towers crumbled to the ground. Officials were calling for doctors and specifically surgeons, and so by the end of the day, I had made my way to Ground Zero with some of the sisters. I saw firsthand the destruction of the towers and, more tragically, human life.

Shortly thereafter, I came very close to giving up the medical profession to pursue the religious life, exclusively, but a conversation with Jesuit Father John A. Hardon changed my mind. He told me that if I didn't find a community that would allow me to keep practicing medicine, he thought that God would feel as if I were throwing away a gift. So, 0nce again, the call to religious life was put on hold.

Throughout my training and practice, I served in the Active Reserve of the U.S. Army Medical Corps, during which I've attained the rank of colonel. Serving the sick, the poor, and wounded soldiers as a surgeon was a triple gift from God, and He entrusted me with an awesome gift that I do not take for granted. I have to admit that what unfolded in my life was not preplanned. "We propose, and God disposes," as the proverb says. Because our Italian-based Little Workers community had experienced the integrity and goodness of the U.S. troops who freed them from German occupation during World War II, I was called back to active military service to support our wounded soldiers, post-Sept. 11, with the blessings of my Mother General. I served first at Walter Reed Army Hospital, and then in Afghanistan as a military surgeon reservist in Operation Enduring Freedom and Iraqi Freedom in 2008. I have actually deployed three times as a reservist since 2001.

When I returned from Afghanistan, the order asked if me if I could retire from the military, and so I did in 2009, after 29 years of service. I professed final vows with the Little Workers in 2011.

I now serve as the superior of the Washington, D.C.-based Little Workers of the Sacred Hearts house, where we run a pro-bono physical therapy clinic and diabetic eye clinic, as well as a pre-school for underserved children. I practice medicine at the Spanish Catholic Center in Washington, D.C. It is a blessing to serve the humble, hardworking people of this community. Fortunately, through my religious order, I continue to help others around the world in need of medical care. After the devastating earthquake in Haiti, I provided relief services to victims near Port Au Prince, and I travel to Africa every year for several months at a time. And so, to this day, I remain an active missionary sister and superior and a board-certified family practitioner and general surgeon.

Mother of Mercy Hospital, Nuba Mountains

My first "tour of duty" at Mother of Mercy was in 2010, and was almost romantic. The rainy season had ended, and the peanut plants were in full growth.

That first time, the hospital was fairly new. There were about 75 in-patients, with a busy crowded outpatient department. Many people had traveled for days, just to see a doctor. If they arrived after hours, they would camp out on the dusty "sidewalks" with other family members awaiting the next appointment day.[3]

The greatest enemy at that time was the malaria-laden mosquito. This in itself was a horrible murderer of the infants and young children. We were actually losing two to three children per week from such infectious diseases. Then there was the latter's ugly twin sister of enteric infections, which causes terrible dehydration from diarrhea. We—all of us, including the nurses and aides[4]—were exposed to some very difficult cases that first go around, and because of that, this "baptism by fire" served, as it were, my adoption papers for perpetual Nuba family membership.

That first mission was tough for the local hospital personnel because they missed Dr. Tom terribly, but after a few days the Nuba folks embraced me as one of their own.

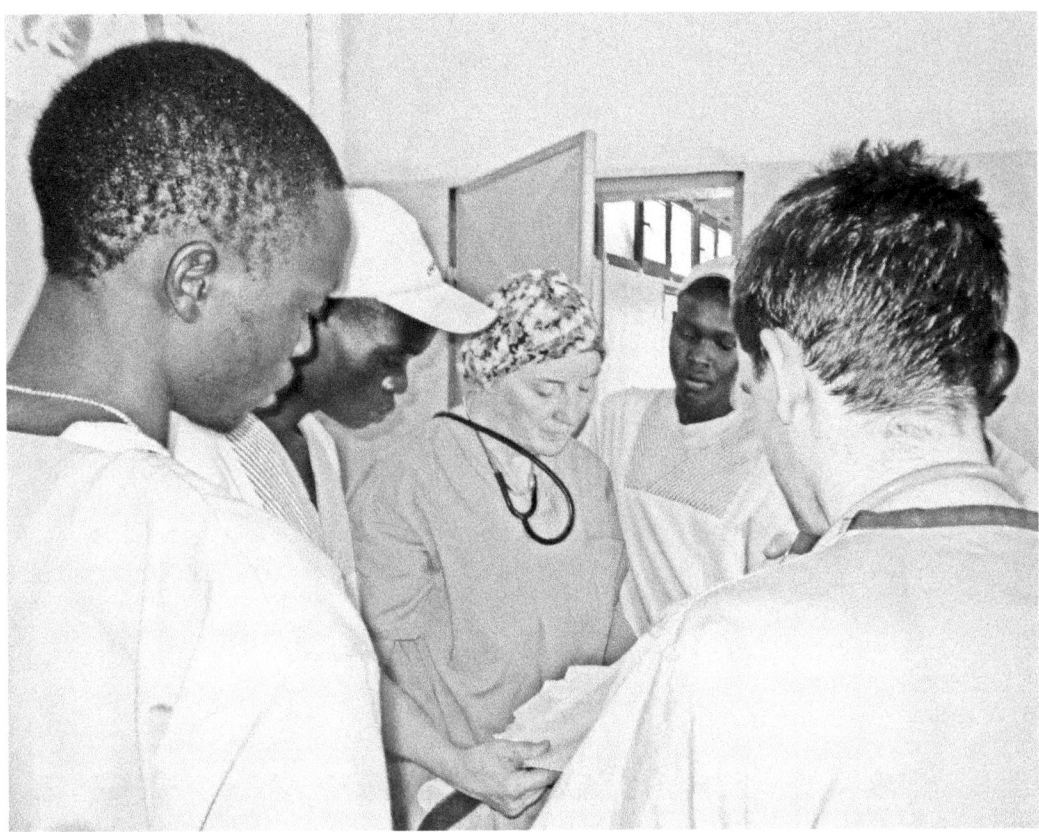

The author making morning rounds at Mother of Mercy Hospital in Gidel, Nuba Mountains, Sudan (Sister Deirdre M. Byrne).

I realized their fear was more of a loss for Tom, and after his first return and their second exposure to me, it was as if I had never left. They are that accepting.

I will never forget the first time I left Nuba after working for about six weeks there. All the workers, hospital cleaners, and cooks stood side-by-side creating a pathway for our truck to drive out of the hospital grounds.... I felt like Atticus Finch in *To Kill a Mockingbird* when Atticus left the court room after a failed attempt to save the life of a falsely accused black man. The upper level balcony filled with poor and humble people who stood to honor a great lawyer who did his best to save the life of such innocence.

My second "tour" in the Nuba began in October 2011. The South and the North had recently spilt into two countries. From the outset there was fear that Khartoum [the North] would become *more* aggressive with the South and that Nuba would be the battleground. It is an oil rich region. And that fear, unfortunately, came to fruition in June 2011.

When I had been there the first time, in early 2010, Mother of Mercy was still receiving mostly non-trauma patients. We were busy with diarrheal diseases, malaria galore, pneumonias and the usual surgical emergencies. But in 2011 life had changed. Now there were serious injuries resulting from the constant daily bombings of the civilian areas.

Even getting to Gidel was now a struggle. The airfield in Kauda, which was a bumpy, crazy twenty minute ride (on a good day) to the hospital grounds, had been bombed. So,

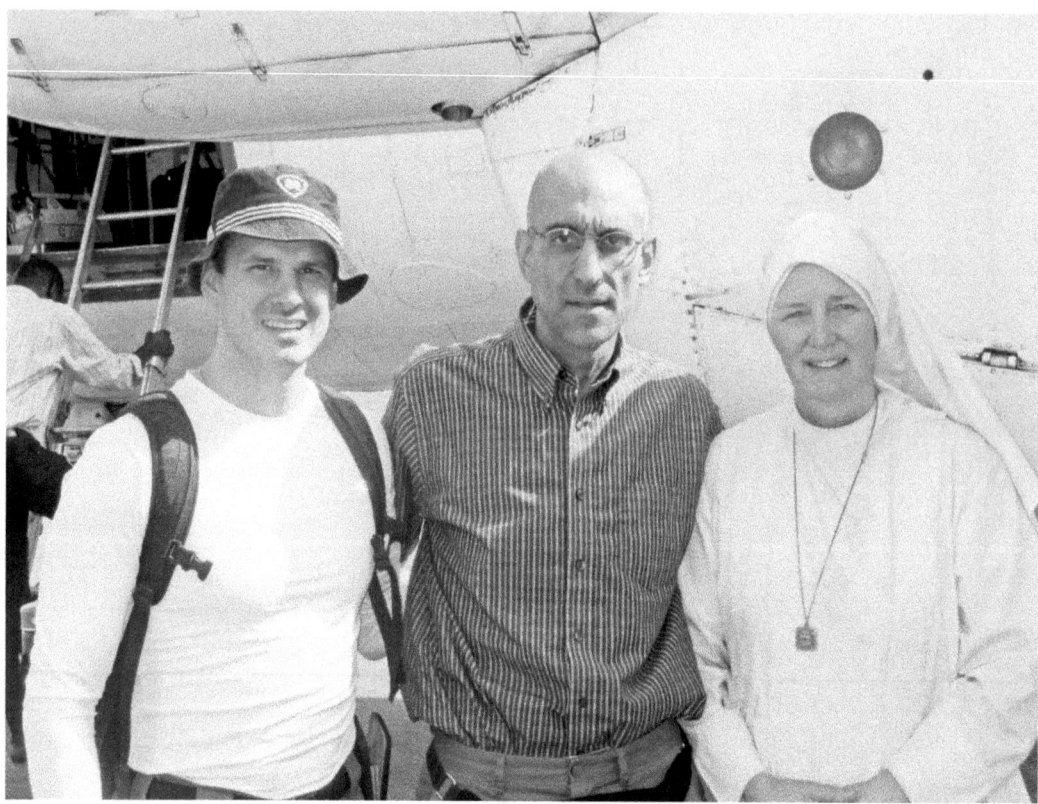

The changing of the guard: Dr. Tom Catena (center), returning to Sudan from a home visit while Sean Wetjen (a first year medical student, left) and the author prepare to leave Sudan (Sister Deirdre M. Byrne).

now one has to fly into the Yida Refugee Camp in South Sudan, very close to the Sudan border, and take a nine or ten hour trip in a vehicle over the dusty, rutted roads.[Editor's note: The Government of Sudan has essentially established a no-fly zone over South Kordofan State (the home of the Nuba Mountains), and no one dares fly in the region, not even the United Nations.]

More than 70,000 refugees had fled Nuba to Yida, a horrible desert journey, which took days by foot. No one owns a vehicle in the Nuba and most don't even own a donkey.

There were, of course, new borders, with border guards separating Sudan from the new nation of The Republic of South Sudan, and that presented its own set of problems. The drive from Yida to Gidel was hazardous not just because of the potholed roads, but because we were easy targets for the North who were known to drop bombs on vehicles. Thank God they had lousy aim.

It had taken me five days just to get to Nuba via the States, and so this final last leg was not easy. In and of itself, staying at the Yida Refugee Camp is not easy; it's not the Hilton.

From North Kenya we took a charter plane charted by the El Obeid Diocese, which carried much needed medicines and food supplies for the hospital and schools that Bishop Gassis has built over the years. The flight involved being strapped into a noisy cargo

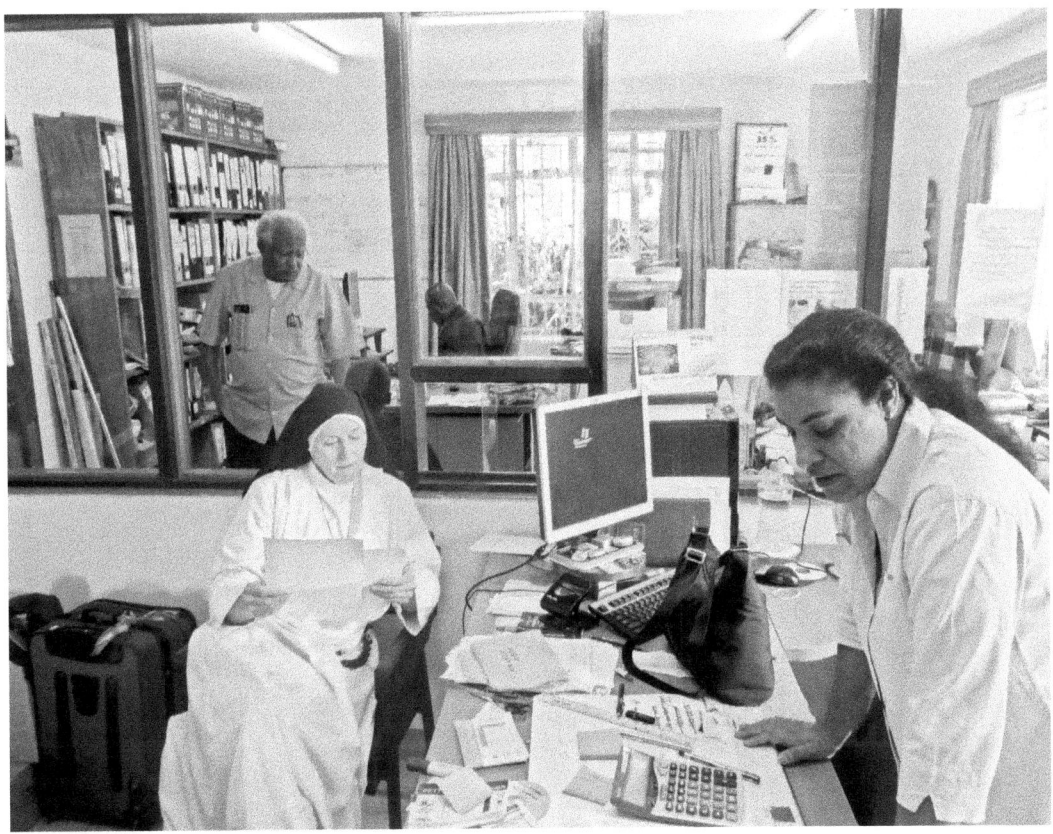

Sharon De Souza (right), Bishop Gassis (standing, background), and the author at El Obeid headquarters (Sister Deirdre M. Byrne).

plane, which took me back to my military days when I was escorting sick patients from Korea to the United States.

Upon arrival in Yida, we stayed at the El Obeid Diocese compound, which is a rat-infested, malarial haven. The only highlight was the "Bishops Throne," which is an outhouse with a wooden toilet seat on a cement stand so older folks like me (and the Bishop) don't have to squat.

Upon my arrival in October, there were over 85 in-patients, with overflow in the hallways. Mind you, there is only one full time, permanent doctor (Dr. Tom Catena) caring for these patients, providing surgical care, emergent and non emergent. A tuberculosis (TB) rehab ward had just gone into operation, providing care for around 20–30 in-patients beyond the routine medical and surgical beds.

My first work day that October was a glorious Sunday morning. I was making quick rounds at the hospital before Sunday mass when a young man approached me with a small bundle in his arms. When he lifted the blanket, cerebral spinal fluid sprouted from the tiny infant's lower back.

"My Lord, Spina Bifida!!! What am I going to do!!! I am not a neurosurgeon!" After admitting the infant to the children's ward, I went to mass and prayed for guidance. This happens a lot to me on mission trips, and Mother of Mercy Hospital was no different. How blessed we are in the United States to have the skilled care for any problem at our

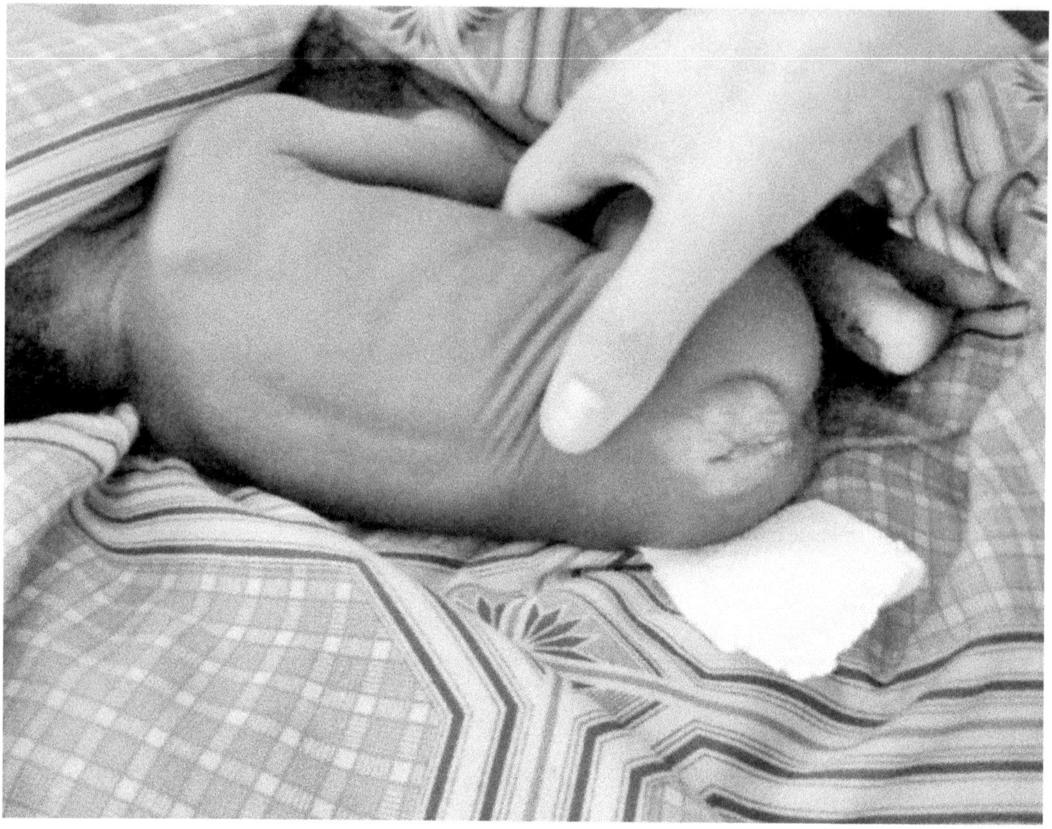

A child who is being attended to following an operation to address spina bifida (photograph by Sister Deirdre M. Byrne).

finger tips, but in the Nuba, I became *the* orthopedic surgeon, *the* GYN surgeon, *the* ENT [eye, nose, throat doctor], *the* urologist, *the* neurosurgeon, *the* pediatrician, *the* internist, you name it! When someone called out or inferred, "We need a trauma surgeon STAT to the minor surgery room," I was off and running to handle the next crazy emergency.

Mother of Mercy has Internet service, sometimes. On this particular occasion, it was working, and thus I emailed a wonderful neurosurgeon I know based in Washington, D.C. Dr. Josh Ammerman. I fully appreciated that I was messaging him late at night DC time, but I was hoping to get some idea of how to tackle the medical issue plaguing this poor little soul whom God gave me as a surgical challenge—as well as reaffirmation that my Georgetown University surgical training did me and this little kid some good. Josh was amazing. He must live with a cell phone next to his ear because he immediately emailed me back, at what must have been about 3 "a.m. ish," his time, sending me what constituted "Spina Bifida Repair for Dummies." That is, he made it seem easy.

And so, after a week of IV antibiotics, we had tackled the problem with great success. God always gives me one case at least, when I am on mission, which He makes it clear that He is the Divine Physician and I am merely his surgical assistant trying to stay out of the way.

It was clear to me, during my first and second missions in the Nuba Mountains, that although I came as a sister-doctor-missionary, I left feeling more and more humbled by

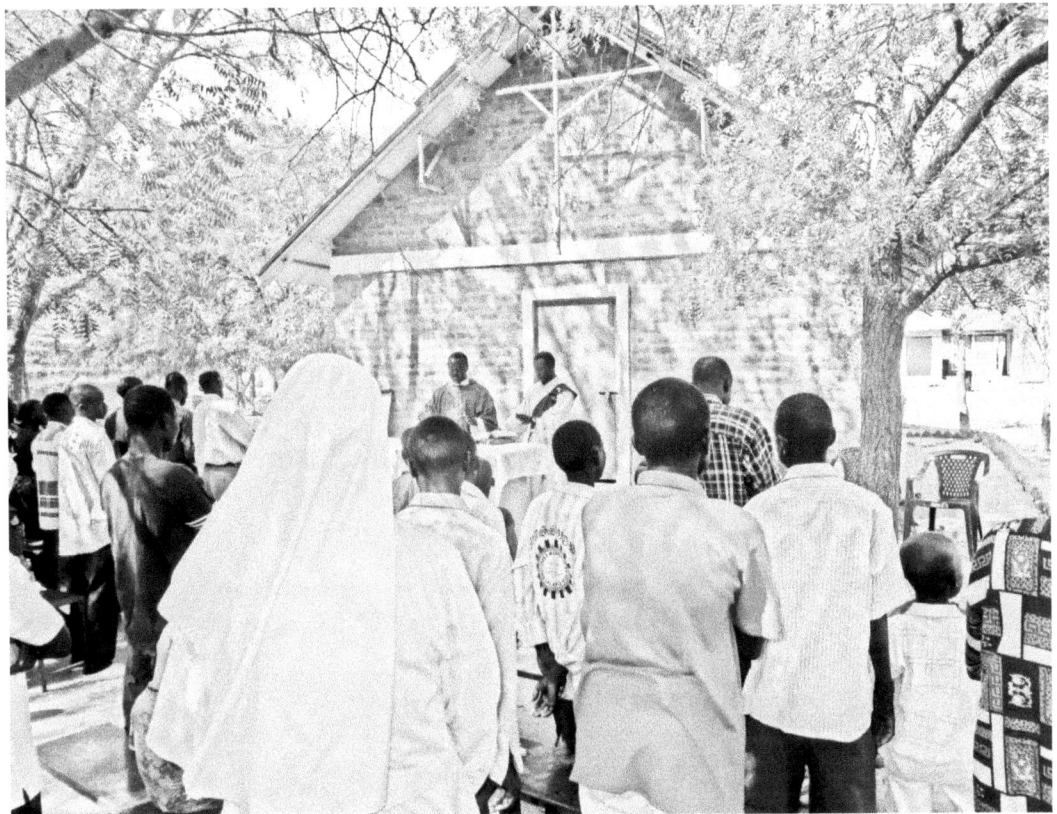

The author at Sunday Mass in the Nuba Mountains (Sister Deirdre M. Byrne).

the strength and joy of the people living there. Where Mother of Mercy is situated, the terrain is dry, desert-like, and it, at times, experiences extremely heavy rainfall—torrential, in fact. It is infested with horrible snakes, scorpions that love to hang out in one's boots, and mosquitoes and the malaria they spread. It is not easy to endure physically, but people are generous and grateful.

My last visit to the Nuba was in 2013, and it was shocking! There were now over 300 patients in the in–patient wards. The number of patients in the hospital was four times greater than when I was there last.

There were patients overflowing in the hallways, and the rear of the hospital was arranged to provide chronic care (i.e., patients with chronic wounds, malnutrition and fractures, and who had had one or more of their limbs amputated). The Nuba Mountains were now being attacked, and we felt like an open target.

The disturbing thing was that many of our victims, now coming in with much greater frequency from villages just a few kilometers away from the hospital, were women and children who had simply been out and about after Sunday church services.

Why the dramatic increase in the number of in-patients? There were two primary reasons. First, Mother of Mercy, which was built by Bishop Macram Gassis of the El Obeid Diocese, had developed an incredible reputation because of the superb medical care administered by Dr. Tom, Sr. Angeline, the Matron, and numerous staff. Second, civilians continued to be bombed by Antonov bombers and continued to suffer from a

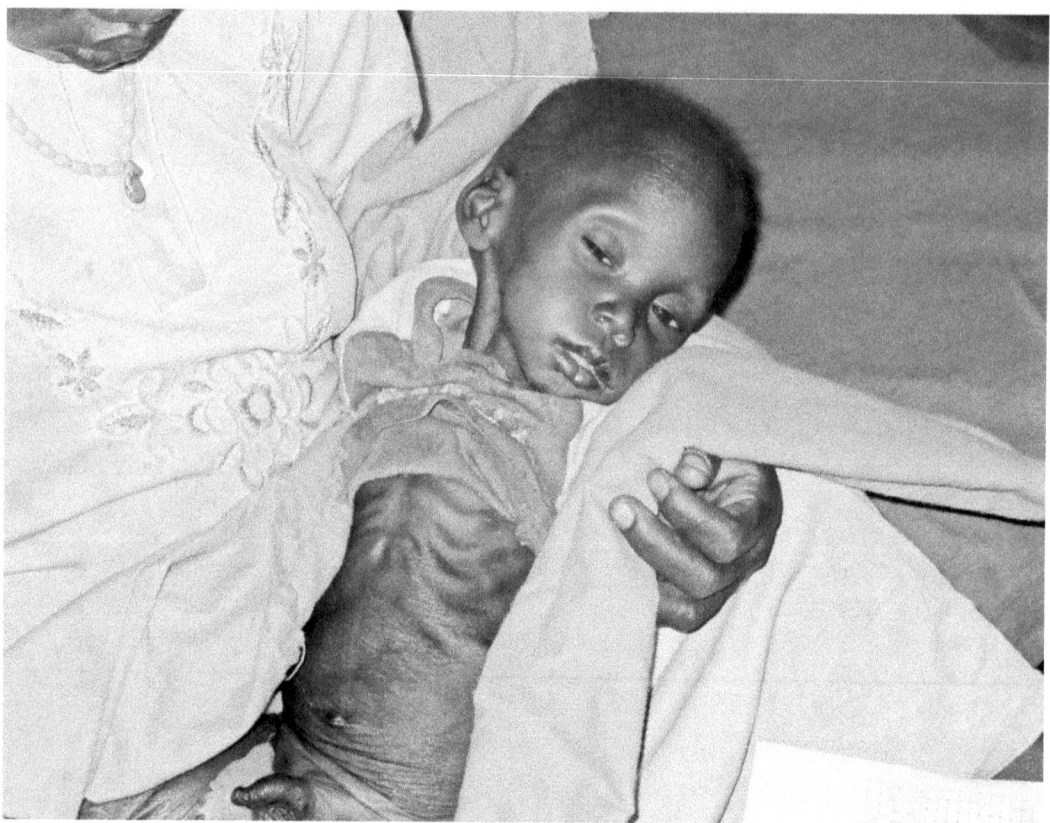

A Nuba child suffering from malnutrition (photograph by Sister Deirdre M. Byrne).

dearth of food, thus the hospital was increasingly inundated with new patients. Furthermore, while the GoS has weaponry that is archaic and dangerous (sharp metal bombs dropped from Old Russian planes) but also attack jets and other modern weapons, the Sudan People's Liberation Army–North is largely equipped with small arms.

One mass casualty I will never forget was when a mother and her children arrived at Mother of Mercy via a rickety vehicle. The children were missing fingers and their mother had half her face blown off, yet was still able to breathe through what appeared to be bloody swollen lips. One of her legs had been sheared off above the knee and her other foot was completely missing. She had sharp shards of metal throughout her torso. I had to use a Foley (urinary) catheter to drain a sucking chest wound filled with blood and air as there was no chest tube available, a common piece of emergency equipment found in any emergency room in the United States. *No experience*—not my days at the Washington, D.C., General Hospital or my three months in Afghanistan during my Army days—matched the tragedies that unfolded before me during those seven weeks in the Nuba.

Bishop Gassis had envisioned Mother of Mercy to be a refuge for the injured for both those from the North and South, but never did he imagine that the hospital would be filled with victims wounded as a result of war. Last year, in May of 2014, the hospital was bombed by GoS bombers. The bombs did not hit the hospital proper, but rather struck the quarters of the hospital staff. Thank God the staff were working in the hospital at that moment, otherwise it could very well have resulted in the deaths of the skilled medical staff, including the doctor and anesthetist. Prior to the actual attack, drones had been flying overhead.

Conclusion

In many ways, Mother of Mercy Hospital is the healing light of hope for the Nuba people. That was the vision of Bishop Gassis and, almost prophetically, this vision has come to fruition.

Indeed, in spite of all the trials, tribulations and seemingly endless difficulties they face, the Nuba have remained strong and stalwart. They are beautiful people who although they suffer much, also love much. Nuba Christians live in peace with Nuba Muslims, sometimes in the same family, and vice versa. And although their traditions are different, for example the polygamous existence of the Muslims versus the monogamous relationship of Christians, the people still get along and are notably nonjudgemental. For me, they are truly inspirational.

Despite all the tragedy and sadness the Nuba have suffered, I have always been amazed at the joy and gratitude that they exude. Each day I would look into their weary eyes and see beyond suffering and victimization, and witness beautiful people who always see their strength in each other but most of all through their loving God who will never abandon them.

In closing, I wish to return to my formative years, and the love and guidance of my parents and the lives they lived. As I mentioned, they both were very devout, and that was the foundation of my calling to religious life and desire to serve others. In that regard, I am proud to note that my brother, Father William Byrne, is the pastor of St. Peter Parish on Capitol Hill and archdiocesan Secretary for Pastoral Ministry and Social Concerns. Thus, he, too, shares a passion for serving those trodden upon.

To this day I remain an active missionary sister and superior and a board-certified family practitioner and general surgeon. During the course of my life I have learned God doesn't always call us to do big things; it's the day-to-day little things we do that help us make God present to others. St. Therese of Lisieux, the patron saint of missionaries, said, "We can do no great things; only small things with great love."

Christ is the servant of servants, and in spite of my human frailties, I aspire to imitate His call to serve. The vocation of sister-soldier-surgeon affords me triple the opportunity to serve, most importantly as the healing touch of Christ and to make Him known, loved, and served throughout the world.

I wake up every day and I love my life. For me, it is not a holy vocation, but a holy vacation.

NOTES

1. One of the fantastic gifts and joys for me about mission work is the opportunity to learn surgical procedures that I would otherwise never do, or learn in a general surgical residency. For example, in 2000, when I was in northern Kenya, I learned how to do open prostatectomies from a skilled Dutch surgeon. That skill carried me a long way during my time in the Nuba Mountains.

Benign prostatic hypertrophy is a common problem in the aging male population here in the U.S. and Europe. A simple surgical out patient procedure or medical therapy can prevent the complications of bladder obstruction or rupture and death. But in the Nuba—and many poor countries throughout the world—where hospitals are few and far between, bladder obstructions can become an emergency. Usually this can be managed with a temporary suprapubic catheter followed by removal of the prostrate gland. For missionary doctors this procedure, along with emergency Cesarean sections (C-sections), are mandatory cases to know how to perform, and ironically they are two cases not formally taught in general surgical residencies, so they are usually learned "on the job."

2. Meaning—a divine call/summons to religious life.

3. On the backside of the ward were other older Nuban men with Foley catheters awaiting their turn to get a new lease on life. Many were on hold either due to the untoward emergencies that "bump them" out of line or because they are in need of blood. It is not uncommon to lose a pint of blood during this particular surgery so it is prudent to have one or two units on hold for the emergencies. But sadly, the lack of blood is always a problem. We lost many a patient due to the inability to acquire blood to pursue surgery.

I will never forget the elderly gentleman who was brought into the hospital with an Open Femur Fracture. "How long has he been this way?" I asked one of his sons. "About a year," one son responded with no apology.

"A YEAR."

His hemoglobin was about 5 mg/dl, which is grossly under normal and certainly too low to operate. He needed an above the knee amputation. But he had already waited a year, so we figured, "We can wait a few more days to acquire blood." This man had four sons, but none would donate a unit blood out of fear of death. Many Africans in this area feel that if they give their blood away they will die. As hard as I tried to explain to them that the bone marrow would replenish their blood and help them overcome their anemia, they refused. We really have no blood bank at Mother of Mercy. What little blood Mother of Mercy can store is saved for the emergencies. Sadly the elderly man with the Open Femur Fracture died soon after admission.

4. Francis, for example, is Mother of Mercy's jack-of-all-trades. He is a college level trained anesthesiologist. He basically does most of what our docs in the United States do (following all of their formal training), and then some. He can intubate, he can do spinals, *and* he will (and has), in the middle of the night, run (while the patient is still on the OR table) to turn on the generator that is outside behind the hospital because the electricity suddenly stopped working. The first time this happened, I was in the middle of a case, the patient's abdomen was wide open, the fan was circulating 100-degree air so we could breathe, and we lost our suction. Francis left in a snap. He didn't even say, "I'll be back in a second!" I, in fact, didn't even realize he was gone. I just knew that the air had stopped circulating and the temperature in the OR was rising. Francis came back in minutes, immediately checking his patient's vital signs and assuring me everything was OK. I wanted him to check my vital signs too when I realized he had left the patient. But what can we do? It was past midnight and everyone else—including some of our night duty nurses—was asleep.

Most of the workers are local Nubans, with barely a grade school education. But Francis and about five other nurses and the lab tech were expats. Most were from Uganda. All are very devout Christians. It was a true joy to work with them.

In the U.S. we live in a world of political correctness, but in the Nuba one feels a closeness to God (even though it is hot as H_ _ _) because the people there do not fear to openly discuss their Love of God, Jesus, Mary and Joseph, and all the saints. Their faith is a big part of who they are. I remember one morning before operating on a young man, he was about to be put to sleep and he asked me, "Doctor, will you please pray with me?" I was very moved by his great faith. He was a Muslim, his wife was a Christian.

A Son of the Nuba
From Forced Exile to My Return as a Humanitarian

George Tutu

I was born in a remote area of the Nuba Mountains called Kurche. It is located in the Moro Hills of the Nuba Mountains. Like many Sudanese, I don't know what day or month I was born. This is why many Sudanese register their birthday as January 1, which is our National Day of Independence. I'm not even sure of the year that I was born, but it was somewhere around 1963.

We had cattle and goats, and grew our own food, but it was like we were living a thousand years ago—houses [tukuls] built with grass and mud, no electricity, no running water, no place to go to the toilet or shower. The first time I ever saw a television was in 1975 when I went to Khartoum. Until then, I had never even seen electricity. In fact, when I first moved to Khartoum, I actually hung my clothes to dry on electrical wires, not realizing the danger of doing so.

When someone got sick, two or three people lifted that person on his bed and carried him to the local clinic. There were, of course, no such thing as ambulances. We lost many people because of that; not being able to get them to the clinic in time.

We had no medicine. If you got sick, you might die or you might live. It was just like that. That's just how primitive our lives were despite the fact those living in Khartoum, the powerful and the privileged, had plenty of funds to create a comfortable life for themselves. In part, that's what led us, the Nuba, to believe that we had the right to fight the Arabs for change.

One of my brothers, Musa, who badly injured his foot, was carried to the clinic. It took those carrying him about two hours footing to OmDurain, where there was a clinic built by missionaries. When they got to the clinic, they found there was no medicine to help him. As they were washing the wound they realized that they had to take his leg. At the time I was around 10 years old.

My father did not put me in school when I was a child, because nobody was aware of the advantages of formal education, plus the first schools in our area did not appear until the late 1960s. Up to around ten years old, I was just a cowboy [a herder] caring for our family cattle.

In the Moro, we were the people of Ei-kam-chang. People believed that the Ei-kam-chang were the ones who controlled the rain. When the rain doesn't come, the people

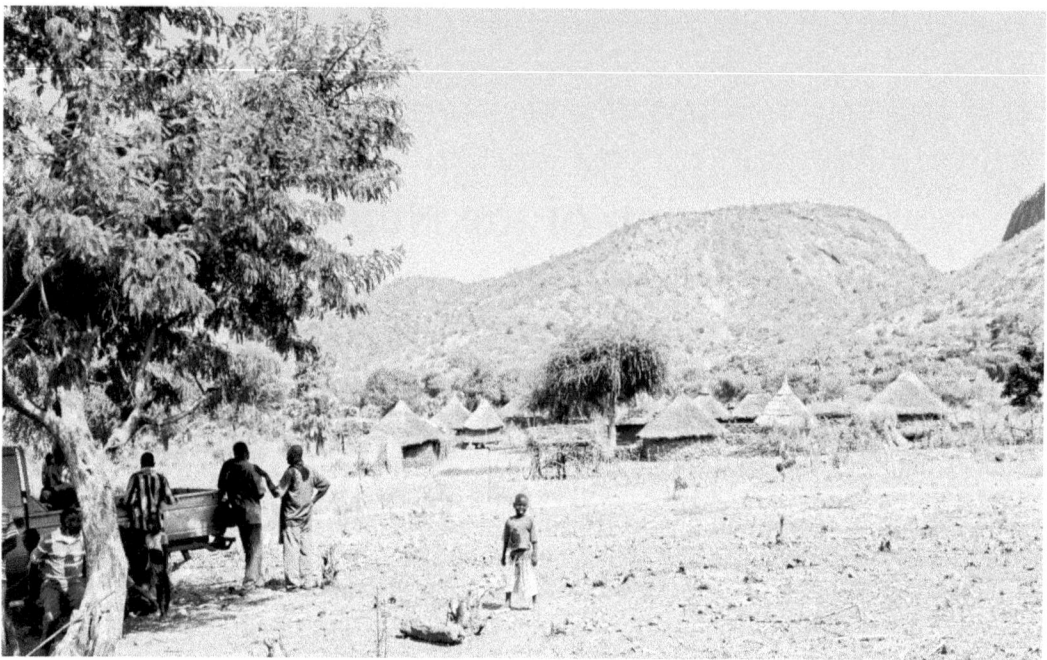

A village in the Moro Hills, Nuba Mountains, Sudan (photograph by and courtesy Slater Armstrong, January 2016).

bring gifts to one of the elders, who is nominated to be the representative to God. He would go beyond the valleys and cry out to God to bring water, while also beseeching the people to remain in their *tukuls*, to take shelter from storms, thunder and lightning.

My family was hit by lightning when I was between five and seven years old. We were living on the top of the mountain at the time, and at the time we were hit by lightening as we were making a sacrifice. My auntie was holding a plate to catch blood from the pig being sacrificed to spread around the compound for my brother who was very sick. He couldn't even talk. This was to wash the evil things away. The lightning struck our family compound, and my brother's room caught fire.

When the lightning struck my brother's *tukul*, we were all sitting around on rocks, and the shock wave was so severe that we all ended up with terrible headaches for two or three weeks. Smoke surrounded our entire compound, and people thought we had all been killed.

While it was frightening and the headaches were terrible, we all believed that God had a purpose—that He was destroying the evil that was in my brother's room and that was causing him to be so sick. And, actually, my brother was healed after that.

Father said, "No one is allowed to cry, let God do what they want to do." This was [predicated on] our traditional tribal belief. We believed in the Creator God, but did not *know* Him, not like one does when one comes to the Lord through Jesus Christ. We believed we were to honor Him.

As I said, we had no medicine, so we went to the village elder to get "washed" with blessed water every week for the headaches.

Each of the five groups of Moro had their own traditions. Today, though, all of the elders who knew these practices of our people have died. Over the past 40 years, most of our people have now become Christians.

We were living on top of the mountain because the Baggara Arabs often attacked our villages and farms. If we didn't flee, then we would be killed or made slaves. To this day, Nuba have to defend their land from the Baggara. They, the Baggara, are connected to the government of Sudan. That is upsetting for a lot of reasons. First, without the help of the Nuba, the Baggara would not have been able to live in the Nuba Mountains. Second, the Nuba traded cattle with the Baggara, who took them north to sell. But then, over the years, the Baggara became cattle owners, and they allowed their animals to graze on our crops, eat our crops, which was our main source of food. And they let their animals stomp on our crops and destroy them.

One day, when I was around 8 or 9 years old, during the harvest time, I was farming with my mom and family, but my father was not there. The Baggara came through, allowing their animals to eat our crops that had been growing for three months. We could not say anything or they would've beat us. We also could not take them to court, because the courts were run by the Arabs. We were not in full war then, but constant conflict. They would kill our people who tried to speak up, who confronted them.

In late 1960, my oldest brother, Butrous, became a Christian. He was the first in our family to come to faith in Jesus Christ. At the time, Butrous was a very famous "stickfighter." He was very popular around the Moro Hills region, as he represented our people in the competitions within the Moro people. Other Nuba tribes wrestle, but in the Moro we wrestled and also had stick fighting. During the last competition, Butrous arrived with his group carrying a cross, followed by five drummers and young ladies who were singing his praises for fighting and encouraging young people to be strong. After he won the fight, he made the announcement that he had become a Christian and would no longer be a stick fighter because there was always the chance he might kill someone. Neither my father nor the community was pleased about this. In fact, they were outraged.

After about a week, my father kicked Butrous out for becoming a Christian. My father had tried to talk my brother out of it, but he was not able to do so. Butrous said there was no way for him to turn back. At the time, he was with the Evangelical Church. He was later baptized in the Episcopal Church.

Butrous had placed a cross on the roof of his tukul, but my father ripped it down and threw it away. Then he kicked him out.

Butrous became very active with youth evangelizing and preaching, and quit working with cattle. Our family looked at him like he was not one of us. This lasted a year or two. All this time my brother was praying for us. By 1968–1969, he had become a very popular and important leader among the youth. At this time, he was writing and singing songs praising Christ.

During this time my father didn't have much to do with my brother. Butrous could come and go as he pleased, but my father and Butrous had no relationship.

I was my father's favorite son to bring hunting. We had some very good hunting dogs that were fast and aggressive. We hunted mostly deer and rabbit. We would talk a lot, and had a good relationship.

In 1973, I traveled to Khartoum to visit my uncle's family. While I was there my uncle made arrangements for me to go to school because there was a Catholic school offering free education for marginalized people, and it was an opportunity my uncle felt that we could not pass up. The school was called The Comboni Catholic Primary School, and it was located in Omdurman.

The school was very good, but every day we departed for home, Arab kids would throw stones at us as we rode home in a lorry. One day, my friend, Yusef, ended up getting hit in the head. (He later became my brother-in-law when I married his sister, Salwa).

The driver of the lorry (a Baggara Christian) went to the headmaster to report the incident. The headmaster was from the Dinka tribe. He told the driver, "If you see them coming again, let the students get out to defend themselves." Eventually, we did that, and the fight was brutal. We ended up at the police station. The driver told the police what had happened, and the police, who were very wise and saw that the Nuba students were injured from the stones, did not punish us. I was about twelve at that time. This is a strong memory in my life up till today.

That area was filled with racist Arabs who followed Sadiq Al Mahdi [the Prime Minister of Sudan from 1966 to 1967 and again from 1986 to 1989, the grandson of the Al Mahdi, who founded the Umma Party, and the great-grandson of the Al Mahdi, who was the self proclaimed messianic figure who fought the Egyptians and the British in the late 1800s]. Sadiq al Mahdi inflamed racism against the Nuba people. And those followers of al Mahdi and their children did not like us, and the children always wanted to fight us.

That same year, the police constantly arrested black people. On the street, all the time, for no reason. Just to harass us. One morning, they arrested my brother, Osman, and his friends. (Osman was helping take care of me in Khartoum while I was in school.) Shortly after they had been arrested I came along and saw a lorry picking up the others and taking them to jail. I stopped to ask one of my brother's friends in the truck if he knew where Osman was, if he had been arrested, too. At that exact moment, the police grabbed me. I told them I was a student going to school.

They said, "We don't care! Why are you here?"

I told them I was looking for my brother.

I told them, "If you bring me to the jail, you will have to bring me all the way back home." I said that because I was so young. So they left me alone.

In 1975, I joined the student movement that followed Father Gabush.[1] He was a Christian and the first priest in the Episcopal Church of the Nuba Mountains. He was from the Nyimang tribe of the Nuba. We had heard about him when we were younger. After I had moved to Omdurman to go to school, I attended the same church that his children attended. (His son was—and still is—a good friend.) Even though Father Gabush was a priest, he had also become a politician, because of the ill treatment of the Nuba by the GoS *and* because the GoS was preventing him from baptizing the people from the Nuba. Also, evangelism was not allowed in general. Even though he became active in opposing the government, he never left his orders as an Episcopal priest.

I, as well as other young people, became a supporter of the Nuba Revolutionary Movement, even in high school. We, in fact, paid membership dues to support the movement.

Back in the 1960s, Gabush had formed The Nuba Mountain Political Association, which he later expanded to the National Sudanese Party (NSP) in 1988. Gabush's aim in broadening The Nuba Mountain Political Association to the NSP was to include all of the other marginalized people in Sudan, versus simply the Nuba, in order to provide them all with a political party that represented their combined interests and concerns.

In 1969, Gabush's life changed dramatically. It had become known that he was extremely keen to overthrow [Sudanese President] Gaafar el-Nimeiri due to his administration's lack of fairness and justice in relation to the marginalized peoples of Sudan. A traitor reported that fact to the GoS' national security office. As a result, Father Gabush fled Sudan and sought refuge in Ethiopia. He was sure Nimeiri wanted him killed, and thus he felt he had no choice but to flee.

In Addis Ababa, Father Gabush began attending the peace negotiations dealing with the ongoing conflicts in Sudan. Nimeiri refused to allow the Nuba to be a part of the negotiations that were seeking to address the issues that ignited the civil war between the government (the North or Khartoum) and the southern tribes, and that upset Gabush. Pushing back, Gabush demanded that the Nuba situation be addressed. That infuriated Nimeiri.

Even though Gabush was not a formal member of any legation, he argued ferociously for more rights for the Nuba. Niemeri ended up applying great pressure on the World Council of Churches to remove Gabush from the hearings. Eventually, the World Council of Churches gave in to Niemeri and removed Gabush from the proceedings. The World Council accused Gabush of being disruptive by insisting on the inclusion of the Nuba in the conversation, even though the Nuba had not been part of the Anyana I movement.[2]

In 1978, Gabush reached an agreement with Nimeiri, and was allowed back in Sudan. While in exile in Ethiopia, Gabush had formed the Nuba Revolutionary Movement, which was to serve as the military branch of the Nuba Mountain Political Association. (The Nuba fought under the Nuba Mountain Political Association until the point in time at which they joined forces with the SPLA in 1983 under the leadership of Yusef Kuwa.) Gabush's Nuba "army" headquarters continued to be based in Ethiopia, where future fighters were trained under Clement Amoda, who is now commander of the SPLA in Nuba Mountains

In 1979, Gabush was once again accused of trying to carry out a coup d'etat to overthrow Nimeiri. He was arrested and held in prison for a little over three years or up to the time Nimeiri implemented Sharia in 1983.

Many young people followed Father Gabush's Nuba Revolutionary Movement, which ultimately joined the SPLA in its battle against the GoS. One such individual was Yusef al Massa, who was from the Moro tribe. He was a nurse at a mental health hospital in Omdurman, which was affiliated with the Episcopal Church. The GoS decided it wanted the Church's building and stole it from the Church. Shortly after that he left for Ethiopia, al Massa joined Father Gabush and entered into the military college in Addis Ababa.

In 1981, the Nuba Revolutionary Movement left Ethiopia for the Nuba Mountains, where Yusef Al Massa recruited 20 to 30 Nuba youth to return to Ethiopia in order to be trained at the Military College. Al Massa also left weapons with a group of Nuba in order to train Nuba inside the Nuba Mountains. That group in the Nuba was also tasked with working to unite the various tribes within the Nuba Mountains. Al Massa was later killed in 1985.

Al Massa ended up walking all the way from Addis to Malakal and then onto the Nuba Mountains, where he began to recruit young people, including Clement Amoda. As I mentioned, Clement Amoda is now the commander of the SPLA in the Nuba today.

Some Nuba reported al Massa to the head of security in Kadugli in September of that same year (1981), and Nimeiri sent the GoS army to defeat the Nuba rebel forces. The battles largely took place inside the Moro area, resulting in the deaths of approximately

30 government troops. Furious, Nimeiri warned the rebels to immediately disband or face the annihilation of the Moro.

In early 1982, thirteen youth were arrested as a result of their involvement with the Nuba movement, and they were transported to Khartoum and imprisoned. The rest of those training in the Nuba left for Ethiopia. In late 1982, they returned and began training and mobilizing a full-blown Nuba army.

At this time, the Nuba military formed an alliance with the Shilluk and Nuer peoples, among other south Sudanese. In early 1983, Nimeiri declared Sharia Law all across Sudan. Because of that, John Garang (who was still with the government army) broke away from the government, and joined the aforementioned alliance. In doing so, he helped to solidify and unite them into one strong alliance, and was elected as both commander and chair of the newly formed SPLA.

Yusef Kuwa served as the first commander of the SPLA in the Nuba Mountains. He had been a teacher and a member of the National Parliament. He left everything and joined the movement, was trained in Ethiopia, and became a commander in the SPLA, and then became the leader of the Nuba at that time.

Around this time, the authorities in Khartoum sought to hang Gabush as a criminal and enemy of the state through the new Sharia system. During the whole trial, none of the black people were working and they all, especially the Nuba, anxiously followed the trial. (At that time the Nuba made up 80 percent of Sudan's armies.) Nimeiri saw these people rising up from every corner of the city and country with whatever weapons they could find, including sticks, to fight for their leader, Gabush. Nimeiri feared the potential uprising, and so the authorities set Gabush free.

In 1984, there was an uprising of all the Sudanese people because they didn't want Sharia Law, which was the majority from every sector, including Arab and Muslim. And so Nimeiri was finally removed from power, and replaced briefly with a transitional military council, chaired by General Suwar ad-Dahhab, until new elections could be held.

Those who had been arrested in 1982 in the Nuba Mountains who were accused of supporting the Nuba Movement, along with many other political prisoners of Nimeiri, were set free during the uprising. A great horde of people overwhelmed the prison and tore it apart. I remember we had a big party, and I was in charge of the event welcoming them home from their imprisonment.

Many of those joined the SPLA, immediately! The people were so encouraged by the uprising they began to fight for their rights. They also realized the only means to do so was to unite with the military opposition to the government, which was the SPLA.

Gabush formed the Sudanese National Party out of The Nuba Movement, and sought to join the democratic elections taking place in the wake of the coup. During the election Gabush won the office of the Nuba representative to Khartoum, but lost the National vote to Saddiq al Mahdi, who became Prime Minister. During this time, fighting was taking place all over Sudan: in the Nuba, in South Sudan, and the Blue Nile.

I was involved with the movement up to when Bashir came to power in 1989. That was when he created the security system that infiltrated the tribes to spy on them. I fled from Khartoum when "security" friends and family informed me that I was being watched by al-Bashir's people and that my arrest was imminent.

Going back some bit, in 1977 I had become involved with the youth program in the Episcopal Church, and continued to be through 1986. In 1978, I also joined Operation Mobilization [an interdenominational outreach organization for missions], and went with a team of about six to seven people to Baba Nosa in West-South Kordofan and also to Abyei, where we shared Christian testimony with Muslims.

After graduating from high school, I had no support to attend university, so after nine years of schooling I began working at the finest hotel in Khartoum, the Meridian Hotel. I worked in food and beverage services. At the same time, I also attended evening classes to study hotel management. I did that for two years.

In 1981, I married my wife, Salwa. I continued to work and attend evening classes. Our first child, my son, Awino, was born in 1982, during our second year of marriage. I now have six children. The rest followed over the next twelve to thirteen years.

Around 1983, while still in Khartoum, I became involved with the Sudan People's Liberation Army (SPLA). This was when Nimeiri was still the president of Sudan. At the time, I joined the Nuba Movement whose commander was Yusef Kuwa. Kuwa had been recruited for that position by Father Gabush. President Nimeiri had aligned himself with the Muslim Brotherhood in response to pressure from the Islamist opposition to move towards the establishment of Islamic political governance. As a result, his government established Sharia Law throughout the country.

The reason I became involved in the SPLA was because of the way the Arabs treated the Nuba people, and because of Sharia Law. Sudan is a very diverse country, with people who are Muslim, Christian, animist, and even some of those who are Muslim or Christian still hold onto animist beliefs. Many of the Muslims are moderate, and even they don't want Sharia Law. One reason, I think, Sharia Law was established by Nimeiri was because of the growth of Christianity among the black people.

When Sharia Law was established, they, the government, began cutting the hands off the black people, saying they were stealing, but often there was no investigation and no judicial proof that any such theft had occurred. Because of that, Sharia Law appeared to be mostly about controlling the black people.

I also joined the SPLA because there was no development in the Nuba Mountains. None! There were very few schools and health clinics, no clean water, no electricity, no toilets, nothing.

At the same time, the government was trying to force us to leave behind our ancestral culture, and to adopt their Arab-Islamic culture. They were trying to force us to change our identity. They even forced us to change our names to Arabic names. (I was informed that my new name was to be Ali, but I did not accept it.) We were not allowed to speak our own languages while in school. We also were not able to move around freely, and we had to be very careful because we could be stopped and falsely accused of something. Also, Christians were not allowed to evangelize.

The Second Sudanese Civil War broke out in 1983 [1983–2005]. The North [i.e., Khartoum or The Government of Sudan] was in a war with the South The Nuba joined in the fight with the South a bit later in the 1980s, both because the Baggara continued to harass us and because both the South and the North brought the war to the Nuba Mountains—began fighting one another there.

In 1984, I was promoted to captain of the food and beverage services, and was sent to Egypt for a short while for further training in hotel and restaurant services. Nothing much happened while I was in Egypt that related to the Nuba Movement. But I was recognized for my skills at my work at the Meridien Hotel, and was quickly promoted.

In 1985 Nimeiri was overthrown in a coup d'état. He was essentially overthrown by all of the Sudanese who were adamantly against the establishment of Sharia law—and that included many people who were Muslim. Niemeri was replaced by a fifteen member transitional military council chaired by General Suwar ad-Dahhab, until new elections could be held three years later.

It was during this time that the government began to arm the Arab tribes in South Kordofan (Miserya, Baggaras, and others) to take part in the civil war. Most of the fighting in the Nuba Mountains was taking place in the Moro areas and the areas of the other eastern tribes such as the Atoro, Kowalib, Lira, and Heiban, where the Christians lived. It was the Christians who were first being targeted.

In 1986, my father came to visit us in Khartoum, in a section of Omdurman, while I was living there with my own family. When we would pray, even blessing food, my father would leave. So we would just leave him alone. One night it happened that the Episcopal Youth group had an overnight gathering near where we lived, and my father heard them singing and playing the drums, and out of curiosity he went to see what was going on. I was not at home, but at work. He stayed there overnight. The next day he came and told me he wanted to be baptized.

As for his turnaround, we believed (and continue to believe) that God was speaking to him, and it was simply his time for God to speak to him. He simply said, "I want to go see Bishop Peter (who my cousin) to be baptized." We were overjoyed that he decided to become Christian. And so my cousin, Bishop Peter, performed the baptism. After this, my father became normal again and more involved with everyone in our family. He joined our family in family prayers and started going to church.

Also in 1986, I traveled to Bradford, England, with our youth choir. Actually, that was the last involvement I had as a youth with the church. After that I was focused on my family, my work, the Nuba Movement and the SPLA.

In 1986, I was asked to remain in Khartoum in order to collect intelligence. During this time, fighting was taking place all over Sudan, the Nuba, South Sudan, the Blue Nile State. Again, I was involved with the movement gathering intelligence, which is what I had been asked to do since I had a position at the hotel that allowed me to overhear the conversations of many powerful people. I remained in that position until Bashir came to power as a result of a coup d'etat in 1989.

A new election was held around 1987, and that is when Saddiq al Mahdi came to power. He created panic amongst the Nuba tribes due to the government troops' murder of a great number of educated Nuba and Nuba leaders during the short time he ruled. This happened mostly among the western tribes, such as the Miri, Kadugli, and Korongu, and a few eastern tribes, such as the Heiban and Lira tribes. This was something that stirred the Nuba to unite and stand against the government and their militia, the Baggara.

The last time I visited home in the Nuba Mountains was in 1988. At the time there was a transitional government, which was preparing for democratic elections. I really wanted to see my mother and father and siblings, and I figured it was a good time to do it, and thus I headed home.

Following the visit to my family, I returned to Khartoum, where I remained involved with the liberation movement, working in intelligence as well as recruiting people to join the movement. It was, of course, very dangerous, but we were doing it discreetly and working to bring the tribes together. We had a secret sign to identify or recognize each other. At the time I was still working at the Meridian Hotel, where I had worked my way up to top level of management. It was a hotel where the movers and shakers used to meet, and thus I had, if you will, access to many "different conversations" by many different people from all strands of society. So, as I listened in on this or that conversation or engaged in conversation with this or that person, I kept track of what I was hearing and anything that I thought was pertinent or significant, I passed on to The Movement. At the time, I also recruited friends from the Nuba who were living in Khartoum and Omdurman.

We were working for the freedom of the black people, who were not free like the Arabs. We believed that we had been denied everything humans were supposed to enjoy, and we greatly desired to change the situation for blacks so that they would feel like human beings.

Ultimately, Saddiq al-Mahadi was overthrown by General Omar al-Bashir and his fellow soldiers in 1989. But things didn't get any better in the Nuba. Actually, they got worse! As I mentioned, the Nuba made up approximately 80 percent of those in the Sudanese Army before Bashir gained power, but once in office as president he replaced all of them with Islamic fundamentalists, thus forming the base and core leadership for *jihad*, including the Popular Defense Forces (PDG) and militias such as the *Janjaweed*.

Though Bashir came to power promising to bring peace, he actually began to prepare for all-out war against the black people, including those in southern Sudan, Darfur, Nuba, and Blue Nile. He increased and advanced war by creating relationships and seeking support from outside Sudan, with the Chinese, Iran, Russia, Iraq and other Muslim countries.

While my family and I were in Khartoum, Bashir began to create cells within different Nuba tribes in order to uncover SPLA members. The spies were Nuba! Some worked within the GoS' national security office. This was in the midst of the GoS making radical changes within the military. The GoS was flushing out all of those military leaders who were not loyal to the National Islamic Front, which ultimately became the National Congress Party.

My best friend, David (whose surname must be withheld due to sensitive security issues in the Nuba today), was arrested along with others in 1990–1991. He was a lawyer. He was ordered to report to security. I told him, "Don't go, these people will kill you!" Still, he went and surrendered. He was charged with supporting the SPLA as enemies of the state, and was imprisoned for two years.

David was not only one of my best friends, but my neighbor, and we worked together in the movement. We were so close I knew I could be the next to be arrested.

Ultimately, I was told by Nuba friends in the NISS (National Intelligence and Security Service) to leave because the government was watching me as I had been accused of engaging in counterintelligence activities. Some of Bashir's spies reported me. So, my arrest was imminent.

Finally, when I was told they were searching for me I chose to leave Omdurman. Sudan. Regrettably, I had no choice but to leave my family behind, but with the plan to arrange for them to join me once I had secured my own safety and established a livable situation.

So before they took any action to arrest me, I took a train to Halfa in northwest Sudan en route to Egypt.[3] As a SPLA supporter I was able to use our underground network that provided support for escapes along that route. I was stopped, however, at the Wad Halfa seaport, where I was to take a ferry to Egypt, because I didn't have the correct papers—that is, my visa wasn't registered in the "security book."

So, I had to return to Khartoum, where I remained for a week in an attempt to figure out how to make a new escape. Fortunately, I met a "security guy" who helped me out by calling his security friends in Halfa and asking them to help arrange for me to leave the country. So a few days later, back in Halfa, I met the same security guy who had stopped me previously, and he granted me passage this time. So, I took the boat from Wad Halfa, at the Egyptian border on the Nile, all the way to Aswan, where I picked up a train to Cairo.

I firmly believe that if we had not had the Nuba Movement, we would've ended up even worse than we did; that is, worse than the second-class citizens that the GoS perceived us as. We would have become more a cross between third class citizens and slaves! No rights and no justice!

We are *only* free because we have been fighting the government. The only work that was available to us in those days was servile labor or serving in the army. And not many were able to attend school beyond high school.

So I made it to Egypt. To Cairo. And I remained in Cairo for five years without my family. There was not enough money to bring my family with me. During those years in Egypt, life was very, very difficult because there was no work available. We had the right to work, but there was no work.

Not even the United Nations helped us Sudanese refugees who had fled the dictatorship of al-Bashir.

The Episcopal Church of Egypt and the Orthodox Coptic Church were able to help us with some small amounts of money (about $3–5/week) to buy food and cover other small needs. Ultimately, they also helped us to find group housing. They also helped me get a job, which provided about $20 a month. I worked for a while with a company making t-shirts. The owner was a Christian, and helped our people a lot.

I, of course, was intent on trying to help support my family back home, but this proved to be all but impossible. In fact, I was only able to send money once during the entire five years I was there. So, in order for the family to exist, we sold our house in Khartoum to the Episcopal Church, which they used for a guesthouse. We used that money to get my family to Egypt.

There were other reasons why it was so difficult living in Egypt. The mental and emotional challenges of leaving my family behind were almost overwhelming; dealing with a racist society as a black minority member was absolutely miserable at times; and living in a two-bedroom apartment with five people and having very limited resources was extremely trying. But that was the situation I was in, and I had to deal with it. During that entire time I remained very active with the Episcopal Church in Egypt.

After I fled Khartoum to Egypt, my father sent my oldest brother, Butrous, to Khartoum in order to help care for my family. That was in 1994. He stayed there for several years until I was able to bring my family to Egypt with me, and then returned to the Nuba Mountains to be with my father.

My father was not very talkative, but he was very involved with the Nuba issues and was a strong supporter of the SPLA. During an attack on our village in 1997, my father attempted to warn our people to seek safety and while doing so he was shot by the militia. He was hit in the stomach, and severely wounded, with his insides torn out of his body. That was how he died.

Life was very difficult in 1997, because while I was now living in Khartoum I continued to hear about the intensification of the war in Sudan—which was actually declared a "holy war" against the Nuba and the rest of the south by the Government of Sudan. During this time not only was my father killed but many other relatives as well by GoS troops and their [allied] militia. These very same forces are still active today, but are now called the Rapid Support Force. They continue to kill and loot, and are intent on destroying the Nuba.

During that period there was great suffering in the Nuba Mountains because neither the UN nor any nongovernmental organizations (NGOs) were able to reach the Nuba to help them. This was because al-Bashir blocked all attempts by humanitarian organizations to reach the Nuba Mountains.

In 1997 I had a dream that suggested I needed to be more proactive, and that led me to form a Christian organization to help both the Nuba who remained in the Nuba Mountains as well as those who had fled from the fighting. I shared this vision with a friend, Gabriel Rema, and together we brought together about 75 Nuba friends, colleagues and fellow refugees in Egypt to help us co-found the Nuba Christian Family Mission (NCFM). NCFM became a Christian community at which we studied, worshipped, and worked together to provide relief and assistance to our brothers and sisters struggling inside Sudan and throughout the diaspora.

We went to both Catholic and Episcopal churches to request assistance, and for a place to meet for prayer, singing, and Bible study. Brian Kane, an American who worked with the Episcopal Church, and who really tried to help Sudanese refugees, led the Bible study. He became like one of us.

We collected clothes from the Orthodox Coptic Church and also collected money in order to rent a container to ship to Mombassa, where the Nuba Relief Rehabilitation and Development Organization (NRRDO) took it from there to the Nuba Mountains. That was our first relief effort.

The Orthodox Church of Egypt also gave us clothes to send home to our fellow Nuba who were now naked, due to twenty years of war. One of our members, Mubarak Butrous, was graduating from their theological college, and so that church was more inclined to help us. He was the first president of NCFM, and I was the first vice president.

Later on, in 1997, the U.S. Embassy in Egypt asked to meet with the Nuba people in Cairo, and we explained our case with the support of evidence: videos and testimonies of the genocide going on in the Nuba Mountains. Ultimately, the UN was persuaded by the United States Embassy to consider our case, to recognize the Nuba as refugees in Egypt. At that point, we began to be allowed to immigrate to places such as the United States, Australia, and Canada, with refugee status. This was accomplished, thanks to the activist efforts of Brian Kane and NCFM, along with the U.S. Mission in Egypt. I was one of the Nuba representatives to the U.S. Embassy.

During this time, I began to complete the process for immigration to the United States, and then, once it was OK'd, to make arrangements to immigrate here with my family. My family had made it to Egypt in late 1997, and in September 1998, we left Egypt for Baton Rouge, Louisiana. We traveled to Louisiana under the auspices of the Catholic Refugees program.

The very first family we met in Baton Rouge was with the Episcopal Church: the Reverend Miller Armstrong, his wife, Mary Ann, their daughter, Dorothy, and their son, Slater. They were already very aware of the situation in Sudan; and, actually, Slater was preparing to travel to Sudan the next year. Slater, who has become a close friend, kindly arranged for me to give talks about the plight of the Nuba people to churches around the Diocese of Louisiana, as well as in Mobile, Alabama, and Dallas and Houston, Texas.

Subsequently, my family and I became members of the Episcopal Church of the Holy Spirit in Baton Rouge, where we remained for eight years until we moved to Denver, Colorado, in the aftermath of the catastrophic hurricane, Katrina, which caused great destruction in much of Louisiana in 2005.

While in Louisiana, we, NCFM, accomplished many things: raising funds for those Episcopal primary school and high schools in the Nuba Mountains, establishing wells in the Nuba, and sending food for those in most need in the Nuba.

In 2002, responding to a specific request from SPLA Commander Abdel Aziz, I personally provided personal and family funds to establish the first teacher's institute to train teachers in the Nuba Mountains (The George Kori Institute for Training Teachers). The school began with almost one hundred students, and one teacher, who was from Uganda, who was paid $200 a month. Commander Abdel Aziz opened the school in 2003, and I visited the school in 2004.

Though the institute lasted only three years, it was very fruitful, as most of the students who attended the institute are now part of the development effort in the Nuba Mountains. When the peace agreement was signed [the Comprehensive Peace Agreement in 2005], the GoS was supposed to take over support for the institute, but it insisted that I hire more teachers and offer enough food to support them. My income was so limited I could not meet their demands, and as a result, they shut it down.[4]

The Nuba Christian Family Mission also hosted The Right Reverend Andudu ElNail, Bishop of the Nuba Mountains and Kadugli, to travel here, to the United States, in 2004 in order to address the situation of the Nuba Mountains, which was just coming to the end of decades of suffering, as a result of both war and genocide by attrition. Both Slater Armstrong and I traveled with Bishop Andudu to Washington, D.C., where we met with Members of Congress and officials with USAID.

After my family and I moved to Colorado, we became active members of Christ Episcopal Church in Denver. Within our first year of being in Colorado, I began working with other Sudanese and U.S. citizens to form the Nuba Water Project. The entire state of South Kordofan had no water system. And the only two places where people could have water delivered were in the cities of Dilling and Kadugli. There, the water was delivered via a donkey cart supply system. That water came from bore hole wells and tank reservoirs. There were no other systems of delivery or water catchments on a larger scale. The rest of us, we shared rainwater with animals! We also dug primitive wells. So this is a large part of why the Nuba fought—for development of an infrastructure that would bring us, the Nuba, into the 21st century, thus recognizing that we, too, were human, just like those in the North, in Khartoum.

Our goal was to move beyond simply drilling bore hole wells, though we recognized the importance of such solutions and that they had their place. So, we sought to find a way to develop reservoirs and other such systems to aid the people. In 2007, we began fundraising, and in that same year, in May, we headed to the Nuba with our first exploratory team. While in the Nuba we met with local governing officials, including the Governor of South Kordofan and the Minister of Water of South Kordofan, among others, which, at times, was difficult because many of the ministers were under the authority of the central government in Khartoum and they were Bashir's people, the very officials/individuals who were at the root of the unfair policies in the Nuba Mountains, and elsewhere (i.e., Blue Nile State and Darfur, to mention but two).

When we toured the largest (and oldest) reservoir at the Miri Dam, we discovered the water in it contained uranium deposits and was unfit for consumption. Ultimately, we were directed by the Minister of Water to build a small reservoir in the village of Bilo, which was to cost between $30,000 and $35,000. We were about to complete the project when the current war in the Nuba broke out in June 2011.

It wasn't until I returned to the Nuba Mountains in 2007 with the Nuba Water Project that I was able to see my oldest brother, Butrous. With great effort we reached my home village, where I was anxious to tend to my mother, who had recently received a terrible cut on her knee from corrugated tin roofing material that was flipped off her home caused by the high winds we have in the Nuba. Reaching her with medical aid was all I could think about until we arrived there after many days of traveling in Sudan. Adding to the agonizingly slow process was the fact that we were held up in Khartoum as we arranged for travel permits.

When we pulled up to my brother's compound, he ran to me, falling into my arms as he began to describe with tears how my father had died ten years ago in his arms. As he wept, he told me he had desperately attempted to push my father's insides back into him, where they had been torn out by the gunshot during the militia attack. Butrous told me that among my father's last words was to ask his forgiveness for the way he treated him when he first became a Christian.

While the Nuba Water Project team has not returned to the Nuba due to the new war, we continue to actively offer aid and assistance in repairing wells in the Nuba by raising funds that we send submit to NRRDO, which uses them to purchase parts needed to repair the wells and water pumps. The latest funds were sent in April 2015 with Dr. Louis Perrinjaquet (who goes by Dr. PJ), a physician from Colorado, who purchased about 200 kits and spare "moving" parts needed to repair the wells and water pumps and helped deliver them. They were delivered to the Minister of Water in the Nuba Mountains who said that the donations would be used to repair many of the approximately 2,000 damaged wells.

In June 2011, when the government of Sudan tried to disarm the SPLA-N by force, renewed fighting broke out in the Nuba Mountains (this was shortly after the southerners in Sudan seceded from the north and formed their own nation, The Republic of South Sudan). I took the initiative to make arrangements to bring some of the very first relief to my people. We raised funds through NCFM, the Nuba Water Project, and the Episcopal churches in Colorado and Louisiana, in order to purchase medicine and food.

I left for Africa in October 2011. In Kampala (Uganda), I immediately went to work purchasing medical supplies, and loading them on a lorry we rented to transport them to Juba (the new capital of The Republic of South Sudan). A medical clinic (Savannah Sunrise Medical Centre or SAS) in Uganda, founded by a good friend, Dr. Robert Muhumuza, who is an American citizen from Uganda, and a gastroenterologist with a practice in Baton Rouge, paved the way in Kampala for us. I then flew ahead of the shipment to arrange for it to be stored in Juba prior to shipping everything on to the Yida Refugee Camp in South Sudan, along the South Sudan/Sudan border.

Before the shipment could be moved from Kampala, though, I received a notice from the Ugandan authorities informing me that we needed a permit that verified that the medicine was legitimate (safe) before it could be transported across the border from Uganda into South Sudan. We also needed official verification that the medicine was what we said it was. Finally, they requested information about the shipment's final destination point. So, I had to fly back to Uganda to handle those matters. It took me a full seven days to work everything out, and as I did we stored the supplies at Bishop Andudu's home in Kampala, which could have led to our arrest due to protocol violations.

Once everything was straightened out and a different lorry was rented and loaded with the supplies, we left for Juba. This time I accompanied the supplies by riding on the truck to Juba. Every security stop along the way we not only had to produce our papers, but to pay "tribute" [graft] to the local authorities.

When we arrived at the customs office at the border of Uganda and South Sudan we were delayed for two weeks as the custom officers there insisted that we pay a $2000 tax to the state of Nimule. Over and over and over again, I told the custom officials that I did not have such funds. No matter how I attempted to reason with them it was to no avail.

One of the officers repeatedly stated that he was unconcerned about the need for medicines in the Nuba Mountains. It was obvious that he was only interested in the graft that he could squeeze from us. When I informed that officer that we represented a Christian organization working to help alleviate the Nuba suffering and that the Nuba should be respected for the role they played in helping to bring about the South's independence, I was blessed that another officer overheard us. He granted my passage for only 50SSP (South Sudanese Pounds), and we made it to Juba with the customs due there. When we arrived in a town 30 miles southwest of Juba, we met with Juba customs officials and left the truck, as Christmas was quickly approaching and businesses were closing for holiday. During this time, we worked to register for tax-exempt status through the National Security office in Juba, which took about another two weeks. After receiving notification of our being granted tax-exempt status, we went into Juba to arrange for storage of the supplies and to arrange for their transport to Yida.

When I arrived in Juba and identified myself to the customs officers, they asked, "Are you the George that contacted us three months ago?!"

I said, "Yes!"

They then asked me how I got the letter of confirmation regarding our tax-exempt status from National Security, and I told them, "God is good!"

Throughout all of this, I arranged with the SPLA–N to have a truck waiting in the Yida Refugee Camp in order to transport the supplies up to the Nuba. Their truck arrived two days after my arrival in Yida. But when the supply plane arrived in Yida, carrying our 300 boxes of medical supplies,[5] we were informed by the pilot that the plane could not land because the airstrip was too narrow. And with that, the pilot turned around and flew back to Juba.

To say that I was frustrated and distraught would be an understatement. I called my wife, who told me it was time to come home.

I told her, "I will not come home until the medicine is delivered to the people."

Next, I spoke with the director of the Yida Refugee Camp, Hussein, and beseeched him to send the entire Nuba community in the refugee camp down to the airstrip in order to create a larger landing strip. And that is exactly what they did. In an amazing display of teamwork and dedication, they enlarged that airstrip and they did so by hand. And they accomplished that monumental task in one day! The next day officials in Juba were informed that the landing strip was expanded and ready for the arrival of the plane carrying our medical supplies.

Two days later the shipment arrived from Juba. The next day, January 1st, we were off to the Nuba with a big lorry (without headlights) the SPLA made available for us. I was informed that the vehicle had been captured from al-Bashir's army.

As we prepared to leave Yida, I was told, "The situation in the Nuba is very different from here. You can expect to be targeted by al-Bashir's air force, his Antonov bombers."

About two hours after we had crossed into Sudan, into South Kordofan State, which is home to the Nuba Mountains, we had a flat tire. As the flat was fixed, which took about three hours, we watched anxiously for Antonovs. The replacement tire was not much better than the flat, but we had no choice. Later, we praised God that it took us all the way to Dar, in the Nuba Mountains area.

About 6:30 in the evening we arrived at a place called Toroga (pronounced Toroche). Nearby a fierce battle between the SPLA–N and the GoS was being fought. We were told that whenever the GoS saw a truck approaching, with its dust trail, they would fire rockets at it. Fortunately, we made it without incident.

About 7 p.m. that evening the lorry got stuck in a small wadi. The driver had made a mistake, crossing at the wrong point, which was impossible to pass, and we could not go forward or back. Not only was the road bad, but we ended up in a very tight spot. A tree was in front of us and there was too little room behind to maneuver back and forth, and thus it took about three hours to work the lorry out of the tight spot.

We had about ten to fifteen people on the lorry, along with the supplies we were hauling up to the Nuba. That entire time, we, all the passengers, attempted to rock the lorry back and forth, out of the rut it was in; and as we did, the local people kept warning us that we were in extreme danger and needed to leave immediately. And they kept telling us to turn our flashlights off, and not to use any light of any kind as it could be detected by the enemy.

We were finally able to dislodge the lorry, but in the process of helping to rock the vehicle back and forth I fell and injured a knee. Since all of our bags and supplies were tightly packed, there was nothing to wrap my knee with.

By the time we freed the lorry up, it was so late we decided to spend the night in the bush. Only one tukul in the entire area was occupied (everybody else had fled), and when we asked the occupants where the nearest SPLA base was located, we were told to forget about that and not to sleep near the lorry in case it was bombed. Not ten minutes later, we heard an Antonov. Immediately, all of us fled for cover.

It was a frightening situation because there was no place out there to really hide. Nothing to hide behind, no holes to jump into.

The Antonov dropped several bombs, but the bombs fell a few miles away so we were not, fortunately, in danger; but still, they were near enough and loud enough to remind us we were in a war zone.

In the middle of the night, about 2 a.m., more Antonovs approached, and again they dropped bombs. But again, the bombs were far enough away from us that we were OK.

It ended up being an absolutely miserable night, and it wasn't only due to the bombings. We had no bedding for sleeping, and it ended up being a bitterly cold January night during which we got little sleep.

We got up early the next morning, about 6:00 a.m., and left without the lorry, which now wouldn't start. Dr Osman al Amin—the Secretary of Health for the Nuba civil society, who had joined us in order to assess the medical needs of the people and to oversee the distribution of the medicines at different clinics—joined me on foot as we set out in search of the closest SPLA base, where we hoped to locate someone who could help us with the lorry.

We arrived at the base about an hour later. There I found many friends, including Commander Abdel Aziz, who joked that my injuries could be attributed to the Antonov. They were all amazed at the amount of time and effort it took to get myself there with the aid, and they celebrated our arrival, along with the recent liberation of al Hamra in the Buram region.

The medicine I had hauled in was designated for use in a local clinic to care for both the rebels and the civilians alike, including children recently wounded by the bombings that we had witnessed from a distance the night before.

Two days later we left for Kurche, where we handed off the remaining shipment for distribution by NRRDO and local church leaders. I then left to visit my family. Upon my arrival at my brother's compound, he, Butrous, said, "What are you doing here? It is too dangerous!" I told him that I had to come bring medicine to our people.

During my visit I witnessed the horrible conditions that my family, as well as others, were living in: no food, no medicine, and people constantly running with children in hand to take shelter amongst the rocks and inside the caves as the Antonovs approached. The bombings were so frequent and so disastrous it seemed that the people in the area weren't even thinking about food, but rather only concentrating on hiding from death.

I thought to myself, "Who can we talk to stop this?"

As I headed back to Yida a few days later, there was fighting near the border. We could hear the bombs in the distance. I was instructed to stay with Commander Abdel Aziz until the SPLA-N troops cleared the area for my safe return. A day later the SPLA-N chased out the Sudanese Army (SAF) from the area. We feared there the SAF may have planted land mines, but we managed to reach Yida safely.

After I arrived home (at the end of January 2012), one of the first things I did was share the story of my trip with the parishioners of St. John Cathedral in Denver. Afterwards, a young lady named Christina, who works with *The Denver Post*, and her boyfriend, Tim, approached me. We ended up setting up another trip to the Nuba for the express purpose of helping to train Nuba to be local video journalists.[6]

That May, I traveled back to the Nuba, and I met up with Christina and Tim a bit later, at the end of May. Not having traveled much in the world, at least not to Third World countries, they arrived with no money, expecting to draw money from an ATM, which, of course, did not exist. Both I, and those I was traveling with, helped them out with what little we had.

Christina and Tim went into the Nuba without me since I was working with Dr. Louis "PJ" Perrinjaquet, and we were heading to Uganda in order to purchase feeding tubes for Dr. Tom Catena, the director of Mother of Mercy Hospital up in the Nuba Mountains. I arranged it so Christina and Tim would travel into the Nuba with Yacoub Kaloka, who was working as the South Kordofan Relief and Rehabilitation Commissioner. While up there, Christina and Tim trained some citizen journalists over about a two week period. Shortly thereafter, they joined up with *Nuba Reports*, the citizen journalists project headed up by Ryan Boyette.

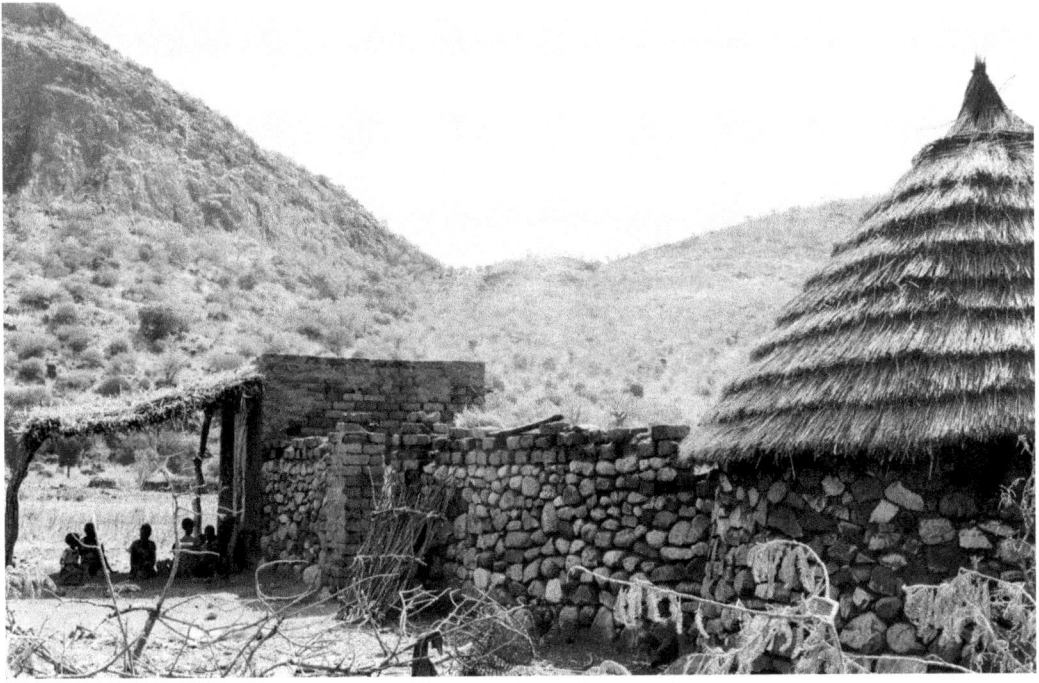

Kurchee Village, which is a stone tukul compound (photograph by and courtesy Slater Armstrong, January 2016)

ENG's Maiden Voyage

The following September (2012), I traveled once again, accompanying John Jefferson and David Hicks on the first of several trips to the Nuba under the auspices of the newly formed End Nuba Genocide Coalition (co-founded by Samuel Totten and John Jefferson). Yacoub Kaloka served as our guide. The express purpose of the trip was to insert food into the Nuba Mountains, where people were suffering from malnutrition to severe malnutrition to starvation as a result of having been bombed off their farms and out of their villages.

In Juba we purchased twelve bags of sorghum and salt, and then traveled onto the Yida Refugee Camp by air. From there, we arranged, through the SPLA, a small pick up truck and a 4-wheeler to transport the food. Since it was the middle of the rainy season, we wanted to be sure we had a four-wheeler with us because sometimes that is the only type of vehicle that can even operate in the rainy, swampy and muddy conditions.

Almost from the start (in fact, just two hours into the journey into Sudan), the truck got bogged down in the thick mud. It wasn't raining, but had rained the week before. No matter what the driver tried—quickly moving forward and then backward in an attempt to rock it loose, slamming down the accelerator to make the truck leap forward, getting all the guys to rock the truck—we remained stuck. For two long hours we tried and tried to rock and jerk, push and pull the truck out of the mud, but nothing worked. Finally, we decided to leave the truck behind, and we began footing it to the closest SPLA–N border checkpoint. (Some of the food was loaded onto the four-wheeler, and transported that way.) That took us another several hours. Finally, we reached the checkpoint at Jau, which is where a former army training camp for the SPLA–N was located, and we spent the night there. Men with the SPLA footed out to the truck immediately, and rescued it (lifting it out of the mud by hand).

Early the next morning, about 6 a.m., we set out again with the truck. But, again, we got stuck. And, again, we left the truck behind and began footing it, carrying all of our personal belongings. We left the truck behind because the roads were so muddy. We feared they were probably impassable so the driver waited until the roads became dry enough to travel. Ultimately, the truck was able to meet us in Dar, but those of us on foot had no idea if that was actually going to be possible or not, so we had decided to press on on foot, not knowing how long it would be before they could drive the truck to where we were going.

We footed all day long, from 6 a.m. to 5 p.m., before arriving in Dar. All of us were completely exhausted. Fortunately, the SPLA–N met us in Dar that evening with our truck and picked us up and took us to a new SPLA base. We arrived there about 8 p.m. The security was extremely tight; and almost immediately, they pointed out where we should take shelter in case there was a night bombing by the GoS. They also assured us that they would awaken us if they heard any aircraft. That night, though, we were not threatened by any bombing.

After the SPLA–N kindly provided us with breakfast and tea the following morning, we continued on our way at about 7 a.m. It was not long before we came across a lady with a small child, both of whom were literally dying of hunger. We prayed for them, and left them some rice and sorghum, and then continued on our way. Several hours later we arrived at Buram.

The area around Buram was suffering horribly. That was understandable as it had been one of the main targets of the GoS' aerial attacks; and as a result, the people had not been able to harvest their crops. We met with the leaders there, and told them what we had with us. They escorted us to a cave where nearly 300 people were in hiding, and we distributed the food amongst them.

Prior to our departure, we left two additional huge sorghum bags for the sheik to further distribute to others in need. It wasn't much, but it was something to carry them over until they could travel to Yida or hold on until further help arrived—if, in fact, any ever would.

Up in the cave with the 300 people, we were shown where a rocket had hit and caused great damage. Fortunately, it had not penetrated the cave. On our way back to the SPLA base, we met a man with two girls, ten years and twelve years, who were heading to Yida in search of food for their family. We asked them how long it would take them to travel to Yida, and they said four days. We asked what they had to eat for the journey, and they said, "We are just walking." At that point we discussed among ourselves how we might help them, and decided we should take them back to the base with us, where we prepared a package of sorghum for them, and then gave them a ride a short ways.

The twelve year old repeatedly insisted that they immediately continue on to Yida so that she could sell her *karkadi* (hibiscus) at the Yida camp in order to raise money to purchase food.

We ended up being in the Buram area for about three days. As we were leaving, we gathered for prayer. David Hicks, who lead the prayer, prayed, in part, on the behalf of the rebels: "God be with you. We know you have been denied your rights, and you are fighting for your rights to survive." In parting, the top officer said that Hicks would be very welcome anytime to return and preach to the SPLA–N's troops.

2013—ENG: Kao Nyaro

In May of 2013, we (ENG) learned from the Nuba Relief, Rehabilitation, and Development Organization (NRRDO) that the Kao Nyaro people were in the most dire circumstances, with absolutely no one entering the area to bring relief. Many were dying as they attempted to make it to Malakal, a large river town along the Nile in South Sudan, in search of food and refuge.

So we took up the challenge to find a way to bring them relief. In the U.S. we raised $20,000, and then with NRRDO's coordination and assistance, we purchased and hauled about 800 bags of sorghum, jugs of cooking oil, some salt and medicines to two areas: Kao Nyaro and Werni. On its own, NRRDO hauled in a similar amount.

Upon our arrival at Kao Nyaro, we were informed that it was the first time in over two years that relief aid had arrived in the region. In all of my experiences, I had never witnessed such a desperate situation. The people had been living mostly on roots and leaves for almost two years. There was no medical clinic of any kind. No schools had been in session as a result of the constant bombing. The GoS army and the Baggara Arab militia had long ago looted all their cattle and belongings, and continued to prevent the people from growing any food in the region. None!

Even as the people had sunk into such a vulnerable condition, the GoS continued to bomb them and carry out raids against them. I am really grateful for the SPLA leadership, because even though they don't have much themselves, they helped the families with what little they had up until our arrival.

I wish to emphasize that while we (ENG) deliver the food to the Nuba people, many individuals, organizations and congregations in the U.S. generously provide contributions that provide us with the means to actually purchase and deliver food to those Nuba in critical need. Among the congregations have been Christ Church in Denver, Colorado; The Episcopal Diocese of Louisiana; and Hope Church in California.

After our flight from Juba to Malakal, we crossed the White Nile River on a pedestrian ferry (which can accommodate a couple of hundred people) in order to transport the food and other supplies from one side of the river to the other. We loaded all 300 of the bags we had with us. On the other side we loaded the bags on a big lorry (some similar to a good sized flat bed truck) we had hired. The lorry transported the bags to a warehouse, which we had also rented. The SPLA–N then arrived with another flatbed-like truck and we loaded the relief supplies onto it as well. Once everything was loaded, we left at about 2 p.m. en route to Kao Nyaro. The first stop was at Kodok, a town, which, back in the 1800s, was a major slave trade center.

On the road to Kodok we passed a UN vehicle. The UN personnel were leaving the area due to the onset of the rainy season. Once we reached Kodok, we continued out into the bush toward Kao Nyaro. The area was not safe due to the fact that the Shilluk (a tribe native to the Kodok area) militia, which were basically serving as the GoS' proxies in the region, were engaged in battle with both the South Sudan Government and the SPLA–N along the border there. Because of that, we were assigned two armored cars with troops for security.

We arrived at Kao Nyaro about 1 a.m. That night we were given a place to stay by the SPLA-N in their compound.

Early the next morning we were awakened by a village full of people seeking the food we brought. There were about 5,000 or more people. They were very desperate. They all looked hopeless [bereft] and sad as they stood there with nothing. They were so poor, so desperate they didn't know what to do with their children, as they had no food for them. None of them talked to us about the constant bombings. They simply, repeatedly, [bemoaned] the fact that they had no food and no water. Most of the people, we were told, were living in caves.

There was little water to drink or cook with. And since they had so little water, they didn't use it for bathing, and as a result, most of the people were extremely dirty. The water hole where they got the little water they had was a long, long walk and a dangerous one. It was so dangerous because of the [presence of the] Arab militia in the area. Also, by footing it to the water hole, they were leaving themselves exposed to the Antonovs bombing the area; that is, it took them away from the protection of the rocks and caves.

I felt overwhelmed by the numbers of people in need. I was very disturbed in my heart and my mind because I had been in several places to assist the Nuba, but I had never seen people so desperate that I was being called upon to help. Because of what I witnessed there, there is nowhere else I feel more strongly compelled to bring assistance by all means possible.

At the same time, I was [thrilled] to hear some of the languages that were close to my language, and I felt like they were my family. I now carry them in my heart and desire to tell others about them [and their plight] in order to urge them to help bring change to the peoples' situation there. I believe that one day the Kao Nyaro will be a strong witness for Christ because of our work and involvement there among them in His name.

As I exited the *tukul* in which I was sleeping, my mind went back to my childhood, remembering stories of the Kao people and how they had remained a naked people (refusing to abide by the GoS' order that all people in the Nuba wear clothes), and that is what I expected to see. I was very surprised when I saw that no one was naked, that everyone was actually wearing clothes. At the same time, it was very sad to see the tremendous suffering they were experiencing due to their overwhelming hunger.

One of the first people to greet me was a very old friend of mine, John Ambde. We had lived together from 1980 to 1982 in Khartoum. The GoS had arrested him in 1983 for his political actions—for working on the behalf of the Nuba. He had escaped during the subsequent uprising (when crowds had attacked the jails and prisons), left Khartoum, and then joined the SPLA.

At one point in time I actually thought he had died, but then in 2007 I heard he was still alive. This, though, was my first time to see him since we were young men, before I married. He told me that he had just arrived from Kurche and had only been in Kao Nyaro a short while before we had arrived. He was on a SPLA-N mission delivering a truck and uniforms to the other SPLA-N troops in the area of Kao. We were so happy to see each other that we spent several hours talking. He has eight children and when I asked him how they were, he said, "We [meaning the men with the SPLA-N] don't talk about how we are living, we just talk about how to protect the Nuba and our own land."

Figuring that he could use it, I handed him about $100. He was so shocked, he didn't know what to say. I told him I wish I had more to give. Then I said, "I don't know what you plan to do with it, but if you wish to purchase some food or other goods for your family then this is what I have to help you do." He went on to tell me that he had heard many stories about my helping our people in the Nuba during my recent trips with ENG. I had to leave him at that point as our team was traveling to Werni.

I felt very sad in my heart for the way the people of Kao were being treated by the Sudanese government. There is nothing there. No services at all: no electricity, no lights, no medical clinics, no medicine. It was just like the Stone Age.

When we arrived in Werni, we discovered they had no water and no food. We were surrounded by around 3,000 people and we only had a small truck with very little sorghum left. We, the members of the team, felt overwhelmed. We had come to assess the situation and to let them know help was on the way, but we were there and we didn't have enough for them despite our presence.

A little child ran up to me and wanted me to pick him up. So I picked him up, and when I did, I mused, "This child is like me! He is *my* child." Then I immediately began thinking: "What do I have? What can I give this child?" I had a cookie in my bag, and decided to give it to him. But when I pulled it from my bag, the other children saw it, and I was immediately swarmed by a thousand hands reaching and crying for a crumb. It is so hard to describe I can hardly do it. *It tears my heart.* And I keep asking myself, "*Why is the UN and the AU treating these people this way. Why don't they help these people?*"

The children don't even have a place to go to school. Actually, there is a building there, which was built by the British as a school for all local youth, but the Arabs took it over and have used it to teach the *Koran*. The Muslim Brotherhood had even renamed the school, calling it the Islamic Center. The local people could do nothing about it as they were under an oppressive and brutal occupation. If they had objected in anyway they would have been imprisoned and/or killed.

As we, Jefferson and I and the others with us, discussed the situation with the people, they described how their family members and friends were dying every day due to a lack of food and water. It was a hopeless feeling. *Absolutely hopeless knowing that here there were people in such great need and no one in the world cared enough to help them.* And it was even more painful knowing that it would not take all that much to really ease their suffering.

We left that evening at about 6 p.m., had a brief visit at a commander's home, and then left for Kao. We arrived a little after 9 p.m. We spent the night there in another SPLA–N compound. The next day we spent several hours distributing the food in Kao. The people were very polite and orderly.

We then gathered all the children around us, and asked them both about how they were doing and what they were doing during this period. There must have been about three thousand kids. They informed us that they had nothing to do. They wanted to be in school but there were no teachers because of the war. They are doing nothing and learning nothing, but they are very willing and desire to be in school. They were all losing precious time in their lives, when they should be learning in school and preparing for life.

We then visited a few *tukuls* during which we heard stories about how dire the people's circumstances had become. How they had little food. No salt, very little sugar, no clothing. How, after they have put long days and weeks and months into growing their food, the Arabs come along with their cattle and destroy the crops—and that if they said anything to the Arabs, they would be beaten or killed. They talked about the difficulty of having no market place such as they have in Kurche. How they were cut off from any communication with the other tribes of the Nuba. And how the Arabs continued to force Islam on them.

We then went to a place called Nyaro and made a distribution there. We assured them that more food was on the way. While there I met a soldier from the Moro, which is where I come from, who had married a girl from the Kao. As we talked I learned that there are some similarities in our two languages. I was able to understand some of the girl's dialect. And actually, the Kao people look very similar to those of us in the Moro tribe.

At the same time, though, as I looked around, it was obvious to me that 98 percent of their lives are primitive. Even in the good times, they only eat two foods: sorghum and sesame. For years, they have even been without those two sources of food since they are not able to farm because of the attacks by the GoS, and so they only eat what they can forage in the bush. It is a desperate, desperate situation.

November 2013

At the end of 2013, in late November, I returned to Kao Naro with Dr. "PJ." We arrived in South Sudan with a little over thirty thousand dollars for food and medicine. We purchased medicine in Juba and shipped it to Malakal. We changed the remaining funds to South Sudanese Pounds (130 SSK), which we carried in a bag. When we arrived in Malakal, members of the local security force asked us what we had in the bags. We told them we were helping refugees in Kodok and Lulu, areas where refugees gathered near Malakal from Werni. Fortunately, we were allowed to go on our way.

We stayed in the local hotel in Malakal, where we were informed by some locals that about 66 people, refugees, had just arrived from Werni and were camped out across the river. Two people had died from starvation on the way, we were told.

We arranged to see how we could help them that day. We took a ferry boat across the Nile to meet them. What we discovered was astonishing. There were actually about 1,200 already there from Werni. They were just sitting under the trees, with no shelter, food or any other supplies. They told us they badly needed sorghum, oil, and salt in order to just exist. We left immediately, along with the group's sheik who joined us, took the boat back across the river, purchased sorghum, salt and cooking oil, and hauled it back across the river to the people. In all, we gave the Werni in Lulu about 60 bags of sorghum.

The next day we rented a boat (on which we loaded medicine) to go down river to Kodok en route to Kao Nyaro. When we arrived in Kodok we visited with refugees who were gathered there from Kao. They did not have any food either. So, we purchased 100 bags of sorghum in the *suq* in Kodok, and transported it via a donkey cart to the refugee area where the Kao had gathered.

We spent that night and the next in Kodok at the Catholic Guest House, a collection of old, worn out concrete houses with no windows, no doors, no electricity. The next two days we spent handing over food to the SPLA–N and local community leaders. Before

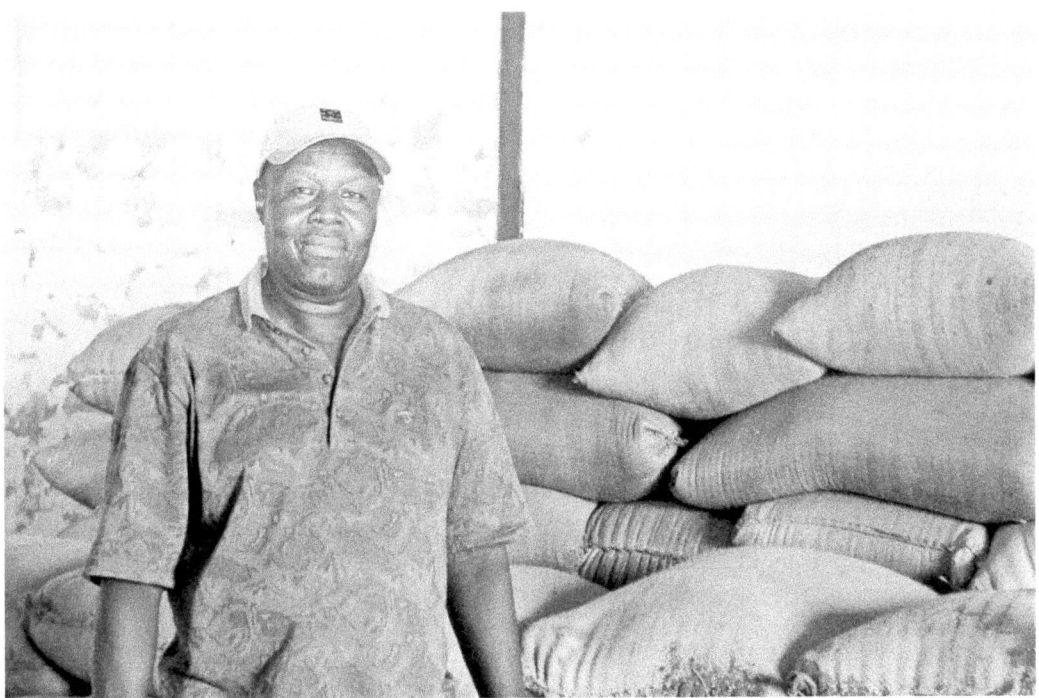

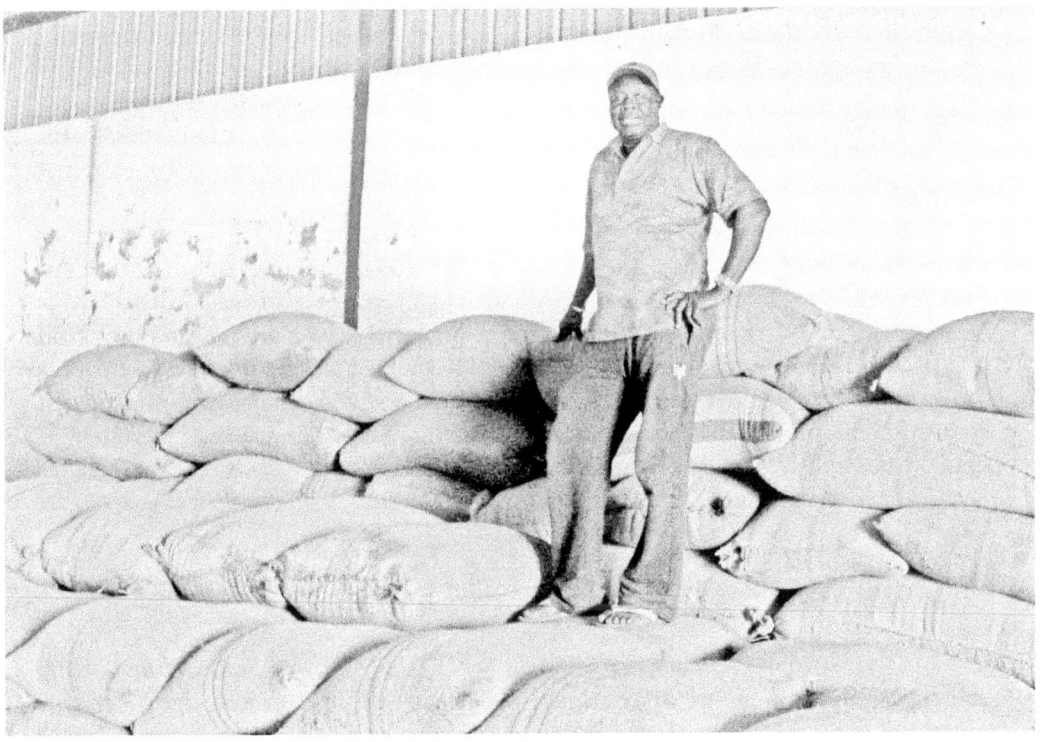

Top and above: The author in front of sacks of sorghum in Kodok, South Sudan, as he prepares to bring relief to the people in the Kao Nyaro region (photographs by and courtesy Tamara M. Banks, May 2014).

we left, we gave them funds with which to hire vehicles and drivers and to purchase petrol so that they could deliver the food, which we had purchased, to the Nuba in those regions I had traveled to on my last trip to the Kao Nyaro.

We then returned back to Juba. Dr. PJ then headed up to Gidel in order to work alongside Dr. Tom Catena at Mother of Mercy Hospital. As for me, I headed back to the States.

May 2014: An Aborted Attempt to Reach the Kao Nyaro

In May 2014 I returned to the region with Tamara Banks, a well known journalist and producer in the Denver (Colorado) area, who had traveled to Sudan on several occasions to cover stories. We arrived in South Sudan about five months after civil war had broken out there. We faced new challenges due to the fighting in the Malakal area, and also in the Kao Nyaro area of the Nuba Mountains. It was our goal to transport food up to the Kao Nyaro ourselves, but unfortunately we had to leave it in a staging area for later delivery by a partner organization due to the heavy rains, impassable roads, and fighting. So we spent the time we had, about a week, in the refugee area of Kodok. We delivered about 80 bags of sorghum to the people there, since they were now cut off from any aid at all.

The situation in South Sudan was extremely dangerous. We could hear the gunfire well into the night as we tried to sleep. We slept with our shoes on just in case those fighting in the civil war attacked the area while we were asleep. We had heard that fighters were advancing on Kodok while we were there, and so it was a nerve-wracking situation for us.

The refugees from Kao Nyaro told us that they had seen a lot of dead bodies floating by in the Nile due to fighting up river in Malakal. They, the refugees, were extremely nervous.

While we were there, we were told by our SPLA–N escorts that if anything happened, we would have to retreat across the border into the Nuba Mountains in order to be safe. That presented yet another problem. If we ended up heading across the border we would be cut off from our rendezvous point with the plane we were supposed to hop for our flight out of Kodok. And actually, we were already worried we might not make the flight due to the onset of the rains, which, we feared, would result in the airstrip being too dangerous to land on due to the swampy mud that the rain always causes. Ultimately, we made it out and were blessed to depart without incident. Once we reached Juba, we headed back to the States.

October 2014

In October 2014, many of us gathered for the Greater Nuba Action Coalition (GNAC) church planting conference in Yei, South Sudan. Church leaders from the Nuba were present, along with many others. At the conclusion of the conference, several of us (including John Jefferson, his wife, a couple of other conference attendees, and I) traveled to Kodok with the intention of carrying out another mission to deliver relief supplies to the people of Kao Nyaro. Upon our arrival we were pleased to find the security situation a bit better than it had been the last time we were there. The refugees had also received some additional assistance from some NGOs. Some of the NGOs had dug water wells, some had delivered a bit of food, and some had even brought tents for the people. The food the refugees had received, however, only lasted about two weeks; and thus, the people there were getting desperate yet again.

We left them with about 60 bags of sorghum. The rest was to be taken to the Kao Nyaro. We couldn't make it to Kao Nyaro, though, as a great amount of water had escaped from the reservoir located between the Sudan/South Sudan border and Kao Nyaro. There was no way we could cross the swamp that had been created by the flood. That was obvious from the lorries that had tried and were stuck and going nowhere.

We ended up spending the night in the bush, on the side of the road, for about two days, with no protection or shelter from the elements. Not only was it absolutely miserable, but we were running out of time to make it back to Kodok for our flight to Juba. In the end, we footed it back to Kodok, which took us countless hours.

I started out a bit later than the others. They were about a half hour ahead of me. As I hurried to catch up with the others, I ran out of water. So, I resorted to drinking water from the reservoir flooding that was in the tire ruts in the road. The water tasted muddy but having had it as a child, it was okay for me, but I wouldn't recommend it to my friends. I asked God to help protect my body. Thankfully, I didn't get sick.

Conclusion

I want to thank all the Americans (U.S. citizens) who have welcomed me and my family to the United States, helped us to become American citizens, and have helped my people through the years. Especially I want to thank those who have worked together with me, and stood with me and my people during the current period of war, many of whom have risked their own lives to help.

I really want to thank the ENG group, and ask that God bless your lives. You are people who not only help my people, but you have a special spirit of the servant heart. I vividly recall, during ENG's first trip, when we were forced to walk nine hours from Jau into the Nuba Mountains; from that time I knew why the people of America are special to people in other countries. May God continue to bless America!

Notes

1. After he had become a politician as a result of the ill-treatment of the Nuba, the authorities told him he could evangelize. Evangelism was not allowed in general.
2. The negotiations were actually referred to as Anyanya I, which was the name of the revolutionary movement of the South Sudanese before the Nuba joined them. The latter had fought for seventeen years against the GoS' army, which was made up of mostly Nuba and which the government used to fight against the southern tribes. It is important to remember that even John Garang, the man who became the leader of the SPLA in its fight against the GoS, had also first served in the GoS' military forces.
3. Halfa is a city in northeast Sudan on the shores of "Lake Nubia" (the Sudanese section of Lake Nasser). It is the terminus of a rail line from Khartoum, where one can catch a ferry to Egypt.
4. In 2013, the South Kordofan Commissioner for Relief and Development, Yacoub Koloka, asked me to consider reopening the institute. My response was that I was already overcommitted with work, trying to bring relief and aid in general to those suffering the renewed fighting.

5. At this point in time, the issue of hunger had not gripped the Nuba Mountains yet, and thus I only carried in medical supplies.

6. This effort actually preceded the establishment of *Nuba Eyes and Ears* (now called *Nuba Reports*) by Ryan Boyette. Some of the individuals trained by our original group later joined *Nuba Reports*.

Confronting War Crimes in the Nuba Mountains of Sudan

Matt Chancey

If people ever take the trouble to think about the nation of Sudan, visions of camels and sand dunes probably come to mind, certainly not the beautiful topographical diversity that I've had the privilege to visit over the last eleven years. But I understand. Growing up in southeast Alabama's *Wiregrass* region, Sudan was about as far from my mind as supporting the Penn State football team. But that would eventually change. Indeed, now, looking back, I can see that much in my upbringing prepared me for the work that has kept me busy for many years.

As a Southerner, I grew up surrounded by the military. A robust patriotism was just part of the landscape. I remember the influence of President Ronald Reagan, and how it formed my childhood image of America as the world's super-hero. Most of my friends were from career military families. The dedication and sacrifices these families made to serve their country made a huge impression on me, and for a very long time, I prepared myself to follow their example and seek a commission.

I was very fortunate to have strong relationships with my grandparents—especially my maternal grandfather—who had served as a fighter pilot in World War II. "Papa" was the quintessential Southern grandpa. He was an old-school, low-country gentleman. A conservative, fundamentalist Christian—and very proud of the fact. Although a descendent of poor tobacco farmers in North Carolina, Papa had a high sense of honor and personal integrity. He always spoke respectfully of his deceased parents, and constantly told stories—instilling in his grandkids moral maxims drawn from Bible stories and personal experience.

But Papa didn't just talk about good principles, he lived them. He served as deacon in his church from 1956 until shortly before his death in 2014. He was involved in the Lions Club and many other charitable organizations and outreach efforts in his community. And he was a faithful donor to every righteous cause imaginable—political, religious, and/or humanitarian.

And there were many other important influences as well. So, contrary to the TV sitcom stereotype of juvenile-acting and irresponsible men preoccupied by sports and entertainment, I had many positive male role models in my life as I grew up. I have three younger brothers, and all of us joined our local Boy Scout Troop, eventually achieving the highest rank of Eagle Scout. But we would tell you that the reason we became Eagles is not because of sheer pluck on our part, but because of the faithful help and encouragement of our scoutmaster, Andy Lewis. "Mr. Lewis" seemed to have a bottomless pit of energy and enthusiasm, and though he invested many years in hundreds of boys, he always made you feel like you were special and could achieve anything you set your mind to do.

Every week for years at our scout meetings, we recited the same oath: *On my honor, I will do my best to do my duty to God and my country and to obey the Scout Law; to help other people at all times; to keep myself physically strong, mentally awake and morally straight.* The Wiregrass is a disaster-prone area, where tornados, hurricanes, and flash floods are almost annual events. So there were plenty of opportunities growing up to practice the Scout slogan of "Do a good turn daily." For example, we lived near the little river town of Elba, which flooded three times during my childhood. Each time, all of us would dutifully join our neighbors and collect food, batteries, ice, and other relief supplies to distribute to impacted residents.

One of my mentors growing up was Mac Newton, a retired businessman who must have been well over 70 when we first met. Mac took a shine to me because we were both active in the local Republican Party, which was still a pretty small club at that time in the "solid" Democratic South. "Uncle Mac" would always greet me with "Hello, Guvnah!" It was one of his ways of trying to get me to think outside of the little world where I had grown up, and a way to express his belief that I could accomplish great things.

I took piano lessons as a child but hated to perform in public. My father, who also played, kept pushing me to perform more recitals, but not because it would help me get over my stage fright. He said he always was nervous when he played in public, but musical talent was a gift. "If God gives you a talent," Daddy would say, "He expects you to use it to bless others. Otherwise, He'll take it away and give it to someone else who will."

So from my earliest days, whether it was through examples I saw in the members of my family, the military, church, or community, serving others was just a way of life. There was no such thing as waiting on someone else to address a problem—especially the government. I was encouraged by practically all those who influenced my life to do my bit to make the world a better place. I was also instilled with the understanding that I had received rights, privileges and opportunities that many others didn't have in the world, and that my role wasn't to horde such gifts, but to use them to help those less fortunate.

Although this upbringing helped prepare me for my present work in Africa, I'm still very much an "accidental activist," and don't pretend to be an expert on the geopolitical history or intrigue of Sudan. I didn't graduate from Harvard University's Kennedy School of Government with a degree in International Politics. What I know, I've learned on the job from the people and the work I've grown to love. As the reader will see, my arrival in this field was through a very indirect path.

In 1995, I left home to take a six-month internship in a law firm near Washington, D.C. I was keenly interested in history and politics, and my new position offered ample exposure to both. This was the beginning of my foray into the complex world of public policy, where I met a lot of interesting people—some of whom would turn out to be lifelong friends.

One person I befriended was a young man named Brad Phillips, who worked as a "Hill Rat" (legislative assistant) in Washington. Brad's passion was foreign policy, especially as it related to Africa. Growing up during the Cold War, his father was involved in public policy and traveled the globe extensively as a geopolitical analyst.

Before the Internet, the best "open source" document that existed to study any given country was a State Department publication known as the Foreign Broadcast Information Service, a.k.a FBIS. One could subscribe to FBIS for every country in the world, and read newspaper, radio, and television (among other) transcripts for any given day of the year.

Brad began reading the Sub-Saharan Africa FBIS at the age of 12. He was particularly interested in Angola and the other Frontline States (i.e., Botswana, Mozambique, Tanzania, and Zambia). At age 15, Brad made his first trip to Angola, which, at the time was home to one of the longest running civil wars in Africa. Then, in 1992, at age 23, he was selected to be an official election observer there. While in Angola, Brad learned that the racist assimilation policy of torture, cruelty, and persecutions, which had characterized the Portuguese colonial regime, had been eclipsed in magnitude by the ruling MPLA government—but with a Marxist ideological twist.

While on Capitol Hill, Brad met Sudanese NBA (National Basketball Association) star Manute Bol. Manute told Brad his personal story and how he had fled persecution by the National Islamic Front (NIF) government in Sudan. Manute's description of NIF policies sounded very similar to what Brad had witnessed in Angola.

In 1997, Brad launched a campaign called the Persecution Project. Initially, it was his attempt to use his background in government and advocacy to raise awareness about the incidence of religious and racial persecution in Africa.

In 1998, Brad's friend Hedd Thomas, who worked for Christian Aid, invited Brad to meet Neroun Philip, then Director of the Nuba Relief Rehabilitation and Development Organization (NRRDO). Neroun shared with Brad his own experiences in regard to the Government of Sudan's targeting and persecution of Christians in Sudan's Nuba Mountains. Ultimately, Neroun arranged for Brad to meet the late Yousef Kuwa Mekki at his offices in Nairobi, Kenya. Yousef Kuwa was the father of Nuba nationalism, and it was he who revealed to Brad that the core of the struggle in Sudan was around the issue of identity.

The information gleaned, and relationships formed, during this time served as the genesis of the *Persecution Project Foundation (PPF)*, which Brad incorporated in 2000, for the express purpose of moving beyond merely reporting instances of persecution to both issuing such reports as well as providing "regular Americans" the opportunity to engage in acts of compassion and relief to the victims.

I was working from home in Shenandoah Valley, Virginia, when I received a phone call from Brad. He informed me that he was officially incorporating PPF, and needed directors to serve on its board.

"What would I have to do?" I inquired.

"Nothing, really," was Brad's response.

I didn't know much about Africa, and had never travelled outside the continental United States. I was thoroughly entrenched in my little American bubble. But Brad was a friend and asked for my help, so I helped him.

And for five years, Brad was true to his word. I didn't do much of anything outside basic company governance. A few scheduled conference calls here and there, some reports and audits to review, etc.

While I wasn't personally busy with the organization during these years, PPF was incredibly busy. This was during the time of "Operation Lifeline Sudan" (OLS), a tripartite agreement between the UN, the NIF, and the SPLM-A rebels. OLS was composed of about 35 major international NGOs working with the UN, and was designed to be the legal framework under which aid would be delivered to people in the war and drought-affected areas of Sudan regardless of their religious or political affiliation.

But what PPF and other nongovernmental organizations (NGOs) quickly discovered was that the NIF—and even some elements of the SPLM–A—were using aid for political purposes. Every day at OLS headquarters in northern Kenya, a UN security briefing was held. All partner NGOs were informed which areas of Sudan were "Red No-Go" zones, where aid could not be delivered. Often, these areas were selected because of security problems. But more often than not, they were off limits because of the NIF's political agenda.

For this reason, PPF made the conscious choice not to join OLS, and, instead, focus on delivering aid specifically to Red No-Go areas. It was this choice that led us to work a lot in an area that ended up on the Red No-Go list most of the time: the Nuba Mountains. But up to this point, I had still not even visited Africa, let alone Sudan.

In 2005, shortly after the Comprehensive Peace Agreement was signed, officially ending the war between the North and South in Sudan, I accompanied Brad on a relief trip. It was my first visit to Africa, and I was going into one of the least developed areas on the continent. I made all the usual mistakes. I packed too much. I looked like I walked out of an ExOfficio catalogue. I was on strong anti-malarial medication, which caused me to have wild, psychotic dreams. I carried around little bottles of hand sanitizer. To the average African, I probably screamed "dumb tourist ready to be fleeced."

The good news about this first trip was that I didn't get malaria. But I did pick up a bug—the Africa Bug.

This rough and wild part of the world fascinated me. I found myself loving the mud and the muck, the constant adventure, the unpredictability of it all. Every day was completely different from the previous. Nothing was consistent or assured. Nothing ran on a schedule

My first trip to Sudan wasn't my last. Although southern Sudan and the Nuba were officially at peace, the province of Darfur was in the throes of an active campaign of genocide by the NIF (rebranded as the National Congress Party) government. Thousands of refugees spilled across the border into the south. PPF began a targeted campaign to provide medicine, safe water, and non-food relief to refugees settling on the border of Southern Darfur and Northern Bahr el Ghazal.

I decided to quit my desk job and devote most of my energy to the day-to-day work of PPF. In January 2011, I moved my family to East Africa. I fell in love with Sudan's fascinating and wild landscape, and I started learning a lot more about the people and the history of the ongoing crises.

A quick Google search will reveal a Sudan marred by violence almost continuously since becoming independent of British and Egyptian rule in 1956. And it's not surprising. Sudan's immense size, its climate, language, tribal, and religious diversity, etc., all combine to create a tinderbox when trying to reconcile regional prejudices and needs through one centralized government.

The result has been instability, economic depression, religious persecution, and vicious civil wars led by a successive line of Islamist bullies masquerading as democratically-elected leaders.

By far, the worst example is Sudan's current president, Omar al-Bashir, who first came to power through a military coup in 1989. Bashir's regime immediately embarked on the well-worn trail of African dictatorships. Under Bashir's reign, Sudan has consistently ranked as one of the most corrupt countries in the world. But it's Bashir's bloodlust for an Arab hegemony which has helped earn him an indictment by the International Criminal Court (ICC) for genocide, war crimes, and crimes against humanity.[1] Many westerners are familiar with the Sunni vs. Shia divide in Islam, but most are not aware that a much deeper divide runs between many "Arab-centric" Muslims and everybody else. An ugly racist undercurrent against the non–Arab population has unfortunately contributed to much of the violence in Sudan.

Bashir began his rule with the continued aggravation of old prejudices between the Arab tribes of his country and the African or mixed tribes. A twin policy of "Arabization" and "Islamization" was heavily enforced in the country, fanning the flames of conflict and accelerating the violence, not just against the southern black tribes (who are mostly a mix of Christian and animists) but also minority northerners, mostly black Muslim tribes, which have no desire to lose their own cultures, languages or identities. This was what the Nuba leader Yousif Kuwa meant when he spoke to Brad about an "identity crisis." Like many blacks in Sudan, he was raised to reject his local culture and ethnicity, and think of himself as an Arab.

The exploitation of national oil reserves hasn't helped matters, because most of the oil fields are located in or near areas traditionally unsupportive of the Government of Sudan (GoS). Bashir's solution has been to ethnically cleanse those areas in a campaign of terror, where the denial of access to food and medicine are as effective weapons, if not more so, as bombs and bullets.

Bashir also employs "militias" which are nothing more than mercenaries given a free hand to rape and pillage. Many local people call them the *Janjaweed*, but the world mostly knows them by the rough English translation "Devils on Horseback."[2]

Bashir's "success" in southern Sudan alone has been credited with two million dead.[3] But that is just in the south. In Darfur, between 300,000 and 400,000 people have died in the last twelve years, and most of the province's population displaced into crowded refugee camps or garrison towns regularly terrorized by local "militias," who use rape as a war policy.[4]

But the area of Sudan which has captured my organization's special attention over the last five years is the beautiful Nuba Mountains in Southern Kordofan State.

The Nuba

As shown earlier, PPF's involvement in Sudan largely began due to our connection with the Nuba Mountains. During the 1980s and 90s as many as half a million Nubans lost their lives, mostly due to a government-sponsored famine.

In my own subsequent travels to the Nuba, I have found the area to be a culturally diverse, but tightly knit and fiercely independent community. Based on my interviews with locals, the acceptance of Islam has been a relatively recent event compared to the rest of Sudan. The Nuba brand of Islam tends to be mingled liberally with local traditions and customs, which makes it a prime target for President Bashir's campaign of "Arabization."

Not only is Nuba religious "syncretism" offensive to Bashir's party, the fact that the Nuba community tolerates a large and growing Christian population in their midst provides the Islamists with even more justification to "cleanse" the land.[5]

The Kadugli Massacre

The latest "cleanse" began on June 5, 2011, just weeks before The Republic of South Sudan became the world's newest nation (July 9, 2011). Bashir was set to lose most of his oil fields to South Sudan, so he rushed to secure what was left. This meant seizing the contested area of Abyei to protect the rich oil fields next door at Heglig.

Abyei town was invaded and secured in May 2011.[6] The fighting in the Nuba broke out a few weeks later. Bashir's army tried to forcefully disarm Nuba fighters who had sided with South Sudan during the previous war. The Nuba would have none of that. So, Bashir's army sacked the capital city of Kadugli and massacred thousands of Nubans.[7] I interviewed dozens of survivors only weeks after the attack began, and they all said the same thing: GoS troops went house-to-house killing people based on three criteria: (1) Ethnic Nuban (i.e. black); (2) members of the Sudan People's Liberation Movement–North (the opposition party comprised of the Nuba); and (3) Christians.

This is when PPF went in. On July 4, 2011, I flew with Brad and a small team on one of the last flights into the Nuba. Bashir had previously ordered all foreign NGOs out of the areas he didn't control, and many complied.[8] But we have never asked the GoS' permission for anything we do, so when the "front door" was closed, we used a "side entrance."

When we landed, I discovered a far different community than the one PPF teams first visited in 1998. There was an actual network of roads (dirt, though they were) and more vehicles, making movement a lot easier. The few years of peace had been put to use, and the benefits of cross-border trade were evident by the widespread availability of daily consumables.

What impressed me most about the Nuba people during this, my, first visit was their strong sense of community. Although Islam is the overall dominant religion, Christianity is in the clear majority in several counties. Dozens of churches dot the landscape on the roads to Kauda (a major town in the heart of the Nuba Mountains). But even where there is much religious diversity, I found blood to be thicker than orthodoxy. I met many mixed families containing Christians and Muslims. And although I did meet some Christians who had been persecuted by their Nuba neighbors, I found more examples of peaceful coexistence.

One good example of this tolerance was seen during our trip, when Brad and I met with the Nuba commander Abdelaziz Adam Al-Hilu. His command post at the time was located in a Christian area, and when word got out that we were in the area, the local church arranged an impromptu welcome service under the protected cover of the mountains. Commander Abdelaziz, himself a Muslim, attended the service with us and was received as warmly by the church as if he were Billy Graham. And the Commander, for his part, joined in singing and clapping along through all the hymns.

The pastor officiating the service was an elderly man named *Kallo* (name changed for purposes of safety/security) who was one of the earliest converts to Christianity from the area. He was baptized as a young man by Australian missionaries who came to the area in the 1950s. When the government ordered all missionaries out a few years later, Kallo continued their work. This made him a target by local Islamists in the government, who imprisoned him during a time of severe persecutions in the 1980s and early 1990s. Kallo was arrested several times and imprisoned for a total of more than eight years, during which time he was brutally tortured. His captors demanded he renounce his faith and produce a list of his parishioners, because they were assumed to be supportive of the SPLM.

Kallo never recanted, nor did he give his captors a list. Amazingly enough, he was eventually released. According to his testimony, his popularity was such that killing him would have made him a martyr, which the Islamists wanted to avoid. But keeping Kallo in prison was also not an option because he was converting too many Muslim inmates to Christianity!

On my first trip to the Nuba, we met with the small local consortium of NGOs still left in the region and began planning coordinated outreaches. This was the start of a campaign to assist the Nuba in the areas of safe water, medicine, and non-food aid to internal refugees. We called it SaveTheNuba.com. And since that time, we've only intensified our involvement.

One of the challenges in an active war zone is the gradual breakdown of infrastructure. We learned that hundreds of safe water well pumps were breaking down for lack of spare parts. So we launched a campaign to repair as many wells as possible. As of this writing, we've repaired nearly 300, many in frontline communities. Water-borne illnesses constitute more than 80 percent of all disease in Africa, so access to safe water is literally a life-saver.

Another area of need is medical. Brad and I had the privilege of meeting Dr. Tom Catena at the Mother of Mercy Hospital in Gidel, near Kauda, on our first visit in 2011. We determined then and there that we would try to help that heroic man as much as we could so he could continue performing miracles for the sick and dying.

In 2013, we began a concerted effort in partnership with the Nuba Ministry of Health to bring in large consignments of medicine to service more than 180 distribution points throughout the "rebel-controlled" areas of the Nuba Mountains, including Mother of Mercy Hospital.

We were told that the Nuba needs 60 metric tons of medicine every year to serve the needs of the entire population. In 2013, we succeeded in delivering eight metric tons. In 2014, we delivered eleven tons. And in 2015, we delivered 33 tons.

A War Against Children

One of my earliest observations was that most people are not political. They are just normal people, trying to live normal lives.

The older generation which lived through the 1980s and 1990s bear many scars—literally and metaphorically—from the intense persecution from the GoS. In 2011, I met an old Nuba church elder whom an Islamist "militia" had stabbed multiple times and left for dead, along with the other men of his congregation during a raid in the late 80s. After the church was burned, the attackers collected souvenirs from the bodies of their victims, including the church elder's left ear.

In 2015, I met a pastor named Yousef, who still bore the scars on his wrists and back from when he was arrested in 1988 and hung from the ceiling by his wrists and beaten. All over the Nuba you can find similar stories of how the GoS treated the Nuba in such horrific ways. And, no doubt, the Nuba suffering through today's travails will end carrying the same with them throughout their lives.

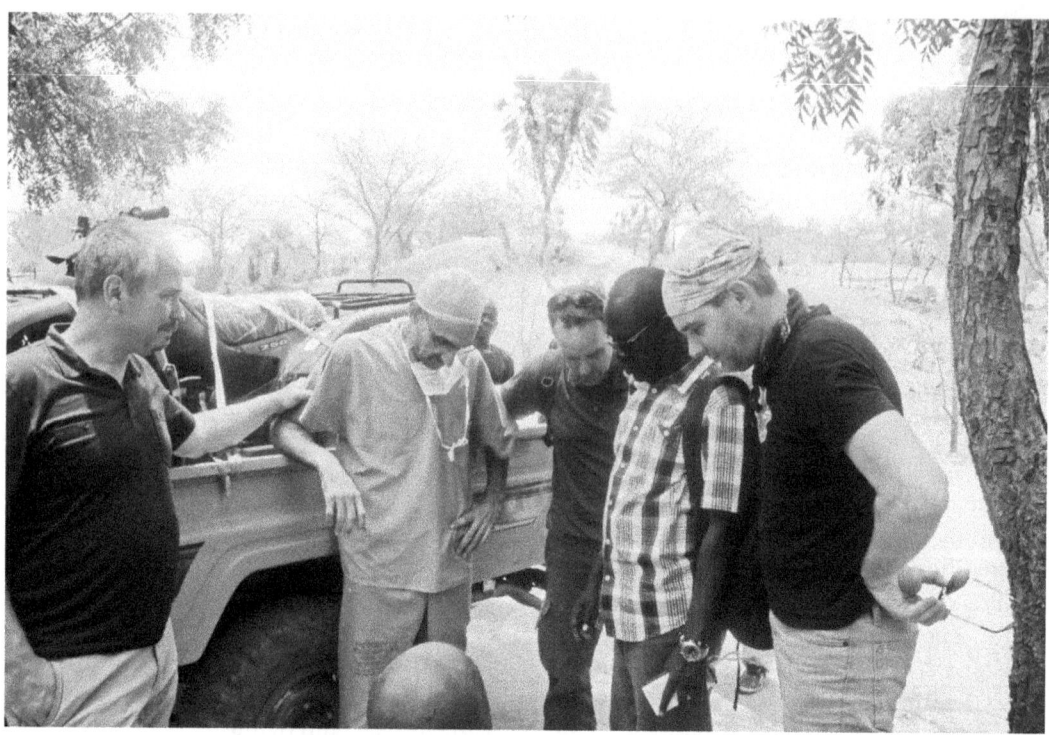

Our group praying for Dr. Tom Catena and his efforts at Mother of Mercy Hospital in Gidel, Nuba Mountains, Sudan (Matt Chancey).

That said, today, it seems, the majority of Nuba suffering in the present war are *little* people. The children.

In the Nuba Mountains, one sees children everywhere. Although an official census hasn't been taken in ages, conservatively, Nuba children under 15-years-old easily constitute more than 50 percent of the population.

The unfortunate reality about a community dominated by children is that during times of war—especially wars of terror—children endure most of the suffering. Most of the sickness. Most of the wounds. Most of the death.

If Bashir's goal is to wipe out the Nubans, children are a big impediment to this policy. Nuba children can be extremely brave. Brad once followed a girl called Reymas up the side of a perilous mountain to a hidden spring in a cave where she collected water for her family ... every day. When they returned to her home, enemy artillery hammered the other side of the mountain, reminding them just how close they were to danger. Reymas could not have been more than ten or eleven years old, but she daily performs duties which would earn most Westerners medals for bravery.

Even though I've been working in the two Sudan's for more than eleven years now, I have never been exposed to more suffering of children than I have witnessed in the Nuba Mountains.

In February 2015, Brad and I were working near the Mother of Mercy Hospital and decided to stop by for a quick visit with Dr. Tom. After greeting us, he took us to see six children who had been brought in a couple days before. What I saw has haunted me ever since: six little figures lying still with most of the flesh shredded from their bodies. The children had been severely burned when their home caught on fire from artillery shelling. The look of pain and misery on the children's faces made me depressed and angry at the same time. A few of the children were heavily sedated just to help them manage the pain. Dr. Tom informed me that most of the children would likely die, but that it could take weeks until their little bodies tired of the constant battle against infection (three children subsequently did die). The mothers kneeling next to the beds could only weep and pray. They couldn't even hold and comfort their little ones! Can you imagine?

The same day we visited the Mother of Mercy hospital, I saw an Antonov bomber flying overhead. I jumped in a fox hole, but was glad to see the plane continue on without dropping its bombs. Unfortunately, though, the plane was on its way to bomb a community we were scheduled to visit the next day.

In fact, the next day we arrived in time to witness the funeral for two women killed in the attack. One of them was Hasha Ali Bashir. She ran to a cave when she heard the Antonov coming, but then panicked as she could not find her two-year-old son, Omar. When she left the cave to look for him, she was hit by shrapnel from one of the bombs and killed instantly, but her unborn child wasn't. *Hasha was 8 months pregnant.* Her family and neighbors could do nothing but watch the little life struggle inside his mother, until the kicking eventually stopped. There was no hospital nearby to deliver the child. The only clinic in the community was closed weeks before. It had been administered by Doctors Without Borders (MSF), but after another one of their hospitals had been repeatedly bombed by GoS forces, MSF decided to pull up stakes and leave, *not just the Nuba Mountains, but the whole of Sudan.*

A few weeks after this incident, Brad was driving through the village of Heiban and was greeted by several children. One of the boys he met was decapitated the next day by a bombing. His shocked father described to Brad the horror of picking up the pieces of his son for burial.

When I happened to visit a refugee community in Delami county, which was being daily pounded by air attacks and artillery fire, a little girl, who could not have been more than four years old, boldly ran up to me with her arms raised, crying out something over and over in her native tongue. Normally, children so young living in a remote area are afraid of "kawaja" (the white man)—and a hairy one at that. When I asked our translator what she wanted, he told me that a bearded white man had come to the village a few months before and told the girl she was so cute he wanted to take her home with him. The girl thought he was serious. So when she saw me, she thought I was the same man and begged me to

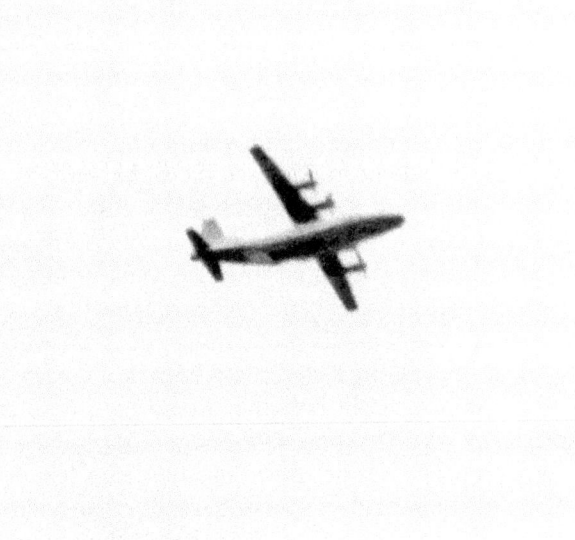

An Antonov bomber flying above the Persecution Project Team somewhere in the Nuba Mountains (photograph by Matt Chancey).

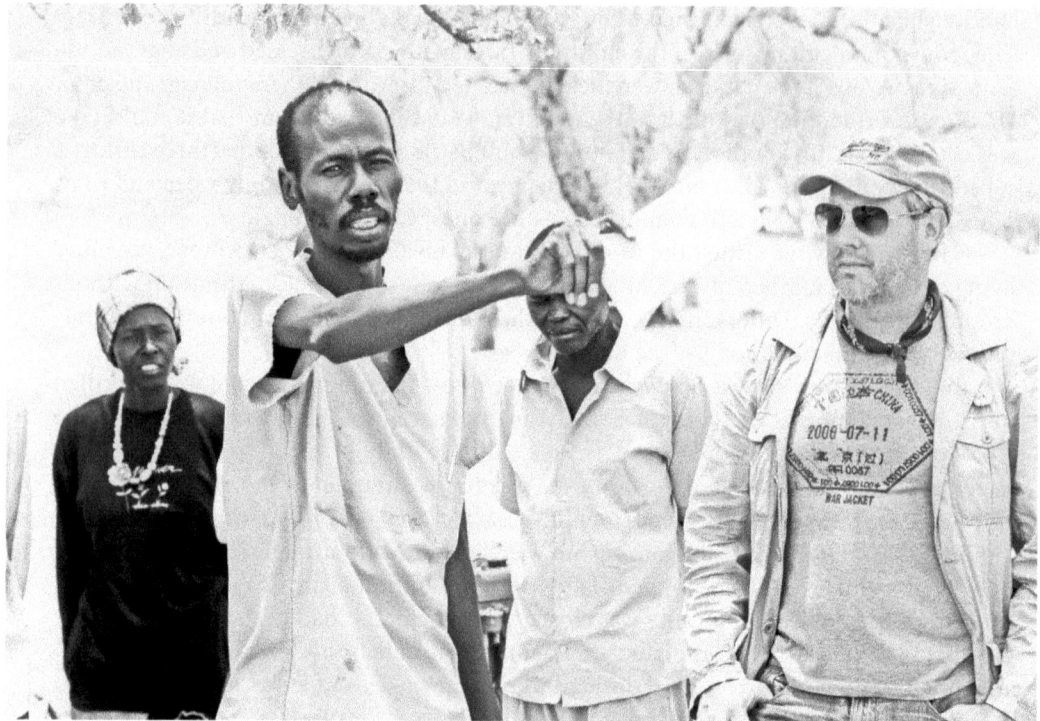

The author (right) with Dr. Ahmed at Mother of Mercy Hospital in the Gidel in the Nuba Mountains, Sudan (Matt Chancey).

take her away from that place. I felt terrible because the only thing I could do was hold her and give her some candy.

Children like this little girl have known no other life than war. I remember being in Kauda talking to a man when we suddenly heard a plane flying overhead. The man's two-year-old son immediately ran and jumped into a fox hole, crying, "Antonov! Antonov!" I knew this child was instinctively responding to the training he had received from his parents, and I thought how terrible it is to have to teach kids how to "duck and cover" before they even learn the alphabet.

Our friend Ryan Boyette, a U.S. citizen who has remained in the Nuba Mountains as war rages and has formed a team of citizen journalists to cover the war, has posted a heart-breaking video on-line (see *Nuba Reports*) of a little boy gasping for breath as he slowly bled out after being hit by shrapnel from a bomb dropped on his village.[9] Watching a child die is about the worst thing one could ever experience, but it has become a regular occurrence in the Nuba, compliments of the Bashir government.

As one might imagine, attending school and learning under war conditions is extremely challenging. PPF assisted one village to build a new model school after the previous one was destroyed in a bombing. The headmaster told us the students have to run to bomb shelters sometimes more than a dozen times a day because there is no way to know if the plane flying overhead is targeting the school or not.

In witnessing all these events, I know I am looking into the very heart of evil. These children are not "collateral damage." *They are the targets of* a sadistic regime hell-bent on wiping them out. And for what? Uncontested political dominance? A pure Arab state? Money?

During the dry months, Bashir unleashes armies of mercenaries from Chad, Mali, Libya and elsewhere to fight along GoS troops in the ongoing ground war against the Nuba. I know this is true, not just because I believe the Nuba soldiers' testimony, but because they've shown me the identity cards taken from the militia members they've killed or captured. This strategy of using foreign jihadists is exactly what Bashir and his cronies did in Darfur more than a decade ago to fuel the genocide there. But the *big* difference between what happened in places like Darfur and the present Nuba conflict is that these mercenary armies have been consistently beaten by Nuba forces since the war began.

Bashir's failure on the ground has led him to rely chiefly on his Air Force. Fast-attacking MiG's or Sukhoi jets work with antiquated Antonov cargo planes converted into bombers, targeting mostly marketplaces, schools, churches, hospitals, and homes—employing banned weapons, such as cluster bombs to inflict maximum casualties.[10] I've stood beside two unexploded bombs lying next to schools (much to the consternation of my wife). *Bashir doesn't want to subdue an army. He wants to depopulate a country. The people*, not opposing political ideologies, are his main enemy. And most of the people are children.

Many policy-makers around the world have been silent about this blatant policy of ethnic cleansing in Sudan. All the while, Bashir's PR machine works overtime to excuse and deny. He discovered a long time ago that he can curry favor with both the U.S. government and the international community by sharing intelligence on jihadist activities (as though Bashir's behavior doesn't qualify) with Western countries in great need of more Arab allies in the "War on Terror."[11]

In fact, according to many sources, the U.S. government has, in the past, made promises to normalize relations with Bashir's government in exchange for cooperation in the War on Terror. The *Washington Post* broke the story a few years ago that the U.S. intelligence community has even been supplying Bashir's own secret service with training and technology allegedly to track extremist elements in his country.[12] To Bashir, of course, the worst "extremists" are people like the Nuba—and those of us who try to help them. The Nuba is one of the areas where our teams must go completely "dark." No phones. How do we know whatever tracking technology provided to President Bashir by Western governments is not going to be used to track us?

Whatever handshake agreements have been made for more normalized relations between the U.S. and Sudan have never *fully* materialized, not because of Bashir's continued human rights violations (which have always been bad) but because of political pressure by the American people themselves, who refuse to ignore the crises in Sudan crisis.

What does it tell us about our nation, as well as other western powers, when it bargains with, cooperates with, and establishes *quid pro quo* deals with someone of al-Bashir's ilk? Is Bashir considered the "new normal" for African governments by the international community? Are we all supposed to adjust our moral compasses so we can ally with one group of sadists to combat another? I believe that these are valid questions for everyone to consider. I don't pretend to have the political solution to the crises in Sudan, but I put little faith in politics these days. My recourse is to repair to my Sunday School days when I was taught "Do not be overcome by evil. Rather, overcome evil with *good*" (Rom. 12:21).

Sadly, the only dependable political ally the Nuba people have is time. Time is running out for Bashir. He's destroying his economy. His endless wars against his own people have essentially bankrupted the Sudanese treasury.[13] Only regular bailouts by his Arab allies have kept the country from spiraling completely out of control.[14]

Outside of garrison towns, the SPLA–N has denied al-Bashir's forces any real grip on the state of South Kordofan (the home of the Nuba Mountains). All attempts at a direct invasion have been repulsed with great loss to the enemy. Nuba soldiers joke that Bashir is their best quartermaster, providing them with most of their arms, vehicles and equipment.

In my visits to the Nuba, I regularly witness the determined efforts by residents to hold on to as much "normalcy" as possible. A civilian government has been installed, planting and harvesting scheduled, etc. Of course, the war is an ever-present danger for everyone, but the Nuba are determined to persevere—and to win.

As for me and my organization, our money is on the children, not their abusers. We can only hope the rest of the world wakes up and follows suit. *But we're not waiting for the rest of the world. We're working now. And we invite others to join in the cause of "active compassion for the persecuted."*

People ask me all the time why I'm working in a place like the Nuba. And in considering the question, I have to say that it boils down to relationships. Over time, you develop friendships with people and they become a part of your community. When your community suffers, you want to help. You can't simply turn away. Some of my friends think I'm crazy to do what I do. But none of them would hesitate to help a friend if a natural disaster struck, or they became sick. I'm not some kind of "action junkie." I've simply made a lot of friends in Sudan through the years, and their burdens have become mine.

I am living proof that you don't have to have an advanced degree in international politics in order to make a difference in the lives of the suffering and persecuted. At Persecution Project Foundation, our advice to concerned people, regardless of their circumstances, is: "*Start* where you are. *Use* what you have. *Do* what you can." *That's what friends do.*

Notes

1. M. Simons (2009). "Court Issues Arrest Warrant for Sudan's Leader." *New York Times*. March 4. Accessed at: http://www.nytimes.com/2009/03/05/world/africa/05court.html.

2. D. Blair (2008). "Sudanese Dictator Omar al-Bashir Faces War Crimes Charges." *The Telegraph. July 14*. Accessed at: http://www.telegraph.co.uk/news/majornews/2403864/Sudanese-dictator-Omar-al-Bashir-faces-war-crimes-charges.html.

3. F.M. Deng (2001). "Sudan—Civil War and Genocide: Disappearing Christians of the Middle East." *The Middle East Quarterly* (Winter). Accessed at: Retrievedhttp://www.meforum.org/22/sudan-civil-war-and-genocide.

4. United Human Rights Council (n.d.). "Genocide in Darfur." Accessed at: http://www.unitedhumanrights.org/genocide/genocide-in-sudan.htm.

5. Eric Reeves (2011). "Abyei and Southern Kordofan/Nuba Mountains Under Siege, Deeply at Risk." Accessed at: http://sudanreeves.org/2011/07/02/abyei-and-south-kordofannuba-mountains-under-siege-deeply-at-risk-july-1-2011.

6. J. Gettleman and J. Kron (2011). "Warnings of All-Out War in Fight Over Sudan Town." *New York Times*. May 22. Accessed at: http://www.nytimes.com/2011/05/23/world/africa/23sudan.html.

7. N.A. Raymond and I.L. Baker (2013). "How Did 7,000 Sudanese Disappear in 2011?" *Global Post*. August 23. Accessed at: http://www.globalpost.com/dispatches/globalpost-blogs/commentary/un-should-investigate-how-7000-sudanese-disappeared-2011–0.

8. E. Reeves (2009). "Khartoum's Expulsion of Humanitarian Organizations." *Sudan Reeves*. March 25. Accessed at: http://sudanreeves.org/2009/03/25/khartoums-expulsion-of-humanitarian-organizations-march-4–2009/.

9. Nuba Reports (2015). "Children Killed as Sudan Increases Bombing Raids." *Nuba Reports.* February 15. Accessed at: http://nubareports.org/bombings-exceed-3000-in-the-nuba-mountains/.

10. Nuba Reports (2015). "Cluster Bombs Hit Homes in May." *Nuba Reports.* June 15. Accessed at: http://nubareports.org/cluster-bombs-hit-homes-in-may/.

11. E. Reeves (2013). "U.S. Counter-terrorism in Lieu of Foreign Policy: The Case of Sudan." October 29. Accessed at: http://sudanreeves.org/2013/10/29/4409/.

12. Jeff Stein (2010). "CIA Training Sudan's Spies as Obama Officials Fight Over Policy." August 30. *The Washington Post.* Accessed at: http://voices.washingtonpost.com/spy-talk/2010/08/cia_training_sudans_spies_as_o.html.

13. E. Reeves (2011). "Sudan's Self-inflicted Economic Distress." *The Guardian.* August 1. Accessed at: http://www.theguardian.com/global-development/poverty-matters/2011/aug/01/sudan-economic-distress-khartoum.

14. *Sudan Tribune* (2014). "Sudan Receives $1bn Deposit from Qatar." *Sudan Tribune.* April 3. Accessed at: http://www.sudantribune.com/spip.php?article50525.

A Moral Imperative
From Conducting Research in the Nuba Mountains to Hauling Food to Those in Most Critical Need

SAMUEL TOTTEN

Introduction

I've been a student of genocide since 1985. The first twenty years of my work in the field was as an autodidact, and one in which I engaged largely in archival work in such institutions as the Library of Congress, the U.S. Institute for Peace, and the Hoover Institute (Stanford University). Over the past decade and a half (2004–present), however, my work in the field of genocide studies moved from research in libraries and archives to field work in Chad, Rwanda, and Sudan, and then onto activism.

As most scholars of genocide studies will attest, a question that they are often confronted with is a variation of: What drove you to study genocide. For most of us, I believe, there's both a simple answer and a more nuanced one. I suppose the same is true in regard to those who turn to a life of activism. It certainly is in my case.

I now live the life of a scholar/activist. Some in the community of genocide scholars assert that the two hats, if you will, are incompatible. One involves, they argue, objectivity, while the other is often generated by passion. Perhaps they're correct that it is ill advised to attempt to be both. Personally, I disagree.

Not a few scholars of genocide pride themselves on being dispassionate. Some even seem to suggest that the best scholars are those who practice disengaged objectivity. To me, both the goals and efforts of such individuals seem oddly disembodied.

As I've said over and over again in debates with so-called critical genocide scholars and others who question the scholar-activist paradigm, it is one thing to take a historical approach to the study of genocide, but when one, such as myself, conducts research in both refugee camps and war zones, where one hears about, sees, and, in certain cases, witnesses the slaughter and death of innocents, objectivity verges, at least in my eyes, on the obscene.

All of this is to say, whenever and wherever innocent people are being beaten down, deprived of their basic human rights, tortured, maimed, and killed, I—as long as I have the energy (meaning, as long as I am in decent health)—plan to continue to put my heart, my mind, and body on the line. If that makes me less of a scholar, so be it. I can live with that.

Formative Years

For various reasons, I hate talking/writing about my formative years. While I was certainly fortunate in a host of ways—a great mother, a wonderful brother, lots of good friends, active participation in wide range of activities (Boy Scouts, Explorers, Little League Baseball, trips to Disneyland, Knott's Berry Farm, Marine Land), a roof over my family's head, plenty to eat—everything seems colored by the painful memories of my old man's menacing brutality.

Almost every single memory of my childhood is, in a way, bruised. My father had a tough and sad life himself as he grew up and as a result he harbored a lot of anger in his heart at the world. He watched his beloved mother suffer for years from a debilitating disease, began giving her shots of morphine when he was in his early teens (his father was a physician and taught him how to do it), and lost his mother when he was thirteen or fourteen. He quit school his junior year and entered the United States Marine Corps in order to fight in World War II. As my brother and I were growing up, he worked as a police officer in a very tough industrial section of Los Angeles. Just as he meted out "justice" on the street in the 1950s to those he and his colleagues arrested, he meted out brutality at home against those he purportedly loved. Even a short list of what he visited on my mother, brother and myself provides readers with a sense of the hell we experienced during my formative years: he hit me in the mouth when I was six years old, breaking my front tooth; he stabbed my brother with a fork when he was ten years old; not infrequently, in a fury, he would overturn our kitchen table during dinner and then jump on my brother or me and pound us with his fists, and when my mother begged him to quit hitting us, he would turn his brutality on her; not infrequently, he would smash furniture in our living room, rip whatnot shelves and paintings off the wall, splintering them and beating us with the broken pieces of furniture; one day he broke my mother's right arm twice—the second instance was upon her return home from the hospital at which time he broke her arm again by twisting her arm savagely and ripping off the cast; more times than I can count, he banged and pounded our heads against the ground—be it against wooden floors or on thin rugs covering concrete floors—and often choked us until we nearly blacked out.

My mother is the sweetest person I've ever met. People love her. She is loving, honest, a great listener, a delight to be with, and largely nonjudgmental. Undoubtedly she has served as a very positive role model. I also had a great Boy Scout master who served as a positive role model and through the years not a few teachers as well.

As I grew up, I came to detest bullies. And when I encountered bullies—particularly those who harassed my brother or my friends—I did not hold back. I would release my built up fury against them, in order to teach them a lesson. Hardly positive, I know; but as the cliché goes, it was what it was.

There are scores of other stories I could relate about growing up under the fist of a dictatorial brute, but I just can't do it.

The U.S. State Department's Atrocities Documentation Project

My desk- and library-bound scholarly efforts took a major turn in 2004 when I was asked to serve as one of the 24 investigators on the U.S. State Department's Atrocities

Documentation Project (ADP), which involved interviewing black Africans who had fled to refugee camps along the Chad/Darfur, Sudan, border as a result of being attacked by Government of Sudan (GoS) troops and their allied militia, the *Janjaweed*, in Darfur. Prior to my departure for Chad, my wife, Kathleen Barta, said, with great prescience, "This is going to be a life-changing event."

Following an ear-splitting and cramped flight in a four-seater plane from N'djamena, Chad to Abeche, the largest town in eastern Chad, we joined the coordinator of the project, her assistants, and a half dozen other investigators at a small compound during which we, the investigators, went through orientation. The next morning four of us were flown south, where a fellow investigator named Brenda Thornton, an attorney with the U.S. Justice Department, and I got out on a dusty plain on the outskirts of the tiny village of Goz Beida, which is just about the most southern point in Chad. The other two investigators, one from England and one from Australia, were then flown to a nearby refugee camp called Goz Amer.

Ultimately, Brenda and I, along with our interpreters and drivers, set up camp on the grounds of a former French colonial compound situated roughly in the middle of the village. A decrepit, plaster building still stood within the compound but it was filthy and stench-ridden, and thus we put up our individual tents a fair distance from the house and slept in them.

Following a meeting with the sheik of Goz Beida, during which we informed him of our work and sought his imprimatur to enter the refugee camp, which was situated on his land, we drove out to the UNHCR refugee camp. The camp, which constituted one of the smallest camps in the region with about 16,000 residents, was a sea of green UN tents spread across a vast area of the desert. Since the camp was relatively new, most of the tents were in excellent repair. In the camp we sought out the *umda* (the primary leader of the camp, who oversaw all of the sheiks), and repeated the ritual we had just completed with the sheik of Goz Beida.

Once we got to work, Brenda and I each took a different part of the camp and worked with our own interpreters (both of whom were fluent in Arabic, English and at least one tribal language). We were charged with asking every interviewee each and every question on the ADP's eight-page questionnaire. Initially, the interviewees were asked to provide basic demographic information: name, date of birth, place of birth, father and mother's names, years of education, profession, marital status, name and age of wife(s), number of children and names and ages of each child. The next series of questions focused on that which prompted the interviewee to leave/flee from his/her village; what he/she had personally witnessed, heard, and experienced from the outset of the attack to the point of arrival in the refugee camp; when, where and how the attack was carried out and by whom; markings on the uniforms of the soldiers and/or militia; whether planes or *doskas* (trucks mounted with machine guns), Land Cruisers, and/or Antonov bombers had taken part in the attack; what, exactly, the perpetrators had said during the attacks; whether the interviewee had witnessed anyone being killed, and if so, his/her name, age, and how he/she was killed and by whom, etc. Generally, the interviews lasted between an hour and a half and two hours.

The first interview I conducted—with a middle aged woman who had been in the refugee camp for nearly a year and had no idea whether her husband and young son were dead or alive, hiding in the mountains of Darfur, living in an internally displaced persons (IDP) camp in Darfur or resettled in another refugee camp in Chad, and had no means to attempt to locate them—has haunted me for years. She had been raped by those who attacked her village, and had not yet had a physical by a nurse or a doctor. She was so humiliated by what had happened to her, she could not speak of the rape directly and thus repeatedly referred to it by saying, "They made me do lewd movements."

Throughout the interview, which was held inside her dusty tent, she spoke haltingly. Periodically, she would fall silent for five to ten minutes or more at a time. Each and every time I reminded her that she was under absolutely no obligation to continue the interview, but each and every time she insisted she wished to be interviewed.

Witnessing the pain in the woman's eyes and voice and her sagging body language set the stage, as it were, for what I was about to face during the course of the interviews with other survivors. What I mean is, it set the stage for the abject sadness I would carry with me as I heard one person's story after another concerning the brutality and horror to which they, their family members and fellow villagers had been subjected to during the scorched earth attacks carried out by GoS troops and the *Janjaweed*.

During one of my interviews in the refugee camp the wind suddenly kicked up, scooping up battered pots and pans, among other items. Swirling, twister-like funnels of dust sprung up, literally turning the entire camp a gauzy brown. With the interviewee, we made a run for his tent. Quickly, we secured all the clasps in an attempt to keep the dust out, but to no avail. Even though it was difficult to breathe, we proceeded with the interview. That evening, and for the rest of my time in the field, I found myself having to clear my throat every five minutes or so, and when I expectorated the phlegm was full of sand. Making matters even worse, the only way I could breathe while sleeping was to create a large pile (comprised of my backpack, clothes, etc.) at the back of the tent and lean up against it, thus sleeping at nearly a 45-degree angle.

Ultimately, after both an internal and external analysis of the data (by the State Department and an outside research firm, respectively), Secretary of State Colin Powell concluded that the GoS had committed genocide in Darfur. More specifically, on September 9, 2004, in a report to the U.S. Senate Foreign Relations Committee, Powell announced that the GoS had committed genocide against the black Africans of Darfur, and was possibly still doing so. (For a detailed discussion of the ADP and the decision by Powell, see Samuel Totten and Eric Markusen's *Genocide in Sudan: Investigating Atrocities in the Sudan*. New York: Routledge, 2006).

Additional Work in Chad

In July 2006, I returned to Chad in order to interview other survivors of the Darfur genocide. With the conflict still raging in Darfur, I decided such an effort would not only help me keep abreast as to what was happening on the ground, but would eventually allow me to put together a collection of first-person accounts of the black Africans' experiences at the hands of the GoS. (In fact, for the next several years I made several trips to Chad, where I conducted interviews in various refugee camps—Gaga, Forchana, Goz Beida and in N'djamena, the capital of Chad. In each location I interviewed approximately a half dozen survivors.)

On that first trip back to Chad, everything was going smoothly until literally just before the small UN plane (a small eight seater) I caught a ride with was about to lift off from N'djamena. Shutting down the engine, the pilot glanced back at us and shouted,

"Something's not right. I'll have the mechanics check it out and we ought to be on our way within 30 minutes or so. Everyone will have to get out but you can wait on the tarmac."

As the pilot pulled up to the terminal, he informed us that everyone had to pull his or her gear from the plane. That accomplished, he taxied over to the mechanic's garage. About 30 minutes later, the pilot was back, had us load our gear and hop aboard. As the plane taxied down the runway a second time, picked up speed and was about to lift off, the pilot shut the plane down once again. "OK, let me see what the mechanics can do. Hopefully, we'll be on our way in an hour or so," he said. An airport official, though, had a different take on it. "No, I'm shutting you down today. The mechanics need to go through this thing thoroughly. No flight today. Come back to tomorrow."

Because we had been informed that the UN personnel had first claim to the seats, I asked the fellow if we would be guaranteed a flight the next day. "Not necessarily," he said. "It depends on how many are booked for the flight tomorrow. Then, any extra seats will be taken by the four passengers with the UN who didn't make it today. The four of you may have to go on different flights; that is, if there are enough seats available on the two or three flights we have flying tomorrow."

Ultimately, my companions and I decided to rent a Land Cruiser in N'djamena and drive to Abeche. To make a very long story short, it took us twenty three hours to travel from N'djamena to Abeche. The first third of the trip we traveled over asphalt roads, the second third over a smoothly graded dirt road, and the last third there was no road to speak of—over large swaths there weren't even any clear tire tracks of vehicles that had gone there before us. The ride was bone-jarring as we made our way over the rocky, twisting, and rutted terrain. During the last third of the ride I did everything I could to brace myself for what I knew would be the next round of punishing head-banging, back-jarring slams against the ceiling of the truck and the metal frame of the door, but my efforts were in vain.

During the dry season, *wadis* are essentially dry riverbeds. During the rainy season they morph into raging torrents capable of sweeping large lorries down river. In Chad, at least, as one pulls up to each swollen wadi there are always three or four fellows standing alongside the road with a long, thick rope selling "insurance." The deal is this: if you purchase "insurance" for $20.00 and your vehicle gets stuck as it attempts to make it across the wadi, the guys guarantee to pull the vehicle out of the swirling water and get it to the other side of the wadi; if one does not purchase insurance and one's vehicle gets stuck then it costs $120.00 to be rescued.

Generally, as drivers pull up to a wadi they not only check out the flow of the water but watch as other vehicles attempt to make it across. If a vehicle makes it across without any trouble then the next driver in line generally foregoes the purchase of insurance, and vice versa. Heading to Abeche we must have crossed a dozen wadis. We never purchased "insurance" and, luckily, never needed it.

To say that it was a relief to pull into Abeche, even though it is a dusty, downtrodden desert town, would be an understatement. Though we were all beat, we had no choice but to check in with the owner of the vehicle who resided in Abeche. After paying him the fee of $400.00 a day, plus the cost of petrol and the driver's salary, we broached the fact that we wished to head to those refugee camps north of Abeche. I was particularly keen to conduct interviews with refugees in such camps as Bahai as I had heard that one might be able to hire guides for travel into Darfur. The owner of the vehicle, however, squelched that plan. "It's too dangerous. We had a driver pulled out of a vehicle last week, threatened with a gun, and then the vehicle was stolen."

In light of the fact that the average person was lucky to make twenty dollars a week in Chad and that we were willing to pay $500.00 to $600.00 a day for the rental of the truck and there were no takers spoke volumes as to just how dangerous the region was. Later I learned that the UN's humanitarian forces in and around Bahai were reduced to a "minimum presence" in early December 2006 due to the heightened danger in the region.

We ended up heading out to the closest refugee camps just east of Abeche: Gaga, Farchana, Treguine and Bredjing. In Gaga, I interviewed a 30-year-old man, who was a member of the Massalit tribe and a sheik. What he witnessed in his village of Hela Zakawka (Darfur) in the aftermath of a major attack by the GoS and the *Janjaweed*, could not but haunt him:

> While I was hiding, I heard the whopping sound of the helicopter, a gray helicopter that was circling, but there was so much shooting I didn't know if it was firing on people or not. When I came out of the trees, I could see the smoke, clouds of it. I decided to return to our village, and as I got closer I saw that about half of the village had been burned down and that some fences and houses were still burning. As I continued on I saw a lot of dead bodies. Some people were injured, shot up, and some dead. Some I could recognize, a total of six. Ibrahim Adam, an old man, about fifty years [old], who had been shot in the leg, could not move. He was crying for water, but I had no water. Abdullah Khamiss, thirty years, was shot in the neck, and when I found him I stayed with him but after one hour he died. Mohammed Gamar, twenty-two years, had been shot in his eye, and the bullet had gone out the back of his head. He was alive, but he could not speak. He died shortly.... Mohammed Ahmed, forty years, had both of his legs badly cut by a knife, probably a *satour* (a knife butchers in the *suq* use to slice meat), and the wounds were very deep. When I found him he was dying and could not speak. Muhammad Yaha, about eighteen years, had a chest wound from a bullet. This man I found already dead. Yaha Adam, another old man, fifty-eight years, was shot in his side, and his insides were hanging out. He, too, I found dead. On that day, fifteen people were killed, but what I've told you is what I remember seeing [Totten, 2010, p. 50].

After spending a week in two different refugee camps—Gaga and Forchana—the group I was with packed up and headed back across the desert to N'djamena. About 45 minutes out of Abeche we reached the swiftly moving waters of the first wadi. We intently watched as several vehicles—one at a time—headed out into the roiling waters, and then, slowly and cautiously, made their way across. Figuring we didn't need to purchase any insurance, we followed suit.

The next wadi was about a half hour away. As we pulled up behind the two vehicles ahead of us, I noticed a camouflaged Land Cruiser off to the side loaded down with rocket propelled grenades (RPGs) around which milled a half dozen heavily armed and menacing looking soldiers.

Again, we watched as the vehicle in front of us entered the wadi. As it slowly made its way through the surging water without incident, we decided to give it a shot, again sans insurance.

We had made it about a fourth of the way across the wadi when we had the sinking feeling (no pun intended) that our Land Cruiser was beginning to sink. At one and the same time, the engine began sputtering, and then died. "Quick!" someone in the back shouted, start it up!"

As the driver ground the ignition in a frantic effort to start the engine, water began seeping up over the floorboard. Within minutes, the water had reached the seats on which we had been sitting. By that time, though, the driver and I were already squatting on the seats. As the water continued to inch its way up, I rolled down the window of the passenger door in preparation to jump into the water with the bag that contained all of my notes/interviews. As everyone in the truck was wigging out, the truck finally came to a rest, but by that time the water was three quarters of the way up the back of the front seats.

As soon as the truck began to settle into the sediment on the bottom of the wadi, three or four guys from "the insurance company" raced out into the water pulling a long, thick rope behind them. They quickly attached it to our back bumper and then hooked the other end to the front bumper of a lorry waiting to cross the wadi. As the truck backed up, it slowly pulled us back towards land.

As I opened the car door to get out, a wave of water, just like one sees in cartoons, poured out of the car, spilling like a waterfall onto the ground. All I could do was burst out laughing, not only at the cartoon-like image but the entire scenario. As soon as I did, the soldiers burst out laughing as well and when I looked up they were giving me the thumbs-up signal. Moments later they insisted that a local journalist who was hanging around the wadi take a picture of me with them. As we all lined up, several of the fellows slung their arms over my shoulders, while still holding onto their weapons in their other hand. So, they went from menacing looking to actually being quite friendly.

Right away, we pulled all of our gear out of the vehicle and hung backpacks, sleeping bags, and clothes on thorn trees in an attempt to dry them out. The Land Cruiser's engine was literally "flooded," and no matter what the driver did, it wouldn't start. After an hour or so it became clear that the driver and his vehicle weren't going anywhere anytime soon, and thus we began trying to flag down a ride. An hour or so later—only about four vehicles passed by that time—a long-distance taxi stopped, informing us that it would be $400 USD to N'djamena. Since we all were flying out the next day there was little we could do about the extortionate fare.

In December 2009, I returned to the camp (Goz Beida) to which I had been assigned during the ADP back in 2004. As I left the village of Goz Beida and headed out to the UNHCR camp, I became confused as I did not recall any of the structures we were passing. Eventually it dawned on me that the entire area was all but completely void of the hundreds of UN tents that had been there in 2004. In fact, there were only about a dozen tents, if that, still standing. I discovered that they were not the original tents but replacements. All of the other tents had been replaced by small compounds, makeshift huts, and small shops. What had been a UNHCR camp had morphed into a village. Over and over again, refugees asserted that they feared they were going to be stuck in Chad for the rest of their lives.

A young woman heard that I was interviewing survivors of the Darfur genocide, and, unlike most victims of rape in Darfur, she sought me out and gently but persistently insisted that I interview her. She also insisted that I include her actual name in recording her story (versus using "anonymous," as many often requested out of fear of being attacked by GoS troops for talking to outsiders). She had a quiet strength about her, but eyes that were heartbreakingly sad. She began by telling me about others who had been raped:

> The Arabs did not want Jugma destroyed because it was one of the biggest villages, and the place where the Arabs could obtain what they wanted and needed. So they forced all of the people [inhabitants] to remain in the village and began raping the girls and women.
>
> Today, there are many children who were born due to those rapes. Some of my family was raped

there. My older sister, who was not married, was raped twice, and both times she had a baby from those rapes. Two babies! Arabs and GoS soldiers did this. Anytime they wanted to rape her, they did. If they saw her in the *suq*, they'd take her; if they saw her along a path and wanted to rape her, they would. And sometimes they even came to my home and took her with them and raped her [Totten, 2010, p. 99].

After speaking about her brothers' reactions to the treatment of their sister and the confrontation they got into with the perpetrators (as well as the subsequent threats her brothers faced), she told me about the nightmare she was subjected to as she and a couple of village women were on their way to a *suq* on market day in order to sell their wares (a load of cooking oil and onions):

I said [to the perpetrators], "Don't take these things."
He [the one confronting her directly] said, "Forget about these things. I not only want your goods but you also."
One of the men said, "We will not only rape you, but impregnate you with a child."
I told them, "Instead of raping me, it is better to kill me."
Immediately, one of the men hit me on the neck with a knife and ripped off my *tob* [a sari-like dress] and sliced off my underclothes with the knife and threw me to the ground and started raping me. The other women screamed and screamed until the men finished.
After all three raped me, they took the [cooking] oil and poured it on the ground. Then one said, "You are rubbish! Get out of here."
As I got up, one said, "We could rape you anywhere. Even in your village" [Totten, 2010, pp. 100, 101].

All these years later I can still see the young woman's face in my mind's eye—just as clearly as if I had interviewed her yesterday in the tiny Oxfam compound where I was staying. While she had a steely resolve not to allow what was done to her kill her spirit, her sadness was palpable. (The aforementioned interviews, along with scores of others, appear in my book, *An Oral and Documentary History of the Darfur Genocide*. Santa Barbara, CA: Praeger Security International, 2010.)

Documenting the Experiences of the Survivors of the Genocide by Attrition in the Nuba Mountains

My initial trip to Nuba Mountains came about in a rather odd way—a classic case of serendipity, really. It was April 2008 and I was flying from Kigali (Rwanda) back to the United States for a couple of days in order to give a talk on the Darfur genocide at the University of Chicago, and we had just landed at the Jomo Kenyetta International Airport in Nairobi, Kenya. As passengers exited I was hoping that very few new passengers would board for the next leg of the flight to Amsterdam. That way those of us already on the plane might have an opportunity to stretch out across the five seats in the middle section of the cabin and sleep the night away.

Not particularly pleased when two gentlemen took two seats in the middle row I was seating in, I pulled out a tablet of paper and began what was to be a full night of work on one of the many projects I was engaged in as a Fulbright Scholar at the Center for Conflict Management at the National University of Rwanda.

To make matters even worse, the two gentlemen pulled out a computer, fired it up, and began watching a raucous movie that sounded not a little mindless. As they watched the film, the two of them broke out in great bellows of laughter, commenting on this or that scene or dialogue. The two of them sounded very much like Cheech and Chong in the middle of one of their infamous party scenes.

The plane was well on its way to Amsterdam by the time one of the two fellows decided to call it a night, closed his eyes, and went to sleep. His buddy, who was sitting next to me, asked, "Do you plan to work all night?" I answered, "Probably." He then asked what I was working on, and when I told him "the development of a masters degree program in genocide studies for the National University of Rwanda," he expressed an interest and began asking me questions. Then he asked where I was going and I told him, "the University of Chicago in order to serve on a panel with Juan Mendez, the Special Advisor to the Secretary General on the Prevention of Genocide, and David J. Scheffer, the former U.S. Ambassador at Large for War Crimes Issues." I then asked him where he was coming from and what he did, and he informed me that he worked for a Christian organization in the Nuba Mountains in Sudan. Now my interest was piqued.

I informed him about my work with the U.S. Atrocities Documentation Project, and how I had been trying to get into Sudan for four years but to no avail. I told him I had come to the conclusion that I was probably blackballed by the Government of Sudan as a result of the book I had published on the Darfur genocide.

He said, "Really close to where I work in the Nuba Mountains there is an IDP camp of people from Darfur. And if you want, I think I can help you get into Sudan without a passport." He went on to tell me how, and I told him I was definitely up for it.

July 2010—First Trip to the Nuba Mountains

Within three months of meeting the fellow with SP, I was stepping off a converted DC-3 military fixed-wing propeller driven plane—which had served as a bomber in World War II but now served as a combination cargo/passenger plane—onto the bumpy dirt field that served as a makeshift runway in the heart of the Nuba Mountains, Sudan. No airport, no air controller tower. No hangars. Nothing.

Grabbing my bag, I simply walked towards the closest town, Kauda. And thus began my love for the Nuba people and the Nuba Mountains.

While in the Nuba during that first visit I met a good number of survivors of the genocide by attrition carried out by the GoS against the Nuba people back in the 1990s.

Gradually, the more I heard about the genocide by attrition, the more compelled I was to delve into its causes, processes, and ramifications. It, the "genocide by attrition," was perpetrated by the GoS against the Nuba Mountains people from, roughly, the late 1980s through the mid-1990s. Furious that the Nuba had joined the southerners in a civil war against Khartoum (i.e., Government of Sudan), the GoS carried out a scorched earth attack against the people of the Nuba Mountains. And, just as it did a decade later in Darfur, instead of solely tracking down and arresting or killing those rebels from the Nuba Mountains fighting alongside the South, the GoS targeted all of the people in the area (females, children, infants, and the elderly, alike). Not only were villages attacked and innocents gunned down, but farms were utterly destroyed or taken over while hundreds of thousands of people were displaced from their homes. Deprived access to their farms, the Nuba Mountains people faced inexorable hunger, malnutrition, severe malnutrition and, in many cases, starvation.

Towards the end of my trip I decided I would return to the Nuba Mountains in order to continue to interview the IDPs outside of Kauda and also begin a project interviewing those Nuba survivors of the genocide by attrition.

June 2011: Second Trip to the Nuba—Rumors of War

In January 2011, I made my second trip to the Nuba Mountains. While there, I learned a lot more about the genocide by attrition in the 1990s, but also encountered rumors of war.

During one of my first interviews with a survivor of the genocide by attrition, the interviewee, a young man with a gentle smile and equally gentle nature, related how his younger sister died of starvation and his mother had all but lost her mind:

> We had nothing to eat but leaves.... We continued like that until the young sister of mine passed away. She died of starvation.
>
> I was about twelve years [old] when my sister died. She was ten years. My mother felt so sorrowful, so bad, she said she wanted to die, to take poison. She did not, though, because of me.
>
> She, my mother, though, still suffers. She is traumatized, not right in the head, mentally. When I go visit her sometimes she is not right. I'm like her guardian, her son, her husband. Life is just like that [quoted in Totten, 2012, p. 27].

Stories such as this young man's were rife as I spoke to scores of people who lived through the genocide by attrition in the late 1980s and early- to mid-1990s.

Shortly after sunset one evening, the compound in which I was staying erupted in excited chatter as knots of people gathered in animated conversation. The upshot was that a notice, in Arabic, had been nailed to a wall of a small makeshift shop in the *suq* in lower Kauda, outlining atrocities that had been perpetrated by GoS troops that very that day against Nuba in Kadugli (the capital of South Kordofan).

Over the next several days word quickly spread that many Nuba were talking about picking up their weapons again against the government. I later heard that almost every *tukul* (or household) in the Nuba Mountains contained a semi-automatic weapon as protection against an aggressive and dictatorial government.

Various individuals, many of whom had either fought along side the south against the north in the Second Sudanese Civil War or had fathers, brothers and/or uncles who had done so, voiced variations along the following lines: "Last time, we [the Nuba] were not prepared to fight, but this time we are!" and "This time we will take the fight all the way to Khartoum."

The people of the Nuba Mountains had recently experienced a series of setbacks that left them incensed and almost aching for war. First, the Nuba had been left out of the Comprehensive Peace Agreement (CPA), an international effort to bring to a close the 22-year Second Sudanese Civil War between the north and south. Part and parcel of the CPA was the option for the south to hold a referendum to ascertain if the people wished to remain part of Sudan or preferred to create a new nation. Since the Nuba had fought alongside the south against al-Bashir and did not trust him—indeed, detested him—they were anxious to break from the north. That was not an option, though, as they were sidelined as a result of political wrangling and compromises made by the GoS and the international community. Second, the Nuba Mountains people believed that the recent gubernatorial election in South Kordofan (the state in which the Nuba Mountains is located) had been rigged, and that that was the only reason Ahmed Haroun, a crony of al-Bashir and a man who had been indicted by the International Criminal Court on charges of crimes against humanity and war crimes for atrocities allegedly perpetrated in Darfur between 2004–2008, had won the election. Third, al-Bashir had threatened to establish Sharia law throughout Sudan, and that was something that the Christians and moderate Muslims in the Nuba Mountains greatly feared.

Each evening thereafter, huge rallies were held out by the tiny UN compound adjacent to the makeshift Kauda airfield. Speakers denounced both al-Bashir and Haroun, and shouted that those GoS spies in the crowd should relay those exact sentiments to al-Bashir.

The tension was such that those in whose compound I was staying had already dug a deep rectangular hole (some three feet by three feet by eight feet) to use as a "bomb shelter" should the GoS begin carrying out aerial attacks against the region.

I immediately knocked out an email about the situation, and fired it off to a host of journalists, newspapers and anti-genocide activists back in the States. Apparently, few to none had any interest in a place (i.e., the Nuba) they probably had never heard of.

Ultimately, Bashir threatened the Nuba people with a replay of the 1990s. Undeterred, the Nuba continued to hold rallies during which they demanded that Haroun and al-Bashir (who was wanted on charges of crimes against humanity, war crimes and genocide for alleged atrocities perpetrated in Darfur) give themselves up to the ICC.

Back in the States: War Breaks Out in the Nuba Mountains

Months later, in early June 2011, I received an urgent email from Ryan Boyette, a buddy of mine who had served for years as the coordinator of the Samaritans Purse (SP) project in the Nuba Mountains. He informed me that SP had abruptly pulled out of the Nuba Mountains due to the recent ground attacks and bombings by the GoS against the civilians in the region. He also informed me that he had resigned from SP as he had decided to remain in the Nuba Mountains in order to both witness what was taking place *and* to write up and disseminate updates in the hope that the international press would pick them up and that, in turn, such reports would impress upon the UN, the U.S. Government, and major human rights organizations across the globe that a disaster was in the making. Since Internet connection was iffy in the Nuba and since it was also dangerous to remain on-line due to the fact that the GoS could target the user, he asked if I was willing to receive and then disseminate his reports to the media and international human rights organizations. I readily agreed to do so.

Day-in and day-out for close to a month, I literally worked around the clock communicating with Ryan and forwarding his updates about both the ground attacks and the aerial attacks by the GoS, including the horrific injuries and deaths civilians were suffering (along with gruesome photographs of the injured and dead) to journalists and major human rights organizations across the globe. Day after day I'd rise about five or six in the morning and work until one to two the next morning.

Over the course of that month or so, I relayed such information from Ryan to, for example, Nick Kristof at the *New York Times,* Jason Straziuso at the Associated Press office in Nairobi, Amnesty International's headquarters in London, Human Rights Watch in New York City, and The Sentinel Project in Washington, D.C., among scores of others. Most not only made use of the updates and helped spread the word about the GoS attacks (including the door-to-door killing of suspected enemies of the state in the town of Kadugli and beyond, as well as rumors of massacres and mass graves), but requested additional information, including specifics that either corroborated or dispelled rumors about what they were hearing in regard to what was taking place in the Nuba Mountains.

At one point, Nick Kristof contacted me and asked if I was willing to knock out an article for his *New York Times* blog. I readily agreed. That piece, "Is Omar Hassan al-Bashir Up to Genocide Again?" (June 18, 2011), read, in part, as follows:

> Omar Hassan al-Bashir, the president of Sudan, is a genocide perpetrator extraordinaire. If medals were given out for such activity, he'd be going for the gold.
>
> In the early- to mid–1990s, under al-Bashir's leadership, the GoS perpetrated genocidal actions in the Nuba Mountains, largely by starving people to death and preventing humanitarian aid from reaching the victims. Not a decade later, Bashir and his henchmen committed genocide in Darfur, carrying out a scorched earth policy that resulted in an estimated 300,000 plus deaths, over two million IDPs, and another 275,000 plus refugees. More recently, just over the past two weeks, al-Bashir's soldiers and hired militia carried out at least crimes against humanity, if not genocidal actions, in the Nuba Mountains.
>
> ... There are also rumors afloat that Bashir is intent on firming up his hold over all regions of Sudan, as he continues to be miffed that southern Sudan, which Khartoum battled for some twenty years in an internecine war that sucked some two million into its deadly maw, seceded from the north. Next month, South Sudan formally becomes an independent state.
>
> As is the case in most violent conflicts across the globe, civilians (women, children, babies, the elderly) suffer most grievously. This is particularly true in Sudan because of Bashir's propensity for targeting an entire population of a region versus solely those engaged in fighting his troops. A colleague in the Nuba Mountains related the following examples to me over a satellite phone the past week:
> - Following aerial and ground attacks by Sudan Armed Forces (SAF), tens of thousands are on the run, seeking sanctuary anywhere they can find it;
> - At least two fresh mass graves were discovered late last week; approximately 1,000 dead bodies filled the one in Kadugli, the capital of South Kordofan;
> - In Kadugli, SAF soldiers and a ragtag assortment of others went door-to-door in search of SPLM/A members and supporters, executing them on the spot;
> - In Dilling, another town in South Kordofan, SAF soldiers and militia hunted down SPLM/A members and supporters and sliced their throats, leaving them to perish in puddles of their own blood; and,
> - In Kadugli, soldiers with the United Nations Mission in Sudan allegedly raped girls and women as the latter begged to be allowed into the UN compound as they feared certain death at the hands of the SAF and assorted militia [Totten, 2011, n.p.].

Alarmed at the new violence in Sudan and the fact that hardly any media were covering the unfolding events, I began knocking out one editorial after another and firing them off to newspapers around the globe. In toto, I authored and co-authored over 40 editorials, which appeared in newspapers (hard copy and/or in digital format) in Australia, Canada, Great Britain, South Sudan, Sudan, and the United States, among them being: the *Arkansas Democrat Gazette*, Canada Free Press, *The Globe and Mail*, *The Guardian*, Huffington Post, New York Times, Reuters[on-line], Seattle Times, *The South Sudan News*, and *The Sudan Tribune*. In the first month I wrote close to a dozen guest editorials, including the following: "Fear Pervades the Nuba Mountains that Sudan Government Intent on Genocide," *Armenian Weekly*, June 13, 2011; "Is Omar Hassan al-Bashir Up to Genocide Again?" *On the Ground* (Nicholas Kristof's Blog), *New York Times*, June 18, 2011; "Cold Blooded Mass Murder," *The Sudan Tribune*, July 3, 2011; and "Open Letter to Francis Deng: Now Is the Time to Prevent Genocide in the Nuba Mountains," *South Sudan News Agency*, July 13, 2011.

Some of the aforementioned efforts and articles caught the attention of a variety of journalists across the globe, which resulted in their quoting me about the tragedy unfolding in the Nuba Mountains: Nicholas D. Kristof, "Yet Again in Sudan?" *New York Times*, June 29, 2011; Jason Straziuso, "Satellite Evidence Indicates Mass Graves in Sudan," *The Guardian*, July 14, 2011, and Geoff Hill, "Human Rights Activists Warn of Genocide in Sudan," *Washington Times*, July 12, 2011.

Beginning in March 2012, I began writing and sending registered letters to various officials in the U.S. Government and the United Nations informing them about the crisis in the Nuba Mountains and suggesting what could be done to stanch the ongoing crimes against humanity and stave off potential genocide. Among them were: President Barack Obama; U.S. Secretary of State Hillary Clinton; U.S. Ambassador the UN Susan Rice; U.S. Special Envoy to Sudan Princeton Lyman; every single member of the U.S. Atrocities Prevention Board (APB); Members in both the U.S. House of Representatives and U.S. Senate; UN Secretary General Ban Ki-Moon; the UN Special Advisor on Genocide Prevention, and on and on. Each letter was signed by at least 45 scholars of genocide from across the globe, and in some cases up to sixty or more. Many of the scholars who co-signed one or more of the letters are among the most renowned in the field of genocide studies today: Dr. Israel Charny (Israel), Dr. Helen Fein (U.S.), Dr. Dominik Schaller (Germany), Dr. Roger Smith (U.S.), Dr. Taner Ackam (Turkey/U.S), Dr. Frank Chalk (Canada), Dr. Eric Weitz (U.S.), and Dr. Colin Tatz (Australia). The letter to Samantha Power, alone, in her role as the chair of the APB, was signed by 66 scholars from eight different countries: Australia, Canada, England, Germany, Israel, The Netherlands, the United States, and Wales.

While Princeton Lyman and several Members of Congress responded to the letters, not a single official with the APB did. One of the letters submitted to the APB was kindly entered into *The Congressional Record* by U.S. Senator Boozman (R-AR).

Concomitantly, I also began sending letters to the United States Holocaust Memorial Council's (USHMM) Committee on Conscience (CoC) about the crisis in the Nuba Mountains, inquiring why the COC—whose mandate, according to the USHMM's website, is "to alert the national conscience, influence policy makers, and stimulate worldwide action to confront and work to halt acts of genocide or related crimes against humanity"—had failed to address the crisis. Letters were sent to William S. Parsons (Chief of Staff of the USHMM), Michael Abramowitz (Director of the USHMM'S Center for Genocide Prevention and contact person for the CoC), and Michael Chertoff (the standing Chair of the CoC). To their credit, they responded to each and every letter. To their discredit, they often failed to address the specific questions posited in the letters. (For a detailed discussion of this effort, see my article entitled "Paying Lip Service to R2P and Genocide Prevention: The Muted Response of the U.S. Atrocities Prevention Board and the USHMM's Committee on Conscience to the Crisis in the Nuba Mountains" in *Genocide Studies and Prevention: An International Journal*.)

A Challenge and the Formation of a Small Team of Activists

In January 2012 rumors began to circulate that either the United Nations and/or the United States was/were contemplating the establishment of a humanitarian corridor in the Nuba Mountains. The rumors continued apace through April but mysteriously and abruptly ended in May. That was when I decided I had to do something, but initially I wasn't sure what that should be. Finally, in late June, I wrote an article, "Obama's Empty Promises to Halt Genocide Leave It to Us to Act," which was published in the *South Sudan News* (June 28, 2012). The conclusion read as follows:

> One has to really wonder what lessons the world—leaders and ordinary citizens alike—has learned from [past genocides]. Even those who espouse such heartfelt sentiments/words/phrases such as "Never Again!" are among those who look away when new tragedies break out —and here I include former survivors of genocide, scholars, and educators at all levels. And if they don't look away, then far too often they stand slack jawed and silent. Neither is admirable; and, in fact, both reactions are unconscionable.
>
> Not one to suggest that others should pursue an avenue I am not willing to undertake, I shall place my name at the top of the list to take part in any of the above suggestions [which included hauling food up to the Nuba Mountains people] that gain traction. *Those willing to step up and be counted and thus avoid the tag of being a bystander in the face of certain crimes against humanity and potential genocide by attrition can contact me at samstertotten@gmail.com* [Totten, 2011, n.p.].

A week or so after the article was published I received a call from a fellow named John Jefferson, an African American businessman and evangelical Christian from California. He said an acquaintance of his, Billy White, an old Sudan hand, now based in South Sudan, had sent him a copy of my article and challenged him to act upon it. His introduction was followed by, "Were you really serious about the challenge and about being ready, willing and able to act?"

"Without a doubt," I replied.

In our brief conversation we agreed to try to put together a small team to begin hauling food up to the Nuba. As soon as we got off the phone we began calling those individuals who we thought would be up for the challenge. Jefferson contacted several fellow evangelical Christians who had spent time in Sudan at one point of time or another, and I contacted several scholars, including Dr. John Hubbel Weiss, Associate Professor of History at Cornell University, who ended up being the only scholar (aside from myself) who was willing to join the effort.

Shortly thereafter, seven individuals took part in a conference call. There was a consensus that we needed to act immediately. Essentially, the members of this new group (which ended up being called, against my wishes, End Nuba Genocide (ENG)) agreed that we would step up and do what the international community and individual nations were not willing to do: (a) first and foremost, insert food to those in desperate need in the Nuba Mountains; (b) raise funds to cover the cost of purchasing food; and (c) spread the word far and wide about the crisis by contacting the media, writing guest commentaries and editorials for newspapers and blogs, contacting and meeting with Members of Congress, and informing anti-genocide activist groups of our actions. We also agreed that each one of us would cover our own travel expenses (the cost of flights, ground travel, accommodations, and food) so that all of the funds we raised would solely go towards the purchase of food for the Nuba.

In May 2012, against my advice, due to the fact that it was the beginning of the rainy season in the Nuba, ENG made its first foray into the Nuba Mountains. The team's truck got bogged down in the viscous mud that is par for the course throughout the Nuba during the rainy season, forcing the team members to load the food on their backs and wearily slog for miles to their destinations. Much to the team members' credit they slogged through the rain and mud and actually got some of the food delivered. Still, it was a lesson hard earned.

December 2012/January 2013 Mission to the War Torn Nuba Mountains

In December 2012/January 2013, I volunteered to oversee the insertion of the next load of food into the Nuba Mountains. The ENG group raised $30,000.00 USD and arranged to purchase 30 tons of food in Kampala, Uganda, and to have it trucked to the Yida Refugee Camp in South Sudan (just across the border from Sudan). From there I would accompany the truck in order to accomplish the mission.

After my interpreter Ramadan Tarjan and I arrived in Juba (the capital of South Sudan), we were informed by the Secretary General of the Episcopal Church of Sudan, who was serving as our intermediary, that the lorry ENG hired was due in Juba within a day or two and would leave Juba on Friday, December 20th and likely arrive in Yida on the 23rd or 24th.

Before heading to Yida, I obtained a permit (the organization that provided me with it must remain unnamed) to travel through rebel-held territory in the state of South Kordofan, Sudan. I also obtained the latest information in regard to both the ground fighting and bombing in the region.

On the 21st, Ramadan and I hopped a World Food Program plane and arrived in Yida about noon. Much to our dismay, the lorry neither arrived on the 23rd nor the 24th. And there was no sign of it on the morning of the 25th. By that time people began kidding us about "Sudan time."

Deciding that we couldn't wait any longer, I purchased close to a thousand dollars worth of sorghum, dried beans, cooking oil, salt and sugar, and we took off for the Nuba at about 10:00 a.m. Christmas day.

After crossing into Sudan, we headed towards Kauda along the dusty, rutted road. Along the way we were slowed down as a result of a series of makeshift roadblocks manned by the SPLA–N rebels. At each of the eight checkpoints, each of us was asked who we were, where we were going and why. We also had to hand over our paperwork (in my case, the permit issued to me, plus a letter of introduction from the Nuba Mountains Relief, Rehabilitation and Development Organization (NRRDO) stating who I was and the purpose of my travel).

As one can imagine, it was a radically different experience in the Nuba this time around, for when I had been there last, war had not yet broken out. In fact, almost everything was different—I could no longer fly directly to Kauda, as the GoS had established a no-fly zone in the region; instead of simply flying into the Nuba without a visa as I had previously, I was now required to obtain a pass from the rebels in order to travel through rebel-held territory; reaching my ultimate destination now meant traveling by truck across the border, from South Sudan into South Kordofan, Sudan, and making my way north for eight to eleven hours along body banging roads versus simply getting off a plane and walking a mile or two into the closest town. Everyone was now hyper vigilant regarding the sight or sound of any aircraft in the sky, knowing full well that they would be manned by GoS pilots who were likely carrying out an aerial attack. When in a compound or speaking with locals near their *tukuls* or in a *suq*, I made a point of always

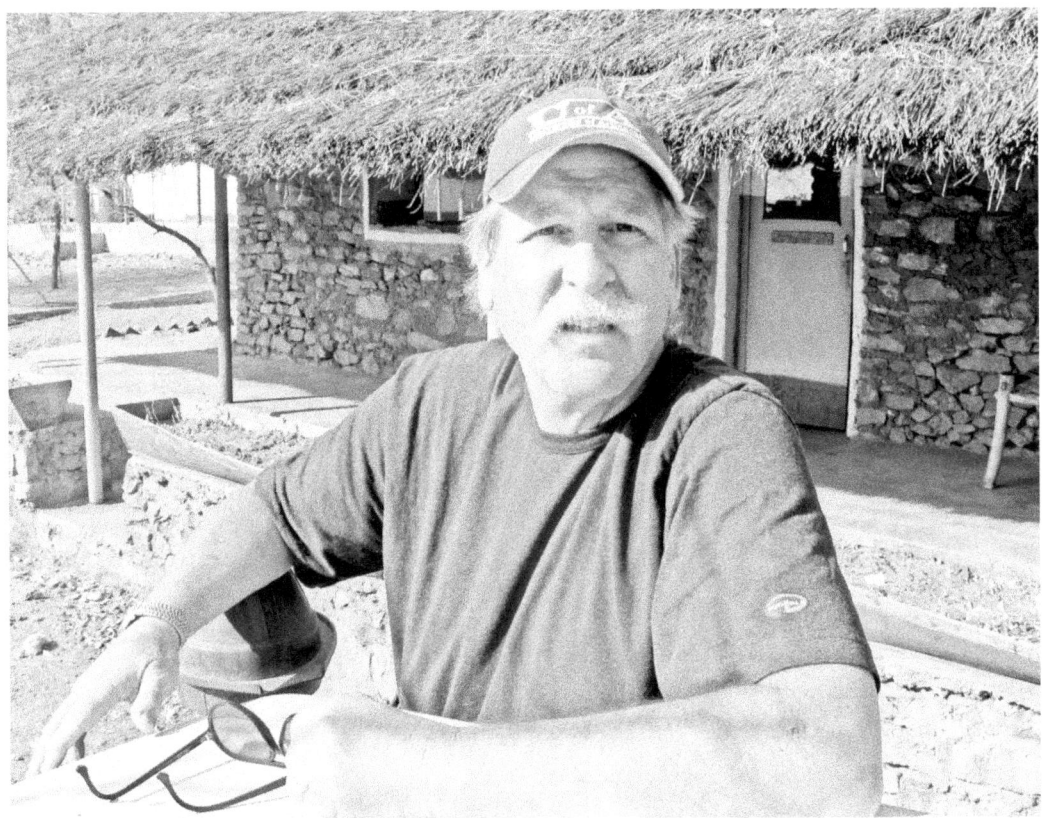

The author in Kauda, Nuba Mountains, Sudan (Samuel Totten).

checking to see where the holes that served as bomb shelters were located should there be an aerial attack. I was well aware of the fact that far too many civilians had not been vigilant enough and as a result had died horrific deaths from the shards of shrapnel that decapitated them, sliced off arms and legs, or caused other grievous injuries.

As we were about to pass through a place called Kurchee, scores of people in their best clothes were exiting a small church. Some men waved us down. One of them was the cousin of Bishop Andudu, one of the major leaders in the Nuba Mountains. He wondered where we were going. When we told him, he suggested that we take a short rest at the NRRDO compound which was up ahead about a half mile.

After we settled under some shade trees in the dusty compound, men—mainly in pairs and threes—began trickling in and taking seats around us. At first, I thought they were simply coming over to offer Christmas wishes, but I soon discovered that on his own volition and without informing us, the cousin of the bishop had called together some fifteen local pastors and informed them about the fact that we were delivering food to the Nuba.

Automatically, the pastors assumed we were delivering the food to them so that they could disseminate it to those in need in the immediate locale. They also assumed that the food was for anyone who was hungry versus, in reality, those who were in most dire need (i.e., those who were suffering from severe malnutrition or worse, did not have access to their farms, had no stores of food to rely on, and/or did not have the financial means to purchase foodstuffs for their families).

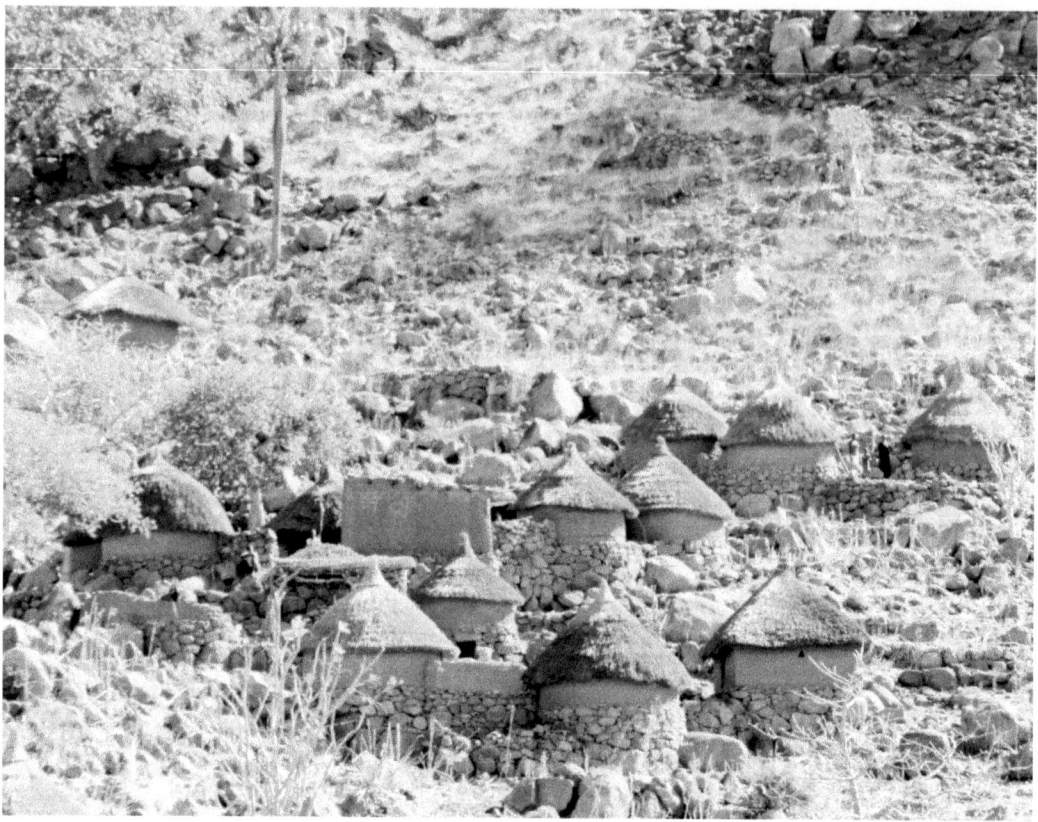

Tukuls (homes) near Kurchee, South Kordofan, Sudan (Samuel Totten).

Intent on making myself understood, I started afresh. The pastors were not pleased with the "revised" message and it caused some hard feelings. In the end, however, following lengthy discussion, we came to a meeting of the minds, which in turn seemed to assuage the pastors. It no doubt helped that I readily agreed to provide the pastors with half of the food I had just purchased in Yida. They said they would split it among each congregation and get it out to those congregants in most need.

That evening, as a number of us were standing around talking in the NRRDO compound, an Antonov came in so low I could make out lettering on its wings. That was my introduction to the fear induced by them. From that day forward, each and every time I heard or spotted an Antonov I made a mad dash for one of the "bomb shelters."

While we were in Kurchee, whenever an Antonov passed overhead and continued south they were met with loud rounds from the rebels' anti-aircraft gun. Suddenly, it really felt as if we were in a war zone. (Be that as it may, the area was not as militarized as I expected it to me. More about this below.)

We decided to wait in Kurchee a day or so for the lorry with the food (we had been told by the locals that no such lorry had passed by in weeks). While waiting I set to work conducting interviews of both civilians and rebels (in regard to the latter, mainly those who had been shot and were convalescing at their family's compounds) about their experiences both during the genocide by attrition and/or the current crisis in the Nuba Mountains.

Several interviews were abruptly interrupted by the sound of the heavy drone of an Antonov. Everyone automatically scanned the skies above. Not infrequently, an interviewee would jump up, yelling, "Get in the hole!" and race towards the nearest one. While most interviews were picked up again, the flow of the interviews had been disrupted and were often difficult to get back on track.

After waiting for four days and still no sign of the lorry with the food, I decided we should head north to Kauda so that we could deliver the rest of the food we had purchased in Yida.

In Kauda, we met with Mr. Daoud Sidiq, Deputy Commissioner of the South Kordofan Relief and Rehabilitation Committee. He informed us that any food to be delivered to the people of the Nuba Mountains should (*and, indeed, must*) go through GAC (a consortium of all local, regional and international groups operating in the Nuba Mountains, which was established for the express purpose of systematically delivering food to those in most critical need in the region). He further explained that GAC conducted needs' assessments, handled the distribution of the food, and conducted both formative and post evaluations of its efforts in order to constantly ascertain whether those most truly in need of food were receiving it and that the food was not being handed out in a scattershot fashion.

Again, the lorry with the food was nowhere to be found. As a result, I decided to

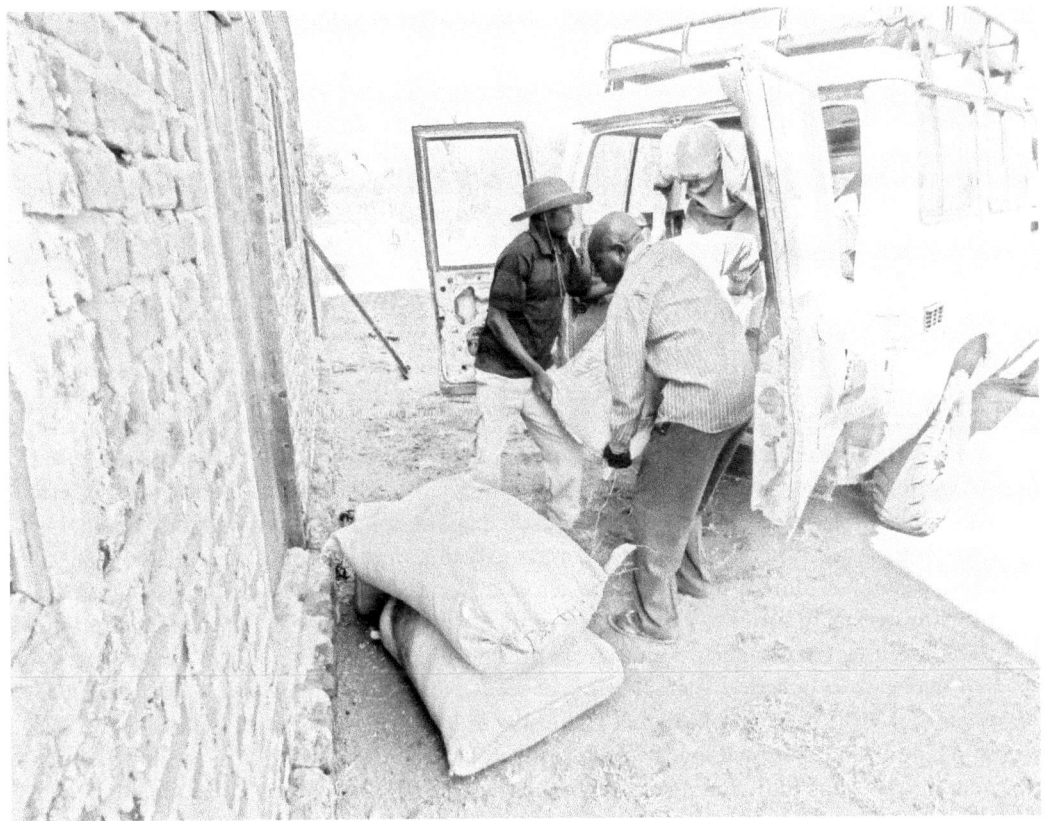

The author's team unloading food for the Nuba people in Kauda, Nuba Mountains, Sudan (Samuel Totten).

head back to Yida (a nine to eleven hour drive) in order to purchase more food so that we could haul more up to Kauda. I figured that since I was in the region and had the cash with which to purchase food I should deliver as much as possible. And thus we did. (As for the lorry, it ended up making it to Yida some three weeks later, two weeks after I had already left for the States. The food, though, was safely delivered to the GAC in Kauda.)

What follows herein are select notes from the report I wrote up vis-à-vis this mission:

Terrorism Via the Skies

Government of Sudan Antonov bombers fly sorties over the Nuba Mountains on a regular basis, almost daily, wreaking havoc. They largely target areas where relatively large numbers of people gather, such as *suqs* (open air markets), schools, compounds of nongovernmental organizations, and farmland.

The bombs are creating terror within the Nuba Mountains, forcing some to seek shelter in caves along the mountainsides, frightening people from their farms, and resulting in horrific carnage. Many have lost their lives to the shrapnel that shears off heads, legs, and arms and/or grounds chests, backs, stomachs, etc., into grisly masses of blood, skin, bones, appearing for all the world as if they had just been processed in a slaughterhouse.

There were some 55 bombings during the two weeks we were in the Nuba. Whenever we were traveling in our Land Cruiser and we heard the drone of an Antonov, we raced to the closest *wadi* and hid among the trees.

The planes flying overhead are a constant and unnerving fact of every day life in the Nuba Mountains.

Food, Hunger and the Potential of a Looming Crisis That Could Be Catastrophic

As we headed up and into the Nuba almost every single person we passed and/or spoke with looked healthy and able-bodied. Put another way, no one appeared to be struggling as they walked along the roads, attended to their cows, pumped water, etc. And while everyone we spoke with complained about not having enough food and being constantly hungry, no one appeared dangerously thin or on the cusp of death from a lack of food. Furthermore, I did not come across anyone who had resorted to eating leaves, roots or insects in order to remain alive, which rumors I had heard in the States led me to believe I would regularly come across in the Nuba.

I began to question the accuracy of what I had read and heard. I also began to wonder if I was naïve thinking that I'd be able to tell by a mere glance that someone was suffering from extreme hunger. I fully realized I would not be able to ascertain whether people were constantly hungry or malnourished, but I had thought I'd be able to detect those suffering from severe malnutrition as a result of their lethargy, weakness, etc.

Once I made it up to Mother of Mercy, the only fully equipped hospital in the Nuba Mountains, the first issue I raised with Dr. Tom Catena, the director of the hospital and the only surgeon in the entire region, was the magnitude of hunger in the region. I figured if anyone could fill me in on the situation it was Dr. Tom, as everyone in the Nuba refers to him. And I was right. Tom—a citizen of the U.S. and a graduate of Duke University Medical School—and his staff have seen the impact of hunger up close. Tall, slim and bespectacled with his hair shaved close to his head and dressed in green scrubs and wearing Crocs, Dr. Tom was a fount of information concerning the issue of hunger in the region: "May, June, July through August, the food situation up here was really terrible. Ninety and more people a day would be lined up outside the hospital doors in search of food, saying, 'We'll do any type of work there is for food.' The malnutrition rates at the time were very high." Continuing, he said, "What most [lay people] don't appreciate is that hunger is not just about being hungry, as bad as that is. It has a ripple effect that can be—and is—devastating. TB increases, pneumonia increases, and malaria is particularly dangerous as a result of sub-nutrition. We see more broken arms. Children are forced to climb trees in search of food, they fall from the trees and break their arms. We actually had to amputate the arm of a small boy after someone had put a tourniquet on his arm [and complications set in]."

Then he added: "The food situation is dire here. People have harvested one sack of produce from their farms, last season they had harvested ten sacks. What we may be looking at this coming rainy season could be a lot worse, especially if people are not able to plant their crops. Not only did we have the constant bombing and terrorizing of people to the point where they were fearful of farming as usual but the rainy season was shorter and thus people ended up with far less food than usual. Many people up here have died from malnutrition. Eventually, bodies just shut down."

The Goal of the SPLA–N

During my informal conversations as well as my formal interviews with both rebel commanders and rebel fighters I was informed that the intent of the SPLA–North was to take the fight all the way to Khartoum in order to overthrow the regime of Omar al-Bashir. When I commented that that was obviously easier said than done, noting that the Second Sudanese Civil War (1983–2005) had lasted some 20 years and resulted in some two million deaths, to a man I was told some variation of: "It does not matter. We are going to do what it takes to overthrow al-Bashir."

"And then what?" I asked.

"We want to replace it with a government representing all of the people, not just the Arabs; one that will respect everyone's basic human rights, including religious freedom. We want a nation where all have equal opportunity. We will let the people of Sudan decide who they want for a leader and how they want to run the country." (Some, usually the least educated, said they had no idea what would happen once the SPLA–N won the war, stating that such a decision would be made by the leaders of the SPLM/A–North.)

My response was, "That, of course, would be ideal, but look at the incredible growing pains South Sudan is going through right now, both in regard to its leadership and the violent and deadly confrontations ripping it apart."

The general response was, "We will be different."

All I could muster was "Hmmmm."

Not as Militarized as I Had Expected the Region to Be

Even with the Antonovs in the air, I was surprised that the region was not more militarized. While we came across gaggles of rebel soldiers hanging around the makeshift roadblocks, the occasional pairs of armed rebels patrolling on foot throughout the desert and *suqs*, and, though less frequently, lorries and Land Cruisers packed with soldiers, the region really did not feel as if it were on a war footing. Those rebels we spoke with, though, told me that the closer to the front one gets, the more heavily militarized the region becomes.

In regard to the latter point, I spoke with an AP photographer who had made it out to the front around December 19th and he reported that for several hours he witnessed helicopter gun ships strafing the area near Kadugli. Furthermore, back in Nairobi (on the 8th of January), I spoke with Ryan Boyette and he told me that several weeks earlier he had taken a group out of journalists out to the front where they witnessed a GoS tank still smoldering from being hit by a RPG and dead bodies strewn all over the desert as a result of recent fighting.

Another ENG Mission

In May of 2013, another team headed into the Nuba Mountains, but this time the starting point was Malakal, a river town along the Nile. The team trucked 25 tons of food into an area (Kao Nyaro) where we had heard that people were literally starving to death. The trip was treacherous in that not only were the roads extremely bad but the temperature ranged between 110 degrees and 115 degrees Fahrenheit, in a region where none of the vehicles have air conditioning. Along the way, the team came across the corpses of Nuba civilians along the dusty road. All had perished from starvation. (For a detailed discussion and description of this remarkable effort, see two other essays in this book, one by George Tutu and one by John Jefferson, respectively.)

May 2014: An Aborted Effort to Complete a Mission in the Nuba Mountains

In May of 2014, I attempted to carry out a second mission on my own, but once I made it to Juba (the capital of South Sudan), I could get no further. Due to both the civil war raging all across South Sudan and the threat of a looming famine there, most non-governmental organizations had canceled their flights into the Yida Refugee Camp, which is where I planned to cross over into Sudan. Locals warned me that it was virtually impossible to drive the long distance from Juba to Yida due to the insecurity in the region. Fighters on both sides of the civil war had carried out horrific atrocities—and were still doing so—and thus I was told, any attempt to make the drive would be tantamount to suicide. After sitting in Juba for five frustrating days in search of a flight to the South

Opposite, top: Rebels ramping up for war—January 2016, Nuba Mountains. *Opposite, bottom:* Rebels just in from fighting the Sudanese Armed Forces near Kadugli, South Kordofan, Sudan (both by Samuel Totten).

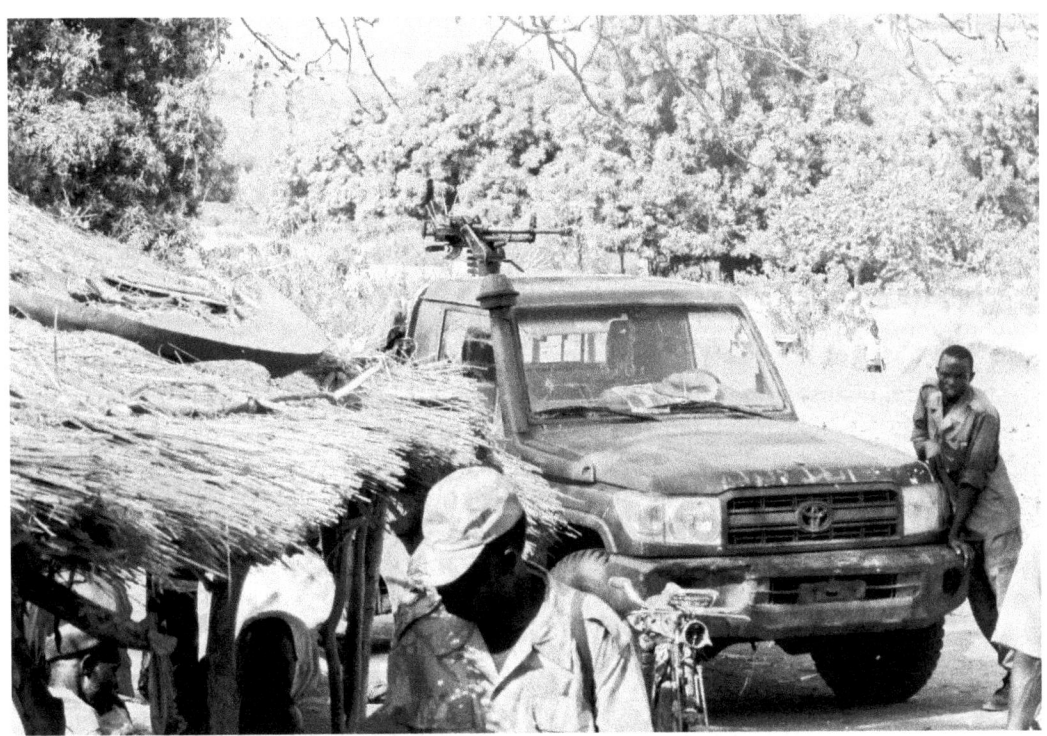

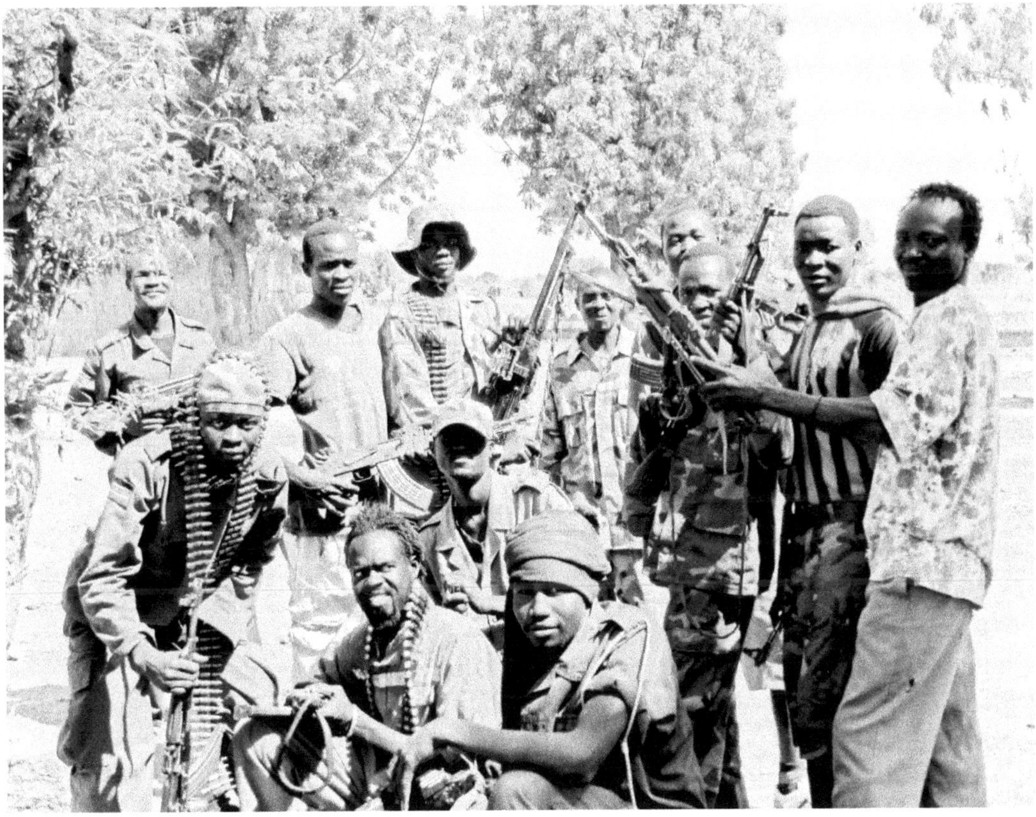

Sudan/Sudan border, I reluctantly called off the mission. Disturbed at having wasted well over $3,000.00 of my own money on flights and housing in Juba, I decided to take the bus to Nairobi: a 31 hour ride across from Juba to Kampala, Uganda onto Nairobi, thus saving 250 plus dollars by not catching a plane.

With the rainy season about to begin in Sudan I had to wait six months until it ended to attempt the next mission.

Resigning from ENG and Working Solo

Ultimately, between 2012 and spring 2014, ENG undertook four missions into the Nuba Mountains for the express purpose of hauling in food. By mid-2014 various members began to branch out and take on different projects in the Nuba Mountains (such projects have included, for example, proselytizing and bringing people to Christ; producing documentary films about the situation in the Nuba Mountains today, with a particular focus on the plight of the Christians in the region; and recording songs and music that the Nuba use to celebrate Christmas). While some of the new projects continued to provide medical aid and/or food, such efforts were secondary. In light of that, in May 2014 I resigned from ENG in order to focus solely on inserting food to those in most critical need in the Nuba Mountains.

December 2014–January 2015: Second Mission to the Nuba Mountains—Delivery of Food to Those in Critical Need

While in the process of obtaining a permit in Juba that would allow me to travel through rebel territory in South Kordofan, I was informed that virtually everyone in the Nuba Mountains was hungry, with many, if not most, eating but once a day. When I made it clear that my intent was to deliver food to those in most critical need, I was informed that I'd find such individuals (a) far from the good size towns, villages and *suqs*; (b) in those areas in closest proximity to the ongoing ground battles; and (c) up in the mountains where they have sought shelter in caves in the hope that they'd provide adequate protection from the aerial bombings by the GoS.

In Juba I also purchased two boxes of bottled water for the trip, which I considered essential since there were rumors that cholera had broken out along the Nile River—just upriver from where I was crossing over the border into Sudan from South Sudan.

On December 3, my interpreter, Alexander Ramadan Tarjan, and I left Juba at 11:00 a.m. on a World Food Programme (WFP) flight (a twelve-seater jet) and arrived in Yida at 1:00 p.m. As our plane taxied down the newly expanded and graded dirt runway in Yida, I noticed a group of people gathered around an even smaller plane (a four-seater). I spotted a fellow unloading something from the plane and called out to Alexander, "I think that's Ryan Boyette over there…. In fact, it is! I can't believe this!"

Ryan, the former director of the Samaritans Purse project in the Nuba Mountains and the person who first welcomed me to the Nuba Mountains back in 2010, was on his way up to the house he built for his new family high up in the Nuba Mountains. (Ryan, a U.S. citizen, has lived in the Nuba Mountains for the past thirteen years, is fluent in

Arabic, and is almost universally known by everyone in the Nuba Mountains.) As soon as I greeted his wife, Jazira, and their little boy, Eben, Ryan and I joyfully greeted one another, and within seconds he asked what I was doing in the region. After I told him, he asked me if I wanted to ride up to the Nuba with him and spend the night in his compound. Since I had not seen Ryan, Jazira and Eben in well over a year and a half—not to mention the fact that if anyone has a solid sense of what is happening in the Nuba Mountains it is Ryan (and this is particularly true since he is the co-founder and director of *Nuba Reports*, a regularly produced newsletter about the ongoing situation in the Nuba Mountains by his citizen journalists' team)—I readily accepted his kind invitation.

Before taking off for the Nuba, I met with the current coordinator of the Samaritan's Purse unit in Yida, and when I asked him if refugees were still pouring into the refugee camp, he said: "It's slowed down a lot. Only about 500 people a month are coming in these days." I quickly did a calculation in my head and thought, "While that may be a lot fewer than in the past, it's still some 6,000 people a year." What I was to discover during the course of this mission was that it's also a fact that each and every month more and more people are being forced from their villages and ending up in internally displaced persons (IDPs) camps in forlorn parts of the Nuba Mountains.

Before heading up to the Nuba, I purchased four thousand dollars worth of food (primarily large 100 pound bags of sorghum, 100 pound bags of lentils, large jugs of cooking oil, and 100 pound bags of sugar) and loaded them on to the Land Cruiser I had rented for the mission (which Ramadan was going to escort up to the Nuba). We quickly discovered that *no one* had any salt for sale. In fact, bulk quantities of any type of food were scarce in the *suq*—which was largely due to the fact that the ongoing civil war in the new nation of The Republic of South Sudan made the long, arduous drive from the markets in either Kampala, Uganda or Juba to Yida both treacherous and often deadly for the lorry drivers. It is also not uncommon for trucks to be hijacked and their drivers left stranded in the middle of nowhere. As a result, there was not only a dearth of food, but that which was available was being sold at sky high prices.

We ended up leaving Yida about three in the afternoon that same day, and reached the Boyette's mountainside home around eleven that evening. During the journey Ryan informed me about the major towns and territory held by the SPLM/A–N as well as the major towns and territory held by the GoS. He also informed me of the ever-increasing use of MIGs and Sukhoi Su-24 attack jets by the GoS to carry out attacks on what they perceived as key towns, along with areas held by the rebels. Along the way, he duly pointed out the burned out carcasses of a couple of NGO-owned trucks that had recently dared to enter the region and had been bombed by the GoS' Antonovs.

Along the way we did not detect any aircraft flying overhead. That was not unusual, though, as many, if not most, of the aerial attacks are carried out against civilian populations from early to mid-morning—and noon at the latest.

The main topic I was most interested in discussing with Ryan as we made our way up to Kauda was where those Nuba civilians were located who were in most critical need of food. He said two places where food was desperately needed was just outside of Kurchee and in a place called Kwalib. He said that those outside Kurchee—that is, those residing in villages closest to the front near Kadugli—often did not have enough food because the various freelance humanitarian groups bringing in food to the Nuba could not reach the area due to the ferocity of the battles.

Toward dusk, a lorry driven by rebels (with a dozen or more heavily armed rebels riding in the back of it), towing a large anti-anti-aircraft gun on wheels, passed us as it headed south. We figured the rebels were on their way towards Kadugli where a ground battle was raging.

After spending a night at the Boyette's mountaintop home, my team—Alexander Tarjan, my interpreter, and Daniel Luti, our driver, a highly educated 27-year-old Nuba Mountains civilian who resides in Kauda with his wife and baby daughter—headed into Kauda to meet with the local commissioner, who we had to see in order to obtain permission to travel to Kwalib. We also needed to obtain a letter of introduction (written in Arabic) from the commissioner in Kauda to the commissioner in Kwalib. Since the Kauda commissioner was in a meeting, Alexander and Daniel decided they wished to get some lunch in the local *suq*. While they were eating, an Antonov flew overhead and everyone—shop owners and customers—scrambled and jumped into one of the holes that now serve as "bomb shelters." The Antonov did not drop a bomb but its appearance was a precursor to what we would face in the coming days.

That afternoon we finally met with the commissioner and obtained the requisite permission and letter of introduction we needed. We then proceeded to the *suq* in Kauda, where we purchased another eight bags of sorghum (each of which weighed about 200 pounds) to add to what we had already purchased in Yida the day before. Once again, though, no one in the *suq* had any salt for sale.

By the time we completed the purchase of the food, loaded it, and headed out to the main dirt road leading towards the town of Heiban, another major town in the Nuba Mountains, the sun was beginning to set. As we pulled into Heiban it was pitch black.

While I was in favor of driving through the night to Kwalib, Daniel was adamant that it would be too dangerous as he said GoS soldiers move at night, and if we were caught by them it could result in our deaths, and if not death then potential imprisonment. Ultimately, we spent the night in Heiban. I was put up in a room at an institute that trained future Christian pastors. The head of the institute informed us that the GoS bombed the area so frequently that all classes for the last several months had been held in the caves of the mountain that loom over the institute. Since the GoS generally does not bomb at night, the students and instructors returned to the campus each evening to spend the night in their respective residence halls.

The next day we got up before sunrise and headed to Kwalib. As we proceeded to Kwalib—which turned out to be a seven hour trip of miserable bouncing and jolting along the worn and pot-holed road—we kept our eyes out for Antonovs and jets. We were all a bit on edge because everything we had heard the past several days suggested that sooner or later we would be confronted with one or the other, if not both.

As we got to closer to Kwalib, the topography changed rather dramatically. Instead of the mountains gradually rising from the flat desert floor in sheer walls of rock and plateaus, the land at the foot of the mountain was "littered" with boulders of all sizes—from the size of bowling balls to mid-size cars. On the ledges of the mountains above, huge boulders sat perched at precarious angles. My immediate thought was: the largest boulders might be great places to crouch against in the event of an aerial attack. Eventually, the dusty road led us to a small, makeshift internally displaced persons camp. After asking around for the local commissioner, we were led to a good sized compound. The commissioner informed us that over the past several months there had been a lot of fighting, along with a lot of bombing. "In fact," he said, "this morning, Antonovs attacked villages near here."

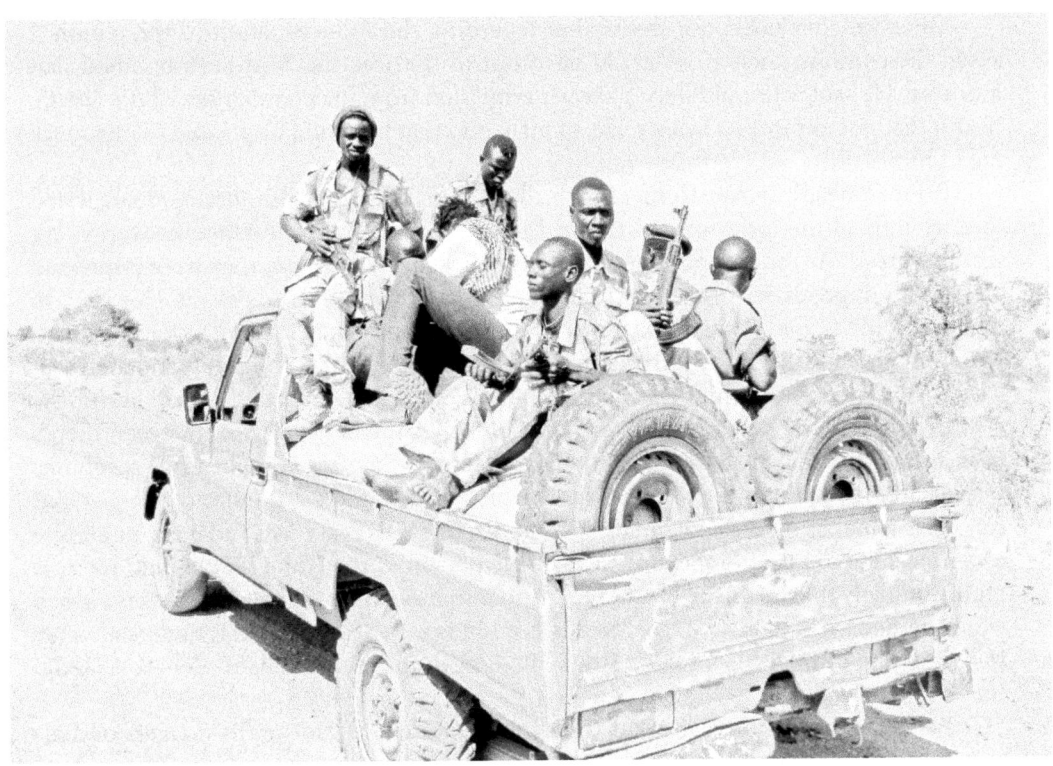

Traveling with SPLA-N in Kwalib, Nuba Mountains, Sudan (Samuel Totten).

He also said that food was at a bare minimum in the area, and that no one had had salt for quite a while. I was later informed by Daniel that people really craved salt and sugar due to the fact that sorghum, which is the main staple in the Nuba Mountains, tastes terrible when not salted or sweetened. Many, he said, have a hard time even getting the sorghum down without something to mask the taste.

Of course, all human bodies need salt. And unlike people in the U.S. (and other First World nations), the Nuba do not eat processed foods, such as canned vegetables, potato chips, pizzas, etc., all of which contain plenty of, if not far too much, salt.

While common knowledge over the past several decades has strongly suggested that too much salt can raise a person's blood pressure, which puts him/her at increased risk of serious health problems, such as heart disease and stroke, what is much less discussed is the impact of having little to no salt in one's diet. In this regard, Harvard Medical School published a paper in 2010 titled "Salt and Your Health: Part I: The Sodium Connection."

> Make no mistake about it: salt is essential for human health. The average adult's body contains 250 grams of sodium—less than 9 ounces, or about the amount in three or four saltshakers. Distributed throughout the body, salt is especially plentiful in body fluids ranging from blood, sweat, and tears to semen and urine.
>
> Sodium is absorbed from the gastrointestinal tract, always bringing water along with it. It is the major mineral in plasma, the fluid component of blood, and in the fluids that bathe the body's cells. *Without enough sodium, all these fluids would lose their water, causing dehydration, low blood pressure, and death* [italics added, n.p.].

Once we concluded our discussion regarding the food situation in the region, I asked the commissioner if we could head out to the area that had been bombed that morning. He said we would need to seek permission from the commander of the SPLA-N unit that was encamped nearby. He, in turn, said that he would be pleased to introduce me to him.

Prior to heading over to meet with the commander, the commissioner suggested that we unload the food we had trucked up in a large, empty warehouse nearby. We readily agreed. As the commissioner and his colleagues looked on, they were impressed and greatly appreciative of the amount of food that we were able to deliver. However, to my eye it didn't look all that impressive as it sat piled up in such a large space. Though I kept my thoughts to myself, the issue gnawed away at me. As it did, I, fortunately—at least for my peace of mind—recalled what Dr. Tom Catena had told me earlier in the year during an interview I conducted with him: "For the better part of the year, there's been no food available in the market, and the few willing to sell their food (sorghum) [are] charging ten times the usual price. The price of one *malwa* (the size of a large paint can) [has gone] as high as 45 Sudanese pounds (US$15)." Forty five Sudanese pounds is a significant amount of money for the average person in the Nuba Mountains, and it is highly unlikely that he or she would be able to purchase more than ten or so cans (which would amount to $150.00 USD) before his/her funds were sapped. That is understandable in light of the fact that the average annual income in the region is equivalent to $348.00 U.S. dollars.

I also attempted to recall what Catena had told me regarding the dangers of malnutrition, which many people in the region are suffering from:

> Malnutrition and its less severe cousin, subnutrition, impair the body's immune system, thus rendering it more susceptible to any disease. Therefore, a poorly nourished person is unable to fight off infection as well as someone who is well nourished. *Simple problems like a simple pneumonia and diarrhea become life threatening in the malnourished. Malnutrition in pregnancy leads to low birth weight babies, who are more prone to disease.* The malnourished mother might produce inadequate quantities of breast milk, thus compounding the problem for the already vulnerable neonate.
>
> *Lack of food also drives people to look for food sources elsewhere—sometimes eating foods which contain poisons or other non-nutritive foods. Lack of food drives children into the trees to fetch wild fruits, with the result that many fall out of the trees, sustaining fractures and head injuries.* We had many children come in with both limb and skull fractures as a result of foraging for food in the trees.

While my recall of such facts tamped down my discontent a bit, it also kept the fire in my belly alive in regard to hauling in as much food as possible to those facing such challenges.

After unloading the food, we hiked over to meet the local commander of the SPLA-N. He and his men were encamped in an area surrounding a dry pond which was protected on three sides by the giant walls of the mountain looming above. Upon our entrance to the camp, we were told that the commander was away but that we could meet with his second in command, a colonel. We were then escorted to a small enclosure closed off with a fence made of tree branches and dried sorghum leaves. Numerous rebels were resting on benches along a table. Shortly, the colonel appeared, and after I introduced myself and told him why we were in the region (to deliver the food) I asked him if he would grant us permission to view the area that had been bombed that morning. He readily agreed, and said that he would accompany us. He then asked if we could travel in our Land Cruiser. I said yes, and then he said he would drive. Six of his men, all carrying Kalashnikovs, jumped on the back of the truck with Alexander. I hopped in the cab, and we took off with the colonel at the wheel.

Within fifteen minutes or so, we reached the area that had been bombed. We got out and walked around the blackened area that had been set afire. I leaned over and felt the ground. It was still warm and smoldering in places. As we looked around I noticed that not a single person was in the nearby village.

The colonel said that he wanted to take us out to several other areas that had been bombed recently. As we drove north, it was eerie as village after village was totally devoid of people. They were, in fact, veritable ghost towns.

Continuing on, we came to a large dry *wadi* whose banks were extremely steep. On the other side of the *wadi* was a forest of trees. The colonel slowed down and then came to a complete stop, and yelled something to his men in Arabic. All of the rebels jumped out of the back of the truck with their weapons at the ready. One rebel crossed the *wadi* and disappeared down the rough dirt track; two pairs of rebels took positions on each side of the truck about ten yards out and walked along with the truck as we moved forward. Finally, two rebels spread out behind us, following the truck. The colonel said that the forest of trees presented GoS soldiers with good places to hide and set up an ambush, and thus he was taking a precaution by having his men on the ground at the ready with their weapons.

Once we crossed the *wadi* and traveled for a hundred yards or so all of the rebels climbed back on board the truck. We then proceeded to drive out to a mesa overlooking a huge valley. As we all walked across the field, the colonel pointed out places (basically holes gouged into the earth) where Antonovs had bombed the area.

At the very lip of a cliff, the colonel pointed to the left and said that the town of Abri, which the GoS controlled, was less than 50 kilometers away (some 30 miles). In the opposite direction, a wall of smoke rose over a mountain range. The colonel said early that morning two GoS jets had attacked a town where the smoke was billowing up, causing extensive damage and the death of some civilians.

On the way back to the rebels' camp, the colonel made a point of driving up and stopping at a series of points where bombs dropped by Antonovs had hit. We pulled up to at least a half dozen such sites. It was uncanny how the colonel knew exactly where the bombs had hit and how he could detect such sites as we were racing and jouncing across the roadless land. The sand covering the indentation of the holes was visibly different from the sand in the rest of the desert. While the desert sand was composed of distinct granules, the sand covering the bomb indentations was powdery. In certain cases, fragments from the bomb sat nearby.

At one hole near the village of Dhera, the colonel informed us that a woman who was a representative of the local council had been killed two weeks earlier. Six or seven large pieces of shrapnel, their edges twisted and razor sharp, were scattered about.

After returning to the rebels' camp, I decided that since it was still relatively early, we might as well head back to Kauda. First, though, I wanted to check out a dusty sad looking *suq* we had passed to see if there was any bulk food (sorghum, lintels, dried beans, salt or sugar) available that we could purchase in order to add to what we had already donated for those need in Kwalib. The first makeshift, open-air shop we approached had five bags of sorghum (100 pounds each), and we purchased them. All of the other merchants demanded such outlandish prices for the bulk food they had available that I refused to purchase it.

We returned to the commissioner's compound and delivered the additional five bags of sorghum, and then hit the road for Kauda. As we drove along the serpentine dirt road across the desert, the wall of smoke filling the sky in the distance appeared like a huge bruise.

As dusk approached and night fell, nerves were a little raw on the truck as Daniel was worried that we might end up coming across GoS soldiers on the move. When we finally made it to Heiban, he was visibly relieved.

Early the next morning we got up and headed back to the Yida Refugee Camp in South Sudan. About two hours out, a jeep-like truck mounted with a weapon with a huge barrel—a weapon known as a Bi-Camp—raced past us carrying four or five rebels. Fifteen or twenty minutes later we came across a borehole where a couple of kids were pumping water. The heat was sweltering and I wanted to soak my head and shirt in order to cool off. At the same time, Daniel decided to get a drink. As we were heading back to the truck I noticed he looked rather bedraggled. "You really look tired." When he answered that he was, I told him that I could take over driving. At first he was hesitant, but when I told him I'd driven all sorts of vehicles—from dump trucks to beach trams to jeeps—he asked, "But on dirt roads like this?" When I assured him I had, he gladly turned the wheel over to me.

About fifteen minutes later, we came upon a large *suq* at a place called Andhulu, which was having its market day. Thinking that we might get a better price on the food if I wasn't present during the bargaining session, Daniel suggested that I park the truck a good ways away from the heart of the *suq*, near a large tree that offered welcome shade from the hot sun, and wait alone with the truck.

Where I ended up parking was near where the rebels in the jeep with the mounted cannon had parked as well. A few rebels sat idly in the front seats but most of the others were nowhere to be seen. Also idling around the area were several camels tethered to trees, while five or six people sat under the nearby tree.

I got out of the truck and stood alongside of it watching the coming and going of the locals. Shortly, about a half dozen people approached me in quick succession and asked if they could have a ride. Some were heading to various villages south while others were heading all the way to the Yida Refugee Camp in South Sudan. I told all of them that we were in the process of purchasing a large load of food and once we loaded it if there was room then I would be glad to give them a lift.

A little later a young man who I assumed to be in his late teens or early twenties approached me and asked where I was heading. I told him we were heading to Yida. He explained that that he, too, was heading to Yida. I asked him why he was heading there, and he replied that he wished to complete his secondary level education. He said that as a result of all of the bombings and fighting in the Nuba Mountains most schools had shut down.

I noticed that the sleeve on his left arm was dangling loose, and thus I asked him, possibly too abruptly, how he had lost his arm. He simply replied, "Antonov." Right then and there I knew I would be giving him a ride no matter how much food we ended up purchasing.

Some 45 to 60 minutes later, Alexander and Daniel returned and said they had purchased six sacks of sorghum at a very good price. I pulled the vehicle over to the shop, and the shopkeeper and his guys began loading the bags of food (again, huge bags, weighing between 150 and 200 pounds). As I stood watching the activity in the *suq*, I noticed a hefty, white fellow a few feet from me taking photos. We introduced ourselves and struck up a conversation, but almost immediately someone in the crowd cried out, "Antonov!"

The fellow I had been speaking with, Brad Phillips, who heads up an organization called Persecution Project (which has humanitarian projects in both South Sudan and Sudan), whipped around towards the main dirt road and yelled, "Quick, let's find cover!" By the time we had sprinted up a small dirt incline leading to the dirt road and were about to cross it, someone yelled, "It's gone! It's going in a different direction."

Relieved, we both commented on how we had heard that Antonvos and attack jets had been active in the region. I actually found it somewhat surprising that the Antonov had not dropped bombs on the *suq* as the GoS generally likes to hit crowded areas swarming with people.

As we headed back towards the truck, Brad asked how much longer I was going to be in the Nuba Mountains and when I told him that I was heading back to Juba and then Nairobi on Monday, he said if I made it to Yida by Sunday he could give me a lift back to Juba in a cargo plane he had rented.

Hopping behind the wheel of the truck again, with Daniel sitting shotgun, I turned around and we headed down the road fronting the *suq*. Daniel pointed to a dirt track in the distance that veered off to the left and said I should take that, but I told him that since we had room on the truck I wanted to give some people a ride. For some reason, he didn't seem open to the idea, but when he didn't provide me with a concrete reason for his resistance I insisted, telling him that at a minimum I was intent on giving the young man with one arm a ride. He acquiesced and I pulled into the area where we had originally parked. When I called to the young man to hop on, it attracted the attention of not only the others who had asked about a ride but many more as well. Minutes later we pulled back onto the dirt road with eighteen passengers on the back of the truck, not counting Alexander who was riding back there as well. One of the passengers, I was to discover, was the Bishop of Debi.

We motored along a dusty track for 30 or 40 miles, moving at a snail's pace most of the way due to the fact the road had been washed out during the rainy season, towards a place called Tonguli, where we planned to drop off the food we had just purchased. As we approached Tonguli, we noticed a fairly large encampment to the right and a water point/pump nearby where several men were sitting under some large trees. Not far from the men sat a tiny makeshift open-air teashop. After pulling to a stop, I announced to everyone on the back of the truck that I had to meet with the local commissioner of Tonguli and that it might take fifteen to thirty minutes or more. Everyone got off the truck and headed over towards the teashop where there was a bench and some rocks one could sit on and rest.

As our passengers got water, Daniel set out to locate the commissioner, who, we had been told, was likely across the road in the large compound. In the meantime, I sat down with a good number of our passengers and chatted with them.

"Antonov!" someone shouted.

Everyone jumped up and scrambled for all they were worth. I jetted straight ahead, almost tripping over a young woman and a young man as all three of us raced down a short incline that led to a large, dry *wadi*. Once we reached the *wadi*, all three of us dropped down on our stomachs, inching as close as we could to the riverbank, and then ... waited.

Several minutes later, we heard people shouting that the plane had passed by. Incredibly relieved, the three of us got up and headed back up the dirt bank to the area where we had all been seated. As everyone came together again, the chatter focused on the close call, the immense relief everyone felt, and how lucky we were that the Antonov didn't bomb us.

Daniel showed up a few minutes later and said that he had located the commissioner. As we were about to head over to the commissioner's compound, the men over by the trees yelled, "Antonov!"

Again, everyone jumped up and headed in various directions. I, again, along with the same young man and woman, headed towards the dirt bank leading down to the *wadi*. But just as I reached the incline, one of the men under the trees yelled, *khawaja* [white man,] quick get down! Get down now!" Against my better judgment, I hit the ground and covered by head and neck with my hands the best I could.

I felt totally exposed and feared that my luck was about to run out. But again, the Antonov flew passed without dropping a bomb. After what seemed an interminably long time, someone called out, "It's gone! It's OK."

As I got to my knees and began to stand up, I saw Alexander starting to get up off the ground near the benches we had been sitting on. In the past—both during this trip and during an earlier trip in 2012–2013—he had been extremely cavalier about seeking safety when Antonovs approached and generally stood around as everyone else scrambled for cover. Both his cavalier attitude and the mocking tone he directed at me for scrambling for cover had grated on me back in 2012–2013, and we had had words about the matter.

"Alexander, what happened to your stance, 'if it's your time, it's your time'?" I called out as I stood up.

Smiling, he said, "This time it was too close," and we both broke out in laughter.

We—Alexander, Daniel, and I—immediately crossed over the road and entered the compound where the commissioner was seated. It was a ramshackle affair that served as home and office. In the distance, a beautiful, large two story stone building sat vacant. It had served as the commissioner's headquarters until he and his staff were forced to move out due to its being targeted by Antonovs.

The commissioner informed us that those Nuba residing high up in the mountains nearby were suffering terribly from a lack of food, and that what we had brought would help stave off the constant pangs of hunger they suffered on a daily basis and would, hopefully, also stave off severe malnutrition.

The commissioner told us that about a mile away was a civic building in which they could store the food until they could get it up to those people in most critical need, or until the people were informed about the food and could come down, pick it up and "foot it" back to where they were hiding in caves.

After collecting all of our passengers, the commissioner and several other men from the area hopped on the back of the truck as well. With many sitting precariously on the railings of the bed of the truck, I slowly pulled back onto the dirt track en route to the civil building.

"Antonov! Antonov!" several people yelled, as people leaped off the truck and made a run for it. I flung open the door of the truck and headed out into the desert trailing behind several other people. As I ran, I surveyed the land for something to hide behind (rocks, preferably) or hunker down into (a large fissure, crevice, or ravine), but to no avail. All there was was sandy desert. Figuring I had already taken too long to locate a place of potential safety—and well aware of the fact that most people in the Nuba Mountains who had been killed by shrapnel had remained upright—I hit the ground and yelled for the two individuals near me to do the same. They both hit the ground immediately.

A few minutes went by and then I heard loud chatter in the distance behind me. Quickly craning my neck around, I noticed that a number of individuals were up and walking back towards the truck. I hopped up and headed back to the truck as well but as I made my way around scrub brush a loud roar of laughter broke out up ahead. Baffled by the laughter, I immediately wondered whether someone on board the truck had played what he thought was a prank. As I got closer to the truck I shouted out over the laughter, "There wasn't an Antonov? This was just…" Someone shouted back, "No, there was an Antonov!" Several others added in quick succession, "It was close!" and "It came right over us!" The laughter, I figured, was nervous laughter or a shared sense of relief.

"Well, whoever saw the plane, good eye!" I said.

A young man in his early twenties said, "Yeah, all eyes on the sky!"

I laughed appreciatively and said, "Exactly! And keep it up!"

As I started to get back into the cab of the truck, I called up to the fellow who had come up with the phrase and said, "You know, that would be a great title for a book about what the Nuba are facing."

(On January 15, 2015, *Nuba Reports* issued a statement that during December 2014, the Nuba Mountains recorded more than 450 bombs, rockets and artillery dropped on civilian targets—the most in a single month since the war began in June 2011. "January shows no sign of slowing down.")

Once everyone was aboard again, we set out again for the civic society building. It only took us a matter of minutes to get there. The dirty and chipped plaster building was a long rectangle divided into three or four rooms. It took three, and sometimes, four guys to lift the huge, heavy bags up and out of the truck and another three or four to carry each bag into the room that was going to serve as the temporary warehouse.

After we said our goodbyes, we got back on the road toward Yida. The rest of the trip took us close to another seven hours. Fortunately, the rest of the trip was uneventful.

After spending the night in Yida, Alexander and I flew to Juba on the good size cargo plane out of Armenia, which had a Russian crew, that Brad Phillips had hired. In the huge cargo space there were only five of us—a Sudanese couple and another Sudanese man, Alexander and me.

Mission accomplished!

April–May 2015 Mission to the Nuba Mountains, South Kordofan, Sudan

On one level, this mission was a resounding success in that four tons of food were delivered to two different groups of civilians in the Nuba Mountains, all of whom are in desperate straits. On another level, though, it was filled with darkness and pain. Ultimately, carrying out this mission was vastly different from earlier ones.

Once we (Alexander, my interpreter and I) reached Juba, we asked around at the airport if any planes were heading to Yida and were informed that a cargo plane was taking off shortly. Just before it took off, we hopped in the hold, which was loaded with huge bags of food from Bangladesh, as well as an array of South Sudanese soldiers and civilians from the Nuba Mountains.

In Yida, we met up with our driver, Daniel, who was waiting behind the wheel of the Land Cruiser I had rented. We immediately headed to the local *suq* and purchased three thousand dollars worth of dried beans, lintels, salt, sugar and cooking oil. As luck would have it, no one had sorghum for sale, which is the mainstay of the Nuba diet, but we figured we'd locate sorghum in a *suq* once we crossed into Sudan.

We pulled out of Yida about 2:00 p.m. that same day and drove straight through to Kauda in the heart of the Nuba Mountains, arriving around 10:00 p.m. After spending the night in Daniel's family compound, we got up early the next morning, and as we motored through Kauda, we came across several individuals we knew who filled us in regarding the fighting in the region. One of them was our buddy Ryan Boyette, the director of *Nuba Reports*.

Each person informed us that our destination (Kwalib) was, indeed, one of the current hotspots in the war between SPLA–N and Khartoum (i.e., the Government of Sudan). In fact, both Ryan and the assistant commissioner of Kauda informed us that in the past week Kwalib had suffered repeated ground and aerial attacks (both from Antonovs and Sukhoi fighter jets), and that a good number of people had fled their homes and villages, with many others having been injured or killed.

As we left Kauda we headed toward Heiban, which, prior to the war, had been a GoS-stronghold. We variously commented on what we were likely to be confronted by as we made our way to and back from Kwalib. Fresh in all of our minds was the rather trying trip in December when we found ourselves constantly screeching to a stop in the middle of the road, jumping out of the Land Cruiser, and scrambling out into the desert in an attempt to locate something that would serve as a protection of sorts.

Just before we entered Heiban proper, we turned left onto the rutted, dusty road that would take us to Kwalib. Oddly, even though it was about 8:00 a.m. not a person was up and about in the good sized town.

Twenty to thirty minutes down the road, a man on a knoll, who had been standing along side several other men, begun running towards us screaming at the top of his lungs. Daniel stopped in the middle of the road, and as he got closer to us, the man, really hyped up, demanded to know why we had not stopped and told him and his companions that a Sukhoi fighter jet had just attacked Heiban. We told him we had no idea what he was talking about, and that when we had passed through Heiban all was quiet. Indignant and obviously not believing us, he raged on and on, and since we had nothing more to say, we continued on our way (all the while wondering where he had heard such a thing and whether or not such an attack had occurred shortly after we passed through Heiban).

Continuing on our way, both Ramadan and Daniel commented on how extraordinary hot it was. Ramadan surmised that the temperature was around 43 or 44 degrees Centigrade, while Daniel guessed it was closer to 42 Centigrade. Forty-four Centigrade would have made it 111 degrees Fahrenheit. (Later in the week, some Nuba asserted that the temperature had reached an outrageous 48 degrees Centigrade, which would have made it 118 degrees Fahrenheit.) I'd never heard a Nuban complain about the heat, but later in the week Ramadan did just that, stating he was so light-headed it took all his strength not to fall down whenever he attempted to walk. As for me, I was miserable throughout the entire trip: constantly sweaty and thirsty as I continued to rely on bottled water that I was sure registered 70 degrees Fahrenheit or higher. By the end of my first week in the Nuba, my tongue had become so swollen I actually had a hard time speaking clearly.

Once we reached Kwalib we drove straight to the compound of the local commissioner. Greeted by a half dozen local leaders, we explained we had purchased and trucked up a ton of food for those civilians in most desperate need. We also explained that we would deliver another ton or two within the next several hours if we could locate other bulk food for sale in the region.

We then listened to what the locals had to say about the most recent attacks by the SAF (Sudanese Armed Forces). They essentially corroborated the rumors we had heard back in Kauda: over the past several weeks Kwalib had been hit pretty hard and pretty regularly by Antonovs, Sukhoi fighter jets, and shelling. Some of the planes, they said, had dropped cluster bombs. Just the day before a family of seven had been killed in a nearby village. Not far from where we were sitting, they told us, a rocket had been shot towards a house but did not explode; the unexploded ordnance, they said, was still sitting in the hole that the rocket had dug out.

Hundreds of people had fled their villages, they said, and were now in roughshod IDP camps spread throughout the region. Many were in critical need of food and medicine.

Once we unloaded all of the food we had trucked up, one of the local leaders informed us that he had a large pile of sorghum at his compound and would gladly sell it to us for a decent price. He commented that his son attended secondary school in the Yida Refugee Camp because all of the schools in the Kwalib area had shut down due to the constant bombing, and that he (the father) wished to send his son some money in order to cover the costs for school supplies and other necessities. As we drove towards the seller's compound, one of the local leaders asked if we wished to see the rocket that had not exploded. I said that I did.

We drove about another quarter of a mile and then got out and walked up a slight hill towards a *tukul*. Only four or five feet from the tukul was a large hole about two feet deep and three feet wide filled with the constituents parts of a cluster bomb—not simply a shell as I had been led to believe. Locals had thrown twigs and branches over the hole and ordnance as a means to keep children and animals from inadvertently stepping or falling into the hole. A man told us that three children had been sitting beside the house when the rocket hit. All three would have certainly been killed had the cluster bombs exploded.

We proceeded to the seller's compound, which was a rocky, head-jarring twenty-minute ride across fields and *wadis* and around other areas that had recently been targeted by the GoS. Once we reached the compound, we purchased what amounted to five bags of sorghum, each of which weighed about 250 pounds each. Subsequently, we delivered the sorghum to the commissioner's compound in Kwalib.[1]

Even though it was late in the day, we decided to head back to Kauda since we figured that was the only place we'd find more food to purchase for other IDPs. Eight, long hours later, we arrived in Kauda.

Word quickly spread the next day, Sunday, that Heiban had, in fact, been attacked the previous morning—shortly after we had made the turn toward Kwalib. At the sight or sound of a Sukhoi 24, three young men in their teens raced towards a hole to jump into. Two of them were already in the hole with the pilot of the Sukhoi fired a rocket, literally shearing the third young man in half.[2]

This was my third trip to the Nuba Mountains during the war and after hearing about the fate of the young man, it was the first time I was really spooked at the thought of even driving down the dirt roads in the Nuba. Daniel, our driver, said that while individuals more often than not hear the slow, lumbering Antonovs heading their way, and thus have plenty of time to either jump in a hole or seek some sort of protection, Sukhois are so fast that they are often on top of a target before one can react, which is why they often prove so deadly. It was not lost on any of us that had we arrived in Heiban just some fifteen to twenty minutes later than we had, we would have been a prime, if not *the* perfect, target, for the Sukhoi. Nor was it lost on us that had the rocket it fired hit our Land Cruiser, there probably would have been nothing left of us to bury.

Despite my dread at getting back on the road, I decided we should head northeast, towards a town called Mindi, only because I had heard that a good number of people had fled to that region following the bombing of their villages and farms. It was my understanding that there was at least one IDP camp just south of Mindi, and that people there were largely bereft of food and medicine.

Just prior to arriving in Mindi, we pulled off the road and asked to be directed to the head of the IDP camp nearby. A man in his mid-twenties, serious and matter of fact but friendly, said that the headman was not available but that he was second in command. He then filled us in on the status of the IDPs: they not only suffered from a dearth of food but they also were without soap or other hygiene products. He added that many youngsters, particularly those five years old and younger, were suffering greatly from malnutrition, and that any help we could provide would be incredibly helpful.

I promised him that the next day we would deliver at least a ton of food (sorghum, sugar, cooking oil, dried beans), along with as much soap as we could afford. He patted his chest with the palm of his right hand and with tears welling up in his eyes, he said, in Arabic: "I do not have the words to thank you enough for your kindness. We will always be grateful to you and those in America who donated the funds to assist us."

Since we were fairly close to Mindi and because it was market day there, I decided we should motor over to see if we could purchase any bulk food in the *suq* for the IDPs. Just as we pulled up and were about to back up under a shade tree, I noticed a camouflaged jeep, with an antiaircraft gun positioned between the driver and passenger seat, racing towards the *suq*, kicking up clouds of dust. Off-handedly, I commented to Daniel, "I wonder what those characters are up to." Moments later the jeep came to an abrupt stop about two hundred yards from us. The rebels, yelling about something, quickly attracted a crowd of 30 to 40 people from the *suq*.

Within seconds, a civilian approached us and said that a young boy had stepped on a landmine, and that the rebels were looking for someone to transport the boy to a medical clinic. Why the soldiers didn't do so themselves, I don't know, and he did not say. Immediately, though, I said we'd take the kid to Mother of Mercy Hospital. As I ran over to the jeep, Daniel pulled up parallel to it. We had to push and shove the crowd out of the way in order to lift and place the boy, who was about twelve years old, into the back of our vehicle.

Checking out the boy's most obvious wound—his upper leg was bandaged and "soaked" with dried blood—I noticed that blood was neither pouring nor seeping from the wound. The boy was still conscious and in obvious pain, but he didn't say a word as we moved him from the jeep to the back of the truck.

I pulled a bottle of water from the front seat of our truck, along with a cloth, and asked a young fellow sitting next to the injured boy to periodically dab the latter's face with the cool water, but not, under any circumstances, to provide him with or allow him to drink any of the water as it could cause him even more harm.

I then told the small group of people who had already boarded the truck—which we later found out included the boy's sister and some close friends—to lift the boy's legs and feet up and place them on an empty jerry can, which was sitting on its side. I explained that was for the purpose of preventing blood from draining into his legs, which could be fatal.

We then set out for Mother of Mercy Hospital, which was an hour and fifteen to thirty minutes away over a very bumpy, dirt road. It was impossible to travel over 30 miles an hour, for if we had the passengers, and the victim, in the back of the truck, would've bounced up and down the entire way. When we came to somewhat smoother stretches, Daniel increased the speed to 50 mph, but such stretches were rare. About half way to the hospital, someone in back knocked on the back window, and we stopped to see what the problem was. We were informed that the village the boy was from was about a mile away and that someone on the back of the truck wanted to alert his parents to what had happened. For some maddening reason, Daniel insisted on waiting in the middle of the field while several people ran to alert the boy's parents versus driving over to the village. After hectoring the hell out of him, he finally drove towards a woman who was running across a huge field towards us. The woman ended up being a close neighbor. The parents had not been at home, but the neighbor said she wanted to accompany the boy to the hospital and thus joined the boy in the back of the truck. Immediately, she hugged him to her breast, pulling his upper body towards her while pulling his feet and legs off of the jerry can. Again, I had to explain why it was imperative to lay the boy flat on his back with his feet and legs raised. The woman looked askance at the suggestion, but finally acquiesced.

It took well over 45 minutes to an hour to reach the hospital. As soon as we pulled up to the gate of Mother of Mercy we informed the guard that we were carrying a badly wounded boy and he waved us right in. I directed Daniel to pull the truck directly up to the entrance of the hospital grounds and I hopped out to notify hospital officials we had a badly injured boy with us. After a few minutes, Dr. Tom Catena approached me and after hearing what I had to say he told me to have the driver pull up over the curb and drive directly into the park-like setting area that serves as the hospital's inner courtyard.

At first glance, Tom thought the young boy was still alive, but when he returned with a stretcher on wheels and bent over the boy Tom looked up and whispered to me that the boy was dead. Stepping away from the truck, he told me that he wished to conduct an autopsy on the boy, and afterwards he would inform those accompanying the boy what had killed him.

I chose not to attend the autopsy, but Daniel did. Later, he informed me that the boy had also suffered a horrific wound to his abdomen; one so deep, in fact, that Dr. Catena was able to shove his entire fist into the cavity of the wound and move it up towards the boy's sternum. As for his leg wound, Daniel informed me that once the bandages were unwrapped, the horrible destruction of the boy's leg was shocking: it had almost been sliced in half, a large piece of bone had pierced the skin, while the rest of the bone had been pulverized, essentially forming a mush-like substance along with the shredded skin, muscle and blood.

As I stood alone in the courtyard waiting for Dr. Catena to exit the autopsy room, a young man in his early twenties, who was sitting on a bench against a wall, called out,

"What is going on?" I walked over to where he was sitting. I noticed he was missing a leg. After sitting down, I informed him about the situation with the young boy. I then asked him what had happened to his leg. He laconically said, "An Antonov."

Once Dr. Catena completed his autopsy and rolled out the body of the young boy, I joined him. Dr. Catena gently told the sister of the boy and the next door neighbor that the boy had perished on the way to the hospital, as well as the cause of his death. Both broke into tears, hugging one another as we lifted the boy back into the truck and then placed a shroud over him.

For some reason, the boy's sister, who had been wounded but only slightly, initially directed us to take the boy's body to Kauda, where their grandparents resided. Some ten minutes later, she knocked on the window and called out that she wanted us to take her to her family's home. Turning around, we headed back across the territory we had traveled earlier. About fifteen minutes into the drive we saw, in the far distance, a man and a woman moving quickly across the dusty barren landscape, the man about 300 yards or so in front of the woman. As we pulled up to the man, who turned out to be the boy's father, he walked to the back of the truck, looked down at his son, and without a word, turned around and walked off into the field alone. When the boy's mother saw her husband heading out into the field alone, she let out an agonizing screech and fell flat on her face, where she remained screaming for the next ten minutes.

For a good while no one approached the mother, and then, once someone did, both the mother and father were helped onto the back of the truck. We then proceeded to Kauda, where we delivered the body of the boy to his grandparents. As each female relative (grandmothers, aunts and cousins) approached the truck and glanced at the boy's body, they broke out screeching. The mother refused to leave the back of the truck and simply started at her son as she, too, continued to wail. No one attempted to provide any solace for the poor woman, and not being able to stand seeing her in such pain, I reached out and touched her hand. She grabbed my hand, glanced up at me, and moved her hand a little higher, latching onto my wrist. (Later, I mused, "I wonder if she is Muslim. If so, touching her hand the way I did was totally out of bounds." Indeed, it would have been impermissible according to the teachings of Islam.) Later that evening, Daniel informed me that the boy would be buried that night, as is customary in the Nuba Mountains.

Ultimately, we discovered that the boy had not, in fact, stepped on a land mine. Rather, he had come across an unexploded bomb near the mango trees he and his sister were going to climb in search of food for their family. The boy asked his older sister what they should do with the bomb, and she told him to leave it alone. Instead, he picked it up and tossed it away from the tree. Then, as his sister climbed up in the tree, the boy began throwing rocks at the bomb, causing it to explode. A classic case of a boy being a boy and not using his head. But also a classic case of the type of tragedy that is not uncommon in a war zone. (It's also likely the boy and his sister would have not footed some five to ten miles to the orchard in search of fruit had the region not suffered from a dearth of food due to the bombing of Nuba farms by the GoS.)

Deeply saddened I was ready to head back to Yida. First, though, the next day, we delivered two tons of food to the IDPs near Mindi. A day later we headed back to the Yida Refugee Camp.

Less than 24 hours later, I passed out in a makeshift shower in the refugee camp and cracked my head against the cinderblock wall. Ultimately, a doctor surmised that not only was I suffering from acute dehydration but had been adversely impacted by the

Mefloquine (Larium), a prophylactic for malaria, I was on, and thus passed out in the shower. When I came to the shower water was pouring down on me, and at first, as a result of the incredible pain all across my lower back and the fact that, at first, I couldn't seem to move, I feared I was paralyzed. But then I found I could move if I slowly scooted along on my butt. I ended up scooting out of the shower, pulling on a pair of under shorts, and then scooting out of the dressing area to a slab of cement outside. After calling for help, I was taken to the compound of Médecins Sans Frontières, where I was placed in their field hospital (a Quonset hut like affair, with huge doors at each end that were constantly open, with some thirty beds). For three days I was attended to by their remarkable doctors and attendants. I was then medevaced to Nairobi, where I spent an additional five days in The Nairobi Hospital. Two months later I am still suffering from chronic lightheadedness and back pain. But such is life.

Once again, this mission would have not been carried out had it not been the gracious and generous donations of genocide and Holocaust scholars, friends and family members, secondary level teachers across the U.S., and other caring citizens.

January 2016 Mission to the Nuba Mountains in Order to Provide Food to Those Who Are Facing Malnutrition, Severe Malnutrition or Worse

What follows are select notes from the report I wrote up about this mission:

January 8th–9th: Juba, South Sudan; Yida Refugee Camp; and Nuba Mountains

As soon as I arrived in Juba, I met with a high level Nuba representative. He informed me that three areas in the Nuba are facing major food insecurity: Sinar, various villages in Kwalib, and Kao Nyaro.

The next day I (along with Daniel Kuti, a friend, who also serves as my interpreter and driver when I am in the Nuba) caught a flight with Samaritan's Purse to the Yida Refugee Camp. Within an hour of reaching Yida, I made contact with the fellow who had driven "my" Land Cruiser down from Kauda, which I had rented for a week. The amount of bulk food available in the *suq* was negligible. We purchased what little we could, loaded up, and, after inviting a half dozen people to catch a lift with us, we were off. Nine uneventful (meaning, no sign of Antonov bombers or Sukhoi fighter jets) hours later we reached Kauda. That night we slept in Daniel's compound, where he lives with his wife and two children.

The Government of Sudan Continues to Burn Nuba Farms and Block Goods from Reaching the Nuba Mountains
(Information gleaned from highly informed Nubans in Juba and corroborated in Kauda)

GoS troops are burning one Nuba farm after another in an attempt to (a) prevent Nuba people from harvesting their crops, (b) create an even more dire shortage of food in the region, and, ultimately, (c) push the Nuba out of the region. At a minimum, such actions constitute a clear case of ethnic cleansing.

While the aerial attacks all across the region have tapered off dramatically over the past several months, attacks on Nuba farms and civilians in those areas bordering the land controlled by the GoS have been under periodic siege by shelling.

The destruction of the farms has not only created food insecurity for those whose farms have been destroyed, but a general dearth of food in the region. In turn, this has resulted in the dramatic increase in the cost of food in the *suqs*, largely resulting in a situation where many cannot afford to purchase enough food to keep their families from experiencing hunger or worse.

Exacerbating the situation is the fact that the GoS is now preventing tractor trailer rigs from carrying goods from the north towards the center and southern parts of Sudan, creating even more hardships in the Nuba Mountains, including a dearth of diesel fuel, regular petrol, soap, and various food items. Again, this appears to be a GoS' ploy to apply ever increasing pressure on the Nuba people to leave the region.

The local police in Kauda have ordered local merchants to cut their price for sorghum by five Sudanese pounds per *malwa*—from fifteen to ten. The merchants, however, have refused to do so; and instead, they have chosen to close down their shops in Kauda and travel to other *suqs* in the region in order to sell their good for the prices they wish. As a result, the supply of food available in Kauda has diminished dramatically, contributing in its own way to the food crisis. While both merchants and buyers could attempt to circumvent the order issued by the police—that is, a merchant could continue to attempt to sell his/her goods at the inflated price to customers willing to pay the (inflated) asking price—but if they are caught during the transaction by the police, both the merchant and the customer could either be fined and/or jailed.

The upshot is that in order to purchase an ample amount of bulk food to transport to those most in need, I was forced to literally travel to three times as many *suqs* in the region as I usually do. Even then, the effort was not entirely successful since bulk supplies in most of the *suqs* were either nonexistent or extremely limited.

Also complicating matters was the fact that I was personally asked by local commissioners not to purchase any bulk food at inflated prices (which often happens when the merchants see a *khawaja* and automatically and exorbitantly increase the prices figuring the *khawaja* won't complain about the inflated prices). The problem, the commissioners explained, is that once merchants are successful at selling bulk food at an inflated price, they often retain the inflated price as the going price for one and all (including the locals, which would price them out of being able to purchase much of anything). The point is, if I ended up paying the inflated price I would have, ironically, ended up hurting people as I was attempting to help them.

On a different note, I was repeatedly told by many in the Nuba Mountains that whenever Omar al-Bashir, the president of Sudan, calls for a ceasefire, which he did back in December, the SPLA–N almost automatically assumes that he has done so for the express purpose of repositioning and amassing his troops in preparation for a major attack. Thus, while it has been extremely "quiet" (i.e., peaceful) as of late in the Nuba, people tend to say, "That's been true up to today. What nobody knows is what tomorrow shall bring."

Almost to a person, what the Nuba believe they are currently experiencing is the proverbial calm before the storm. In other words, while most are enjoying the current "quiet," it is a "nervous enjoyment" and/or "a nerve wracking peace," and that is because most are positive that the storm (a major attack) is coming, sooner or later. They believe the attack will involve a great number of troops along with a barrage of artillery shelling, and repeated aerial attacks by Antonovs and Sukhois. Many believe that the assault will be an all out attempt by the GoS to take over "the center"—meaning, an attempt to take over Kauda, the largest town in the region controlled by the SPLA–N.

The morning of January 9th I met and spoke with Mr. Kamal Malah, Coordinator of the Nuba Relief and Rehabilitation and Development Organization's (NRRDO) health project. We met in a tiny, dirt-floor café constructed of tree limbs and branches.

Immediately, we began to discuss the issue of food insecurity in the region. In part, Malah stated the following: "Three areas where people are in dire trouble are Kao Nyaro (in the east); the villages of Sinar, Mundi and Ngarto (some 40 kilometers from Kauda); and various areas in Western Kadugli (along the front of the major ground war)." This corroborated exactly what I had been told in Juba by a high level official from the Nuba.

When Malah began going into specifics about the plight of the people in Kao Nyaro, he became extremely emotional and his voice broke: "When you see them...." Pausing, he began to tear up and said, "It is so terrible.... They are. I can't even speak about it...."

We sat in silence for several minutes, and then he continued: "You see them, and you know what they are suffering. Many are dying from starvation."

After pausing momentarily, he said: "Those areas —Kao Nyaro, and where you plan to go, Kwalib, are split off from the rest of the SPLA–N controlled areas, and because of that the people are not able to access food. Their farms have been burned by GoS troops. And now the GoS is blocking people from traveling to the *suqs* to purchase the little amount of food they can afford. And those areas are not reachable by individuals, humanitarians, such as yourself, because you would get killed trying to make it across GoS-controlled territory."

"So, how do I get the food to them?"

"You will need to deliver it to the commissioner in Kwalib, and he will have to get word to the people in those areas that are ... that are like islands, sitting all alone surrounded by GoS controlled territory ... that food is available for them. And at night, those people in those villages without [food] will have to sneak over to where the food is and then sneak back, footing it back to their villages, while hoping they will not be detected and killed."

January 10, 2016, Late Morning

Hauled food to the IDP camp in Sinar, a small village about 30 to 40 kilometers from Kauda. About 450 families reside in the camp. Over the past year, the IDPs have been forced out of their villages by the GoS and chosen to settle in Sinar. Without access to their farms or stores of food and with few jobs, food insecurity has been a major issue. (This is the same group for whom I provided food, cooking oil and soap to last April.)

Upon meeting with several sheiks and a few others (boys and men), I was informed by the leader of the IDP camp, a sheik named Yacoub, that because sorghum was now so expensive to purchase in the *suq* (it had more than tripled in price, he said, since I was last there in April), most families in their community were extremely short of food and many people, especially children, were suffering from malnutrition or worse. Another man, in fatigues, to whom everyone showed deference, asserted that there were at least 60 to 70 such children. Another man asked us if we had any of "the chocolaty" medicine" (i.e., pluppynut, a highly nutritious paste/food for those suffering from malnutrition) that we could give them. I stated that we didn't, but that we could transport the children in need of such to a clinic where they would surely be provided with some.

Several men spoke up and complained that the closest clinic, which is located just down the road in Mundi, did not have any medication other than that for pain. I told them that I planned to see Dr. Tom Catena in the afternoon and I would speak to him about their concerns. We also promised that we would return the next day with more sorghum and salt.

I then asked if they were in need of anything else. One man mentioned that they desperately needed soap, as none had been available in the *suq*. Another commented that a lot of children had been extremely ill, and they felt it was due to a lack of cleanliness.

Shortly, we were shown to a large compound with several *tukuls,* where a group of boys (teenagers) and men unloaded the food we were delivering to them: two tons of sorghum, a large bag of salt and a jerry can of cooking oil.

As we were preparing to leave, Yacoub asserted that their situation had changed very little (i.e., not gotten any better) over the past year as they has only received one other donation of food and medicine from another humanitarian group—that is, over and above what we had delivered in April 2015. That other donation had been delivered in August, he said, by Samaritan's Purse.

Yacoub said he didn't have much hope that anything would change in the near future. A lot of the IDPs, he said, wished to return to their farms, but it was impossible since the SPLA-N now used the area as a base of operations in order to rebuff advances by GoS troops.

January 10, 2016, Early Afternoon

That afternoon I headed over to Mother of Mercy Hospital in Gidel to see and speak with Dr. Tom Catena When we first sat down with Tom under some trees, he commented on the "schizophrenic" situation in the region—how it had been "calm" (no bombings) but at the same time people were on edge sensing that fighting might resume at any moment. The word was that since December there had been a major shifting and amassing of troops by both the GoS and the SPLA-N.

After catching up, I told Tom that one individual at the IDP camp had claimed that 60 to 70 children were suffering from malnutrition. Tom told me that that didn't sound right. "In fact," he said, "one of our visiting doctors, Ingrid, goes to the clinic in Mundi every second Thursday, and if that were the case she certainly would have heard about it by now. And if she had heard about it she would've gone to the IDP camp to check out the situation." To him, it sounded as if a false rumor had sprung up and the people had accepted it as the truth. He told me he would let Ingrid know what was said and that she could look into the matter.

When I mentioned the complaint about the purported lack of meds in the clinic in Mundi, Tom said that the clinic was operating under the auspices of Mother of Mercy and he knew for a fact that it was fully stocked with meds and that those who claimed otherwise were ill-informed.

Continuing, I told Tom that several individuals in the IDP camp had asked if we were carrying any of that "chocolaty stuff," i.e., pluppynut. Tom said, "You never know if people want it for children who are truly suffering from malnutrition or want it for themselves. And not necessarily because they are suffering from malnutrition or are particularly hungry but because they like the taste of it." Then he added, "Even if they [the adults] are suffering from malnutrition, the pluppynut manufactured for use with children is not the correct formula for use with adults." Two lessons learned and worth remembering, I thought.

When I mentioned that I had met with Kamal Malah and that he had told me about a dramatic increase in teen pregnancies in Yida, Tom, who is very mild manner, got really worked up and said, "I don't know why they don't shut that damn refugee camp down. It is going to destroy—it is destroying—Nuba culture. The people need to leave that place and get back here and just deal with the bombs. Too many people are sitting around doing nothing and that is becoming their way of life. Or, in the case of the kids, they end up doing things that will just make their lives that much more difficult. Really, the place needs to be shut down."

January 11, 2016, Morning

We returned to the IDP camp near Sinar. Initially, we met with a couple of sheiks and informed them that we had delivered a couple of tons of food the day before and that we were back with more. After thanking us, they guided us to the same compound where we had unloaded food yesterday. Again, several male IDPs unloaded the gigantic and incredibly heavy sacks of sorghum (roughly a ton's worth), salt and the jerry cans of cooking oil.

Subsequently, we were invited to meet with several sheiks and a half dozen other men. The meeting was held in a common area used for meetings, under three huge mango trees. Seating was comprised of long, thick tree branches anchored by short thick wedges of wood in the form of a Y. Right away I raised the issue of the purportedly 60 to 70 children who were suffering from malnutrition. One of the sheiks asked if I would like to see the children and meet with their parents. I said I would. A couple of the teenagers were asked to locate those parents with children who were suffering from malnutrition and to bring them and their children to meet me. Within about five minutes seven sets of mothers and their children were standing in front of us. (One of the sheiks commented that they could only locate a fraction of the mothers and their children as most of the others were out tending their fields.) It was then that I saw exactly what Salah had described to me the day before.[3]

Before I exchanged a single word with any of the mothers, I noticed that one of the children, a baby (who I was ultimately told was roughly two years old but who looked like an infant,) could not raise his head upright. That is, his head lolled to the side and remained there for the next half hour.

Another child, about five years old, sat in his mother's lap and as he did his legs swung to and fro, but when his mother lifted him up onto his feet and attempted to get him to walk he began screaming and his arms and legs flapped spasmodically about.

As the mothers and the children stood in front of us (a couple of mothers held their babies in their arms and a couple sat down and rested their children on their laps), I began to ask the mothers about the health of their children. One mother who was holding her child in her arms said that the child, again quite small for his age, had begun crying all night long about a month ago and had not stopped since.

Ultimately, I offered to take the mothers and their children to the closest medical facility, which was the German Doctors' Hospital in Lewere. Only one of the mothers accepted the offer, the one with the baby who cried all night along. The other two mothers said they had to attend to other matters.

January 11, 2016, Afternoon

After driving the mother and her child to the German Doctors' Hospital, Daniel and I spent the rest of the day traveling from one *suq* to another in search of diesel fuel for the Land Cruiser which we needed to make the long trip to Kwalib and back the next day. All we could locate was enough to partially fill the tank. That automatically prevented us from heading to Kwalib. While we could have made it from Kauda to Kwalib and then back to Kauda, we would not have had enough to make it back to Yida.

January 12, 2016, Morning

I made a point of meeting once again with Kamal Malah, the health coordinator with NRRDO. I wanted to share with him what I had heard and learned at the IDP camp the day before and what (Dr.) Tom Catena had to say about what I shared with him.

When I told Malah about the baby who could not seem to raise its head, along with the fact that the mother refused a ride to the German Doctors' Hospital, he said, "I am not surprised. It's harvest time and when it's harvest time all the people are concerned about is getting their plants harvested."

"But … but…," I said, "her baby is not well at all! Anybody could see that. Not only dramatically underweight but, like I said, it can't even lift its head up."

"Yes, but no matter what the situation is, most are solely focused on getting their crops harvested. They fear that if they don't do it now and wait and then a big battle breaks out or the Antonovs begin to bomb again on a regular basis they will lose everything! Everything! And then their entire family is in jeopardy, because no one will have anything to eat—or at least not enough to eat. So that is the number one priority."

Continuing he said, "So, if one child dies … well, they feel they have no choice but to get the crops in."

January 12, 2016, Late Morning

Late this morning we met with the Commissioner of Heiban County, Mubark Bolis. The previous evening Daniel had bumped into Bolis in Kauda and Bolis had said, "I hear you are working with a human rights investigator." Daniel informed him that the information he had was incorrect and that, in fact, we were in the Nuba to deliver food to those most in need. Bolis told Daniel that he wanted to meet me and that we should be at his office prior to noon the next day.

Upon meeting Bolis, he kindly welcomed me to the Nuba, and thanked us for the work we were doing. Initially, he simply wanted to know what we were delivering and to whom. Then he inquired about our previous missions to the Nuba. He said that the next time I was in the region I should visit him at his main office in Heiban, and that he would assist us in way he could.

During the course of our conversation he mentioned that he had just met with high level military officials about the critical need to get water out to the SPLA–N troops who were out in the field, far from any boreholes, setting up perimeters as they prepared for a potential attack by the GoS.

January 12, Early Afternoon

This afternoon we traveled to a *suq* in a place called Talatah, about twenty kilometers from Kauda, in order to purchase two to three more tons of sorghum. On the way we continued to come across one *doshka* (a Land Cruiser pick-up with a mounted machine gun in the bed) after another, along with the bivouacking of scores of rebel troops in the bush. I'd never seen any such activity during my previous trips to the Nuba.

In the *suq*, a manned *doshka* was parked in the center of all the activity. Heavily armed SPLA–N personnel also made rounds of the *suq* on foot. Again, this was distinctly different from what I had witnessed previously.

We quickly discovered that none of the merchants had any bulk sorghum for sale. As a result, we put the word out what were in search of—bulk amounts of sorghum, lintels, dried beans. Ultimately, we located two gentlemen who said they had a ton's worth of sorghum back in Kauda that we could purchase. We agreed to purchase it but when we went to pick it up, the gentlemen failed to show. That was most unfortunate as we were planning to deliver that food along with three other bags of sorghum we had stockpiled back at Daniel's compound to Umduram.

That night, about 8:00 p.m., the guttural rumbling of a plane rent the air. Everyone in the compound jumped up and began heading towards the compound's fox hole, but then someone noticed that it was a drone. Since the GoS has essentially established a no-fly zone over the Nuba, any plane in Nuba skies means it's either an Antonov bomber, a Sukhoi (fighter jet), or a drone. The first two wreak havoc, while the last one conducts surveillance and collects data. While everyone was relieved that the plane was not an Antonov or a Sukhoi, the fact that it was a drone was still somewhat unnerving as the common assumption is that its presence likely presaged the coming of a new battle.

January 13, 2016

We left Kauda at 5:30 a.m. en route to the Yida Refugee Camp. It was the first time on this trip that we've been totally vigilant in regard to listening for and scanning the skies for Antonovs and Sukhois—meaning, we had become a bit casual since it had been so quiet.

Since we could not make it to Kwalib due to the petrol situation, we decided to head to the Umduran to meet with Farouk Musa, the executive director of the locality. A year ago we had dropped off several tons of food which Musa had promised he would get to those in the far reaches of the locality who were facing serious food insecurity.

Upon our arrival at Musa's compound, we found it deserted, and there was no sign that anyone had been there recently. We also noticed that the tiny tea stand across the road was gone. We flagged down a fellow who was riding by on a camel and he informed us that due to the increase in bombings, the area got so dangerous that Musa had moved his office to Kurchee. (This was the area where Antonovs had flown overhead three times in less than a half hour when we were last there.) So, we turned around and headed to Kurchee. There we located Musa and he informed us that those who had not fled from their villages in Umduran were in dire need of food, particularly those along the border separating SPLA–N-controlled and GoS-controlled territory. He and the half dozen or sheiks who met with us were extremely pleased when we informed them that we had two tons of sorghum, a jerry can of cooking oil, and a huge bag of salt that we wished to donate to those in most critical need.

About ten minutes after we left Musa's compound, we entered a small *suq*, which looked deserted in comparison to how it usually looked. Daniel decided to check to see if anyone had diesel fuel for sale. After an unsuccessful attempt at locating any petrol, we entered a tiny dirt floor café made of tree branches and Daniel had tea and bread for breakfast. As he waited for his tea, he told me he had come across a fellow in the *suq* who worked for Samaritan's Purse whose face was badly injured. The fellow had told Daniel that a day earlier he had been heading south on a motorcycle and as he approached a roadblock just north of Kurchee he noticed that the fellows standing along each side of the road allowed the rope, which served as the roadblock, to drop to the ground. Figuring he did not need to stop he retained his speed, but just as he was about to pass the men, they yanked on the rope, drawing it as taunt as they could. Despite his desperate attempt to stop he hit the rope at neck level, flew off his motorcycle and landed on his face. Before he was able to get to his feet, three men had surrounded him and began punching and kicking him. When he screamed at them, one of them yelled, "Don't you know what this is? It's a roadblock." The victim screamed back, "I know, but no one is beaten at a roadblock." They continued to beat him, and then dragged him into a tukul not far from the road, where they continued to beat him and threaten him with death. Just as he thought he was going to die, another man entered the *tukul* and those beating him immediately ceased their attack.

The upshot is that Daniel and another fellow in the café, who happened to be a police officer, wondered aloud who the culprits were, whether they would even be around should someone attempt to locate them, and, most significantly, mused that it sounded like the culprits were not Nuba but possibly SPLA from South Sudan, who had volunteered to fight alongside the Nuba against the GoS. It was actually a good guess for it is common knowledge that many of those fighting in South Sudan today regularly engage in criminal acts as part and parcel of their daily lives in the extremely corrupt, highly volatile, and deadly region. At one and the same time, the Nuba rebels are known for being polite and honest.

I commented that while I had been threatened in various ways by soldiers and rebels in Chad, Kenya, and South Sudan, I'd never been harassed or threatened by the SPLA-N, and had never been forced to hand over money or goods on demand.

Daniel said that upon his return to Kauda he was going to report the incident and do everything he could to see that the powers that be conduct an investigation. We all agreed that the last thing the Nuba needed was a bunch of criminal elements infiltrating the SPLA–N. Especially if they were from South Sudan, where beating, robbing, raping and even killing people with impunity had become a sickening way of life.

The rest of the trip was uneventful, and five hours later we pulled into the sprawling Yida Refugee Camp. Another mission accomplished.

On a personal note, almost every time I am in the Nuba Mountains I seem to contract this or that malady. This time around, ugly, painful sores popped up on my forehead, neck, stomach and back, accompanied by a raw throat and a piercing headache I could not get rid of no matter what I did. The upshot is that I ended up seeing three doctors back in Fayetteville (my general practitioner, a dermatologist, and a tropical disease specialist), had several vials of blood drawn, was put on four different medications, had a sonar scan of my liver, and have been referred to a gastroenterologist. My plan is to return to the Nuba Mountains in early May, just prior to the onset of the rainy season. Once the rainy season sets in it lasts through November, at which time it is all but impossible to traverse the swampy and thick, muddy "roads." It is also a period when people have to rely on the food they've harvested and stored, and if they have little to none then they are in great trouble.

NOTES

1. As we were unloading the sacks of sorghum I noticed that Brad Phillips, the fellow I first met in the Nuba back in December 2014, was sitting under an awning talking with various local leaders. We greeted one another, and then went our separate ways. The primary reason for mentioning Phillips is that he ended up spending the night in Kwalib, and experienced something rather remarkable. More specifically, in his monthly newsletter *Africa Messenger*, which his foundation, the Persecution Project, publishes, Brad wrote the following:
On my last trip to the Nuba, I visited a displaced community living at the base of a mountain. The people had abandoned their village because it was within shelling range of the Sudan Armed Forces. Where they live, there are no wells, but a small spring was found high in the mountains, inside a cave too small for most adults to enter. So, everyday, a small group of girls carry plastic jerry cans on their heads and climb the mountain. I had to see this, so one morning I accompanied them. It took us two hours to reach the cave, then the girls filled their containers and began the longer journey back down.
I could not believe the courage of these girls. I heard no complaints. They showed no fear. They cheerfully went about their work—alone, in an active war zone, climbing [the] mountain several times a day to get water for their families in hiding. After our trip down the mountain ended and we sat to take some lunch, the Sudan Armed Forces began shelling the other side of the mountain where we had just been climbing. We counted 40 shells striking the mountain over the course of an hour, shaking the ground beneath our feet [Phillips, June 2015, pp. 1–3].

2. Ed Lyons, who works with the Persecution Project, was up in the Nuba Mountains in April 2015 when we were, and he writes, in the "Africa Messenger" (a publication of the Persecution Project) that he actually attended the boy's funeral: "One of my grimmest memories from this trip is of attending the funeral for a boy from Heiban. We had just passed through Heiban the day before on our way to a place called Delami. Soon after..., a Sukhoi jet from the Sudan Air Force swooped in and rocketed the town, killing 13-year old Khalid. Khalid was entering a foxhole with his brothers when shrapnel cut him in half. His father was forced to pick up the pieces of his son for burial" (Lyons, 2015, p. 2).

3. Ryan Boyette was recently interviewed by PM (Australia) (March 2016), and had this to say about his latest experience regarding malnourished children in the Nuba Mountains:
I was in my Land Cruiser and I saw a couple carrying a young child. They frantically waved me down and so I stopped to speak with them. I told the man, quickly before he said anything, "I'm going north. I can't drive you. You're going south." He looked at me with great disappointment and I realized something was very wrong and I asked him, "What's wrong?" And he said, "My child has died on the way."
They had been carrying their child for three days, walking, trying to reach a refugee camp and on the last day the child had died of malnourishment and the father was just carrying the child. I said, "Okay, please get in the vehicle. I can bring you to Yida, so you can bury your child."
And when they got in the car—the mother who had been so strong up until the point she got into the car—you could tell that it was the first time she had sat down and rested for three days, and she just started crying in my car.

REFERENCE

Harvard University (2010). "Salt and Your Health, Part I: The Sodium Connection." *Harvard Men's Health Watch*. October. Accessed at: http://www.health.harvard.edu/newsletter_article/salt-and-your-health.

Sojourns Through Worlds of Suffering

JOHN C. JEFFERSON

All good stories have a beginning, middle and end. Sudan stories are no exception, but they are different in that they have an uncertain beginning that stretches back farther than memory because everything that happens in them is predicated upon another time, place or person that directly impacts them. To try to begin understanding even one's own personal experience in Sudan and how it started is to enter into an infinite regression. The middle of every Sudan story is murky, hard to pinpoint and packed full of powerful sensory and cognitive events that first make indelible impressions on one's psyche, only to be immediately replaced by others just as, if not more, powerful, until all that remains is a cacophony of sounds, images, imaginings and interactions with a people and culture too diverse and complex to comprehend at any given moment in time.

As for the conclusions to one's personal Sudan stories, they never really come. That is, just when you are ready to write your epilogue, memories flood back and you find yourself succumbing to the sweltering heat of the lowland swamps, fleeing the dust storms caused by the desert winds, shrinking from the blinding equatorial sun, and being overwhelmed with the smells of burning grasses, wood, roasted meat, and yes, raw sewage flooding your nostrils. What sounds like a million simultaneous conversations on a stock exchange trading floor floods your ears, and the outline of a tall dark man wearing fatigues and flip-flops carrying a Kalashnikov slung across his back obscures your view of a radiant orange sunset.

The story of my experiences in Sudan—and, more specifically, the Nuba Mountains—though unique, is unable to defy this paradigm. Indeed, Sudan stories, like Sudan's people, and Sudan itself, will always amaze, befuddle, delight, confuse, amuse, awe, shock, disgust, impress, and enlighten you, all the while challenging convention and resisting definition.

Strange Beginning

The murky beginning of my Sudan story began in 1998, when I was running a youth hostel in Tel Aviv, Israel, and a couple of daring British travelers who had been staying there for a couple of months decided one day to leave some of their gear in storage and set out for an adventure to the war-torn country of Sudan. That really captured my imagination!

First Trip into Sudan

The first time I, myself, traveled into Sudan was in 2004 on a medical mission to the Blue Nile state. At the time, I didn't know one Sudanese state from the other. In fact, all I knew was that I was going to Sudan, into an active war zone, with a *crazy* Christian doctor, who was the founder of the mission organization running the trip; an ex–Special Forces commando; a Buddhist, who made a small fortune working at Microsoft; a Vietnam vet who happened to be an elder at my church, and various other "eccentrics." The organization was called Medical Teams WorldWide, which had been founded the previous decade with the vision of addressing the needs of the neediest people in the toughest places across the globe to reach. True to his calling, the founder, Dr. Alan Kelley, traveled to war-torn Sudan regularly to meet the needs of desperate people, just like those I was destined to encounter on the trip I was about to undertake.

Because of Dr. Kelley's reputation among the Sudanese with whom he had worked, he was requested to return to Sudan in order to help those people who were suffering from malnutrition and death from outbreaks of measles, along with other opportunistic diseases. Despite the formal invitation by the SPLA[1] command, it was still necessary to pack everything we'd need to serve the people and sustain ourselves for over a week. (The team consisted of eleven Americans and two Sudanese translators.)

One of Dr. Kelley's close contacts and confidants, a missionary originally from Great Britain named Joe Jones, who was nicknamed "Indiana," picked up our group at the Nairobi International Airport and took us to the Methodist Guest House in the Kileleshua section of Nairobi, where we unloaded bag after bag of medical equipment, boxes of medicine and various other supplies for the mission. (Dr. Kelley spared no expense in making sure he had everything he needed for the two-week mission, from medicines to MREs.[2] There was even a battery and solar charging system for the vaccination refrigerator waiting for us at the home of Mr. Jones, who would also accompany us.)

Sitting around the guest house the evening of our arrival and not feeling quite like going to bed, I decided to go to the storeroom and inventory the gear, which consisted of over 20 duffel bags of supplies and equipment. I was mesmerized by all the "junk," and thought it would be a good idea to number and tag them. The doctor gave me permission to do so, and soon my effort turned into a group activity, with a listing of the contents of every single piece of gear, et al. Tellingly, I thought the exercise would simply make it easier to locate this, that or the other—little did I know how important the list would become down the road.

A plane large enough to transport the team of about nine of us and several tons of Unimix, a nutritive formula for those suffering from starvation, as well as all of our gear and many, many cases of water, was chartered to get us to Sudan. We, first, traveled from Nairobi to Lokichoggio, a town in northwestern Kenya, bordering Sudan and Ethiopia. Upon our arrival there, our group divided up into two groups, each staying at a local hotel built especially for the flood of UN and other humanitarian organizations moving in and out of Sudan in the heyday of programs such as Operation Lifeline Sudan (OLS), which like many other well-intentioned efforts at helping the people of places like Blue

Nile, eventually petered out. Along with OLS and its funding, most of the relief organizations died off leaving only a couple of NGOs (non governmental organizations) and faith-based groups to cobble together a relief effort for those people in desperate straits who were still suffering in the aftermath of the twenty plus year Second Sudanese Civil War (1983–2005).

From Lokichoggio (Loki) we flew for three hours at low speed and low altitude en route to Sudan, much of the way skirting the Ethiopian side of the border to avoid Government of Sudan (GoS) radar detection or GoS spotters At this point one might ask, "Why would anyone take such risks and where does one find a pilot and plane for such a journey?" The legacy of OSL, which provided aid to much of Sudan's war torn region (but not the Nuba Mountains) in the 1990s, still had a remnant in the economy of various logistics companies willing to fly over and/or into dangerous areas like this. The pilots they recruited were mostly Ukrainians with Afghan War experience. They were just as likely to fly a humanitarian mission, as they were to fly a bombing raid on innocent villagers. Luckily I didn't find that out until we returned. I did notice their seemingly utter disregard or concern for safety. While we were on a fueling stop, I marveled as I watched the pilot precariously pump jet fuel from a metal drum into the plane's tank while balancing a lit cigarette between his lips like it was a toothpick in a banjo player's mouth. The fumes were so strong I couldn't get within twenty feet of the mechanical hand pumping operation, even if I had wanted to do so.

Ultimately, we arrived in the "city" of Karmuk, which was very hot, humid and eerily underdeveloped, where most of my interactions with locals were confined to people who worked in and around the Samaritan's Purse hospital compound, the hospital itself and those members of our team (i.e., drivers, translators, and security guys).

Rusted hulks of tanks, jeeps, trucks and chunks of metal too mangled to even imagine what they had been were strewn across the ground. White-washed, single story, mud brick buildings with peeling paint and chunks of stucco missing from their outer sheaths were the only signs of development, along with scattered water pumps and the occasional string of electrical poles devoid of wires. We were told to avoid traipsing around the area, both off the worn paths or in the nearby hills, as undetonated landmines from the previous war (the Second Sudanese Civil War) continued to shear legs off of unsuspecting people.

A tour of the clinic and immediate area around the town reinforced the sense of desolation of the place. The 50-bed facility serve a population of roughly 150 thousand people, adding weight to the people's argument that they had been intentionally neglected by the GoS.

Our guide, Dr. Atar is a local hero, who, despite being educated in Khartoum and Cairo, refused to leave his people. He was somber, but hopeful despite the circumstances, strong in his determination and conviction to stand by his people in Blue Nile State (an area, like the Nuba, currently under attack by the GoS), and resolute in the hope change would eventually come, but prepared to face the ultimate sacrifice if not. Over a decade later, Dr. Atar is still the only doctor based in the region, which is still at war after a brief five-year hiatus during the time of the Conditional Peace Agreement.

So there we were, dropped off by a plane crew in Karmuk, behind the battle lines, essentially in the middle of nowhere. The only communication was via satellite phone.

As Dr. Kelley started preparing us for the next phase of the journey—the hourslong truck ride into the bush to the remote villages in the interior—he started to ask for things we couldn't locate. With every bag opened, some things were apparently missing, but how?

Exhausted and hungry after our grueling day of flying and schlepping equipment and supplies from one place to another, we made a meal from our MREs, and then as we were getting ready to bed down still unable to locate all the gear, the question—"Do we have all of our bags here?"—arose. Immediately the list I wrote up came into play. Ultimately we were able to deduce that four bags were missing. We assumed we must've left them in Loki. Some of the contents were essential to the medical programs we aimed to help: stethoscopes, batteries, a generator, and an assortment of medicines. Without all the equipment in those bags, our mission would have been severely compromised and too many compromises had already been made on behalf of these people, mostly by the international community, which was for the most part ignoring their plight as evidenced by twenty years of unchecked civil war.

The list allowed us to ascertain, exactly, what we were missing. Using our SAT phone, Dr. Kelley was soon in touch with the charter company in Loki, as well as the guesthouse where we had stayed the night before. In the rush to leave the morning of our departure, four of the bags that had been secured in the hotel office were apparently left behind. As fate would have it, there just happened to be another charter capable of delivering the four bags, whose routing was close enough to Karmuk to make an emergency stop the next day.

On Mission

Finally on our way, we traveled in a huge truck, which the rebels had commandeered from rampaging GoS forces. The rebel soldiers were accustomed to riding in massive fast moving vehicles designed to move items, not people, such as this, and knew where and how to stand without falling down and hurting themselves. Those of us from the States didn't.

The rebels were used to moving men and materiel all over the region, but not Western men (a different breed from the battle hardened SPLA soldiers) or medical equipment, which was even more fragile than the Western men. In the back of the truck, along with rebels and villagers, we had bags of Unimix, duffel bags filled with supplies, camping gear, and cases of bottled water. It was an extremely bumpy and highly uncomfortable ride. Picture those numbered balls bouncing around inside the glass globe for the lottery.

Our primary goal was to get to a series of villages and start a vaccination program for the children, who were highly susceptible to death from measles outbreaks, as well as a host of other opportunistic diseases stemming from severe malnutrition. In addition, Dr. Kelley planned to see as many patients as possible, dispense medicines, and help people learn about rudimentary health maintenance, sanitation and sanitary practices in a place where there is no infrastructure and many and varied ways to come down with various illnesses, some of which could prove deadly.

We bivouacked in a town called Mayak, where the doctors (another was Dr. James Okamoto from Seattle, who had been working with Dr. Kelley for several years now) conducted the first clinics. It was approximately 120 degrees, and we had to carry all of our equipment from the camp to the only buildings in town where we could see patients.

Malnourished children and protein-starved adults, many with infections from wounds, were everywhere.

All the civilians we came into contact with, of course, were potential targets of the GoS, who were routinely being driven from their homes, denied any form of humanitarian aid, and completely cut off from the world.

Despite the hardships and obstacles we faced, during our eight days in the Blue Nile State—traveling to the villages of Mayak, Wadega and Daimen Gazien—we were able to immunize 1,550 children for four diseases (measles, mumps, rubella and meningitis), treat 500 people for a variety of conditions (i.e., fevers, flu, infections, malaria, pneumonia, parasites, allergic reactions, burns, and lymphoma cyst removal), and help initiate the reversal of starvation for about 500 children, all at a cost of $65,000. From this experience I was able to see how a small organization, with a fearless leader, could overcome incredible odds to get equipment, supplies and humanitarian relief into a war zone without any loss of life and, in the process, possibly save hundreds, if not thousands, of lives.

Reflections

I never envisioned myself as a foreign missionary. I also didn't envision myself focusing on Africa, much less Sudan, for any type of work. At the time I went on my first mission trip, I was learning Spanish and much more inclined to consider doing mission work in South America. The trip to Blue Nile changed all of that.

To be completely honest, I was at first shocked by the fact that we spent an incredible amount of energy and resources to help a Muslim group. While that may seem harsh, I always saw Sudan as the story of Christian people being persecuted by a radical Islamic government. Though a strong element of truth exists in that notion, I was to discover there was a lot more to the story than what I had thought. Actually, I'm still discovering the complex nature of the conflicts in the region all these years hence.

What I discovered on that first trip was that the Muslims in the Blue Nile State were just as much victims of their government as the Christians and animists were in the south. Indeed, they were just as hungry, just as marginalized and in as much danger of potential "extinction." I also found out that not a few had been Christians at one point, but due to being coerced, often through force, they had "converted" to Islam.

I also began to learn that anyone residing in rebel territory was as good as a rebel in the eyes of the Government of Sudan. The fellowship and sense of camaraderie I experienced in building relationships with the people of the Blue Nile would carry over to the Nuba Mountains when I would eventually head there several years—actually, just shy of a decade—later.

South Sudan

As stated earlier, my trip to Blue Nile was in 2004, one year before the Second Sudanese Civil War ended. It would be another three years before I'd return to Sudan, this time to the South, during the pounding out of CPA (Comprehensive Peace Agreement).

More specifically, I traveled to the towns of Rumbek and Torit, respectively, in order to attend a pastor's conference and church planting mission. It was during the time in Rumbek that my commitment (and calling) to Sudan took a key turn.

After spending a day with the pastors at the training center, I marveled at the degree of congeniality and openness of the men in attendance. All of them had seen war, dislocation, death, and suffering—many on a regular basis. Some had fought in the military, others had been refugees in neighboring Uganda and Kenya. As we were standing in a circle chatting and discussing the day's events, I started to mentally recede from the group. It was as if everyone around me went silent while an inner voice told me my laughter and joy was different than that of those around me. It was a sobering reminder that despite the common ground we all had established at the conference, my evolving Sudan story was not a Sudanese story. The closest comparison I can think of to capture the distinction that had formed in my mind is the difference between a child watching a Memorial Day parade and his grandfather's actual experience on the battlefield during World War II. My conscience was forcing me to recognize what they had been through to get to this point and what it had cost them. Every single one of them had, at one time or another, left behind family members, livelihoods, their homes. All had faced drastic conditions and impossible choices. One of the men, Ding, had been a Lost Boy, who had traveled by foot between Sudan, Kenya and Ethiopia, all the while witnessing various friends die along the way or be abducted by both rebel and government soldiers. Another, Dima, had taken on the gigantic burden of caring for his brother's wife and five children after his brother had died. He faced a constant, ongoing, struggle to figure out how to support them all. A third, Ruman, had spent years fighting in the bush before becoming a chaplain and a civilian pastor.

Ultimately, I could only respond to my personal musings by promising I would never leave or forsake these people, even if war returned to them. The magnitude of the commitment I made to myself scared me at the time, because the threat of a return to a war footing was looming. Years later I would extend my commitment to the Nuba people as well, though at the time I knew almost nothing about them or the degree of importance regarding their role in securing the tenuous peace for South Sudan.

A couple of days after the pastor's conference had ended, while having dinner, I met a man from the region known as the Nuba Mountains. All I knew of the place was that it was in the North, and that its destiny in the unfolding peace process was not as clear as the region in the South. I had also heard of foreign missionaries being killed there. As I sat with this man and listened to his stories of brutal oppression by the regime in Khartoum, I naively asked him why they, the Nuba, didn't start a social movement to raise awareness of the situation in order reach those outside of the Nuba Mountains, as well as create what would amount to a "civil rights movement" within Sudan. If the situation in Sudan hadn't been as dire as it was, I think he would have chuckled at my naiveté. He did tell me in no uncertain terms there was no option for a program of civil disobedience in Sudan akin to what happened in the United States in the 1950s and 1960s. Any protest, he assured me, would be met with certain and immediate death. This was yet another sobering reminder of how uninitiated I was when it came to Sudan, and how little I really knew about it.

It would be another five years before I made my own way to the Nuba Mountains to wage a "protest" of my own against the Government of Sudan for its ill-treatment of its own people. The interactions with the pastors at the conference, my personal and silent commitment to stand by the Sudanese people, my experience in Blue Nile State during the war, and this random conversation with a pastor from the Nuba Mountains during my second trip to the region, all played a part in moving me inextricably towards an alignment with the plight of the Nuba.

Miriam's Story—First a Spark, Then a Flame

Between 2007 and 2012 I didn't think a great deal about the Nuba Mountains, but rather spent my time going on short-term mission trips in the southern part of the region, which would become The Republic of South Sudan in 2011. Some were medical- and humanitarian-oriented, others purely for the purpose of sharing the Gospel and helping to strengthen churches in the region following the long, deadly years of civil war and religious oppression by the GoS.

Upon returning from one of these trips in 2012, I chanced upon an article by Nicholas Kristof of the *New York Times* about the plight of a Nuba woman named Miriam.[3] Her story was gripping as it vividly conveyed the absolute desperation of the people of the Nuba Mountains. Kristof not only described how this woman, before fleeing out into the bush, grabbed an automatic weapon and began firing aimlessly as her village was being attacked, but also described the condition of Miriam's fellow Nubans who she was trying to protect. He reported that during a trip he had taken into the region, people were reduced to eating leaves, poisonous roots, and tree bark to stave off hunger. I was shocked. As mentioned, I had just left the country to the immediate south where there were mangoes falling off the trees and plenty of other food available. Now, being back in the States, I wondered how I could have missed even hearing about so much suffering happening just a few hundred miles away. I asked myself: "Were these not also the people to whom I had made a commitment never to leave in the lurch, even in the face of war?" I had made that silent commitment standing in the midst of several pastors from the new South Sudan, but weren't the same "Sudanese" people suffering in the Nuba Mountains? Indeed, as I was to discover, the Nuba had fought side-by-side with the people from the South in their struggle against the government of Khartoum. Thus, I felt the only answer to my own question was an unequivocal "Yes!" But then, I became frightened.

First Trip into the Nuba Mountains

Dr. Kelley's example was not only laudatory, it was inspirational. It helped me realize what was possible, even in the face war. My efforts would build on the work of people like Alan Kelley, but unlike the doctor who acted alone and built an organization around himself, I was more inclined to partner and surround myself with people like him. That's exactly what I set out to do in initiating the formation of what eventually became the End Nuba Genocide (ENG) coalition, whose mission was to get immediate and direct aid to the Nuba people, and "tell the world" what was happening to them based on first hand experience. It was June and the pace of my Sudan story was picking up, running like sand through an hourglass, but every grain of sand seemed to represent another dead Nuba.

By September of 2012, almost a year after the start of the new war in the Nuba Mountains, I was headed to Sudan on a plane from my home in the San Francisco Bay Area. I was used to the route I was to take through the Netherlands and then Nairobi onto

South Sudan, but this would be the first time I'd ever set foot in the Nuba Mountains. I didn't even know if there were truly mountains in this region because I'd never seen anything I would truly call a "mountain" west of Ethiopia during my earlier trips to Sudan, though I knew there were some peaks scattered about. My experience of Sudan was mostly hot, flat, and terrain that was sometimes forested, sometimes covered with thick bushes.

My sense of entering the Nuba was a mixture of the possibility of facing potential danger along with curiosity, trepidation, and a religious fervor to reach persecuted peoples forgotten by the world. It was a volatile cocktail of emotions and motivations that temporarily blinded me to the real risks of entering a war zone, especially after so many years of enjoying the relative safety of peacetime South Sudan. And the latter didn't even factor into the looming issue as to how I and those traveling with me were going to manage our mode of travel. There were still a lot of unknowns even at the late stages of this mission (meaning, while actually on the way to Africa), which was largely due to the sense of urgency to reach the Nuba, where more and more people were said to be dying by the second.

Call to Action

It is said desperate times call for desperate measures. Whether or not this is attributable to any particular individual or not, it certainly rings true, especially during a period such as the beginning of the war in South Kordofan in June 2011. Stories of atrocities committed against civilians under attack as if they were armed combatants themselves were starting to become commonplace. My sense of urgency to find a way to help these people led me on a path straight into the Nuba Mountains. But I knew I couldn't go alone; I had to find help.

I started with the most likely candidates who possibly knew what was happening on the ground in the region, missionaries. During my years of going back and forth, I met quite a few missionaries who either resided or worked in various parts of South Sudan or had projects there but operated from the United States, Canada, Europe or another African nation. However, time and again as I inquired about who was operating in the Nuba, I was met with a blank. Little seemed to be known about the plight of the Nuba—at least among those I was speaking with, and no one I knew was engaged in any missions there due to the violent nature of the conflict. There was also a humanitarian aid blockade there, pretty much unheard of in the civilized world. Despite this fact, I was able to find one person who was not only focused on the Nuba Mountains, but ready to go there. I contacted him, Samuel Totten, a scholar of genocide studies based at the University of Arkansas, Fayetteville, and after a brief phone call, I knew was starting to make progress on responding to the promise I had made years before to do something about the heartrending images in Nick Kristof's story of Miriam that continued to haunt me.

On Our Way, September 2012

Totten and I agreed to form a group/team by contacting individuals who we each thought might have an interest in taking action to prevent what appeared to be the incipient stage of another genocide by attrition, which the Nuba were subjected to by the GoS in the 1990s. Through my missionary contacts on one end, and Totten's contacts with genocide scholars and human rights activists on the other, a small group of six individuals was quickly formed. We initiated our efforts by holding regular conference calls to discuss goals and objectives, formulating a plan, and potential strategies.

The "A Team" that was formed was small, but extremely focused and well connected: Slater Armstrong of Joining Our Voices; Mark Hackett of Operation Broken Silence; David Hicks of e3 Partners; George Tutu; and Dr. John Hubbel Weiss of Cornell University. One member in particular, George Tutu, a Nuba, was very well connected within the Nuba community, both in the U.S. and abroad. Many years earlier, George had formed the Nuba Christian Family Mission (NCFM), with the specific purpose of serving as a Christian aid and development organization for his people. Tellingly, he had also spent a relatively large portion of his life on the run from the government of Sudan and was familiar with the risks associated with even bringing humanitarian aid to the people the GoS was trying to destroy. Ultimately, we formed what became the End Nuba Genocide (ENG) project. This small, fledgling organization without a 501(c)(3) designation, operated on a shoestring budget by us—all nonprofessionals in the area of humanitarian relief and mission work—eventually conducted numerous missions to the Nuba Mountains, delivering over 120 tons of grain and $10,000 worth of medical supplies. Altogether, over the course of the next three years, we raised over $125,000.

Stepping Up and In

The Treaty of Westphalia ended years of bloody religious and political conflict in Europe in 1648, but ironically, and inadvertently, set the stage for leaders of "sovereign" nations like Sudan to carry out horrible atrocities against its own people with impunity. It is within this context that war is being waged in Sudan, with the bombing of civilian targets and moratoriums on all foreign humanitarian aid in both the Nuba Mountains and the Blue Nile State. Thus, any attempt to help malnourished and war ravaged communities in the state of South Kordofan, which is home to the Nuba Mountains, constitutes a violation of, at least Sudanese law, if not international law. The upshot of the aforementioned treaty that freed thousands of Europeans from death, hunger and the depredations of war is, now, today, essentially allowing" for all those hazards and more against the Nuba people. Despite such obstacles, we immediately began to plan how we could, initially, get five tons of corn soy blend (a nutritive grain) to the Nuba people as quickly as possible. As we saw it, we were obeying a higher law, operating over and above the principles of international law, while—at least in our minds—not violating it, much like the law of aerodynamics doesn't nullify but rather overcomes that of gravity. Be that as it may, we would soon be up against the combined forces of nature and man in trying to deliver hope (and food) to the Nuba people.

Roadblocks

Over the course of my years working with various ministries in South Sudan I had become familiar with the Sudan People's Liberation Army (SPLA), and had had various interactions with its members, the rebels. Though I don't specifically remember encountering any Nuba people in those early years, I came to understand the integral role they (the Nuba) played in the South's struggle against the GoS. It has even been said the Nuba were among the best fighters within the SPLA. It seemed ironic that the men who fought so long in the struggle that eventually opened the door for the South to obtain its freedom would ultimately be forced to remain in the North—and not only that, but in a situation in which they would become increasingly isolated as a result of the changing dynamics in international politics, including a U.S. government which was softening its stance in relation to Khartoum's criminal and murderous actions.

The Nuba was now in a battle for its very existence. And part and parcel of that was the GoS' refusal to allow NGOs to deliver humanitarian aid to the region, which was slowly but surely, along with the bombing of civilian farms, creating a humanitarian disaster. Under these conditions, our fledgling coalition connected with one man that could tip the balance in our favor.

At the outset we decided that not every member of our group needed to go on every mission. We figured that different guys might be able to make one mission but not another, depending on his situation at work or at home. We also thought it was wise to have at least one of the guys back in the U.S. who could serve as a liaison in case the team needed help.

An Ideal Partnership

Early on, it was decided that those on the team who would undertake this first mission would be me, David Hicks, and George Tutu. A young fellow named John, a member of a church I attended, Hope Church, and one of the early and most ardent supporters of the ENG coalition, also came along. Sam Totten volunteered to head up the second mission, which was to be carried out several months down the line.

As we began plans to purchase the food, have it hauled to the border of South Sudan/Sudan, and then transported into the Nuba Mountains, we also initiated contact with the humanitarian branch of the Nuba government in exile (The Nuba Relief, Rehabilitation and Development Organization or NRRDO) to ensure our efforts didn't run afoul of their plans and efforts. Operations such as these were (and are) delicate in terms of timing and logistics. Furthermore, tight coordination with authorities was of the utmost concern. We didn't know it at the time, but on our initial foray into the Nuba Mountains we would ultimately be traveling with one of the best people to know in the region, not only a representative of the humanitarian wing of government in exile, but a former military commander who was accorded great respect by almost everyone we encountered along the way. Jacoub (whose surname must remain secret due to reasons of security) had an austere, intense look about him. He seemed like he had the weight of the world on his shoulders. He also seemed to be able to look right through you, into the heart of a man, and tell whether he was up to the task at hand.

Once Jacoub made the decision to help us, he led us, and when we thought it was almost too tough to continue, we all ploughed on, taking each new step to prove to Jacoub we could do it and/or not to let him down. In his own inimitable way, he frightened, intimidated, inspired, comforted, humored, and, ultimately, carried us in order to make it possible for us to achieve our goal. When our vehicle got bogged down in the muddy muck resulting from the onset of the rainy season, Jacoub, despite having recovered fairly recently from a bout of malaria, literally marched us across the border, first leading the way, then taking up the rear so that no stragglers would be put in jeopardy during the two day, 35-plus kilometer trek across extremely difficult and dangerous terrain.

Determination

When we arrived in the Yida Refugee Camp along the South Sudan/Sudan border, our small team of four had become an advance team in the sense that our food shipment was still en route from Kampala (Uganda). As luck would have it, we mistimed our arrival in that we were met by the initial rains of the rainy season in the region. (In fact, it would not be until several weeks after our return that the bulk of the food would make it to its destination in Nuba Mountains.) We knew of no other relief efforts, and thus we figured that even the relatively small amount of aid we planned on delivering would perhaps be more than the people we encountered would have seen in a long time.

So, with the rainy season now upon us, and the options for entering the region very limited, we had to face the stark fact that we were 32.2 kilometers (20 miles) from the South Sudan/Sudan border, and more than *another* 40 kilometers (or some 24 miles) from the nearest population inside of Sudan. Figuring we might not be able to get the five tons of food from Kampala in time to insert it before the rains made it virtually impossible to even hike in, we had to make some quick and critical decisions. One of the first was to purchase 1,000 pounds of food along the border in South Sudan.

Though clouds are usually a relief from the blazing equatorial sun, as the rainy season approaches clouds signal the end of the ability to move easily over the unpaved "roads" of the Sudan. While we planned our approach, light rain fell intermittently. Our whole mission hinged on one thing: getting into Sudan. Two of the limiting factors impinging on our ability to accomplish our mission were (a) the return dates of our flights to Juba and then back to the States, and (b) the torrential rains which we knew were coming sooner or later—it wasn't a matter if they were coming, but rather a matter of when they were coming. While I still had my day job back in the States to consider, even those with more flexibility had nonrefundable tickets, which would result in their paying hefty penalties should they miss their flights. The latter was not really an option since the effort had already been an exorbitantly expensive endeavor for all of us.

Ultimately, we were forced to wait while our Nuba partners attempted to find a vehicle capable of making the trip. Thus, the precious few days we had to spend in the Nuba, should we even make it there, were ticking away. As painful as the thought of not getting in with the 1,000 pounds of food we had with us was, it was more painful to think about returning home to our friends, family and supporters having failed to reach our goal.

Finally, after two days of waiting, still not certain we would be able to actually get into Nuba, we were informed that a vehicle was not available. So, we formed a new plan. With hundreds of people streaming into the camp every week, we *knew* there had to be a way to reach those areas where the refugees were coming from via foot. This is where Jacoub came in. He told us he would go with us, and thus we ended up following the same path that the refugees flowed down but only in reverse; and not only along the same path, but via the same mode of transportation: footing (as the Nuba say). Going into an extremely difficult and potentially deadly situation such as we were facing could be seen as either incredibly foolish or incredibly brave. We were neither. We were with Jacoub, and the confidence he instilled in us was probably not unlike that of the hundreds of men he led over his career in the SPLA.

Be that as it may, entering an active war zone is still fraught with dangers and risks. Though we got a lift to an area close to the border, the vehicle got stuck on the road in what would best be described as a small pond. And thus the footing began, with each of us carrying a pack that weighed in at approximately 70 pounds. The 70 pounds included our tents, cooking equipment, water, personal food, camera equipment, survival gear (headlamps, water purification, first aid kit, etc.), Christian literature (bibles, tracts), and gifts for children (candy).

Since we were as much on a fact-finding mission as a humanitarian mission, whenever possible, we periodically stopped and talked with people along the way. By doing so, we were attempting to informally document the effects of the war on the civilian population.

One group of people, in particular, caught my attention: a family of children. The oldest of the kids may have been in their late teens, with the youngest under ten. The children informed us that their parents chose to not take the long journey (over 100 kilometers or 60 miles) on foot from their village to the refugee camp (Yida). For me, that really spoke to the severity of the situation the Nuba were facing: stay and risk starvation or death from above (bombing), or leave and take a journey filled with risk and uncertainty, which will end in a refugee camp in a neighboring country. Knowing a bit about African cultures and familial ties and being cognizant of the fact that children are

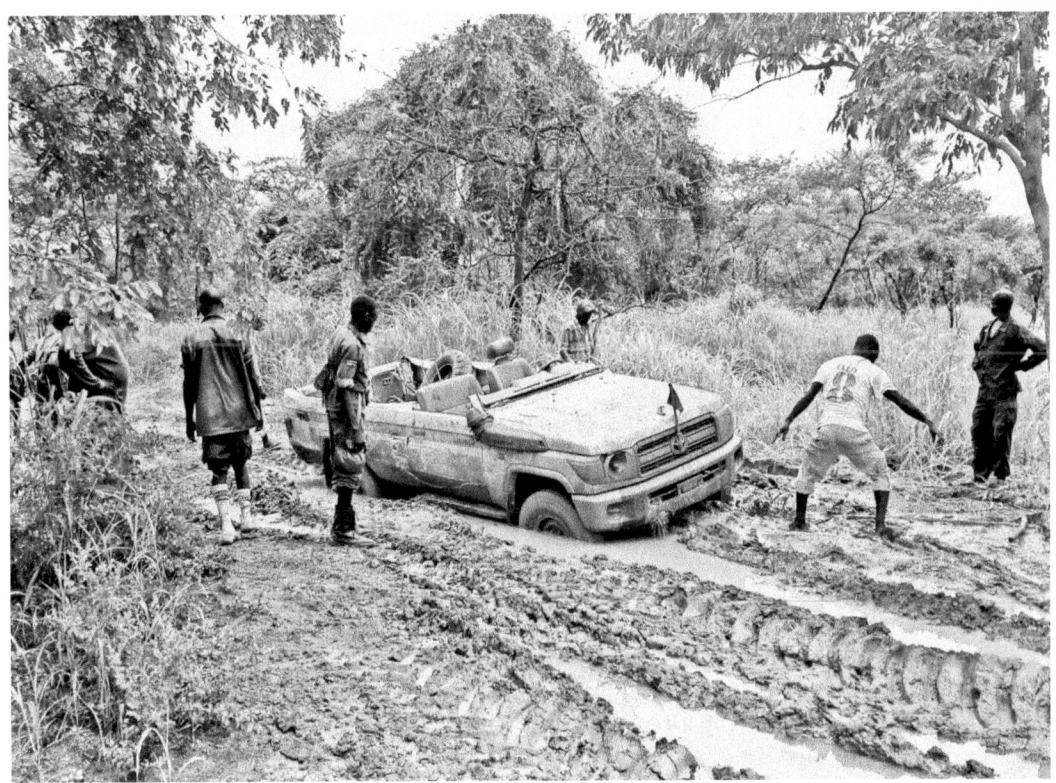

Road conditions in Sudan make for tough travel in the rainy season (John C. Jefferson).

an insurance policy and much needed source of help in simple, agrarian and subsistence farming communities, I asked myself what it took for this family to make the decision to split up the way it had. Was it to give the children a chance for more reliable food, water, education and health care? Were the parents too weak, too old, too afraid to make the journey, or did they feel compelled to remain behind in order to protect their homes and whatever mean possessions they had? Continuing on, we gained more and more insight into the plight of the Nuba as we "swam" upstream against the tide of refugees fleeing the Nuba Mountains.

There was actually a lightness to our step as we headed away from the disabled vehicle that bogged down a few miles south of the border. Though our packs were heavy, and we had already broken into a serious sweat, first, simply getting our gear out of the truck, and then, beginning to hike along the road next to thorny thickets just waiting to catch every piece of skin and fabric that came within a millimeter of them, we were at least on our way to our destination. And that felt good, especially after what seemed to be an endless wait.

As the temperature soared into the triple digits, we quickly became exhausted; and as we did, each and every step became more difficult. The weight of the packs, the loose, sandy soil of the roadway, the buzzing flies, the thorns and the blinding sun with no shade wears quickly on the uninitiated man from the West.

Once at the border, we attempted to make a realistic assessment of our situation. We were still in South Sudan, but ahead of us was a marsh of tall reeds and bush land, with deep rutted tire tracks and muddy paths going in a myriad of directions disappearing into thickets and rushes. For once, I welcomed the inordinately long bureaucratic processes at an African border crossing. We were essentially passing into a no man's land, so our main issue was whether or not we would be able to get out once we were in.

We had hired a young man with a quad runner to help us carry our gear, but it became clear rather quickly that we had too much to expect him to carry. Thus, we hired a couple of additional "vehicles" to help transport our precious little foodstuffs. Two bicyclists were willing to carry sugar and salt, and a motorcycle carried a couple of additional bags of grain. We would tell the people when we got inside, this represented the vanguard of a bigger shipment to come.

As we set out for the first time with nothing but our destination before us, we marched in silence along the muddy tracks, stopping several times to get our bearings, as if we were a freight train leaving a switching station and trying to locate the right tracks north. The humidity seemed to increase as the radiant energy from the ground met the hot air. As the treads of my companion's boots became thick with mud, I realized the Sudanese making the trek in flip-flops had the right idea. I had already put on my Tevas (a brand of sandals designed for wet environments like kayaking, perfect for marshy Sudan). (I ended up being the only one without blisters as a result of wearing the Tevas, but ended up with scores of tiny bites on each ankle from some kind of invisible insect.) We marched on and on this way, having started out around midday, and arrived at a small checkpoint in the interior just before nightfall.

That night the swarms of mosquitoes were absolutely miserable, so we bedded down quickly after sunset, having already filtered several liters of water and prepared and ate our dinner of boiled Thai noodles. The day of walking with the hot sun above and the deeply rutted, swampy, bush trail beneath, our feet had taken its toll. We all knew, though, that Sudan had a lot more punishment to deal out on the road ahead.

The next day, in fact, was a brutal test of endurance. We hiked almost the whole day, part of it without water, eventually stumbling into a small military outpost and village. There we refreshed ourselves by sitting with some of the "rebel" soldiers under a group of trees and partook of some drinking water one of our team members was able to procure somehow. The latter was the first to arrive at the outpost as he had gotten a lift on a quad runner due to a severe case of dehydration. After he was dropped off, the vehicle continued to shuttle the grain, sugar and salt to the outpost, while the rest of us who were not as close to collapsing, marched on. To exacerbate matters, along the way, in addition to the imminent threat of being bombed, we were told that not too long before bands of militias had been terrorizing people fleeing to Yida.

As we periodically stopped to interview people streaming southward towards the refugee camp, we heard story after story of bombings, whole villages without food, and attacks on civilians by GoS soldiers. These lucky ones had had to brave the same elements we were now facing: little food or water, inadequate clothing and no shelter at night. All feared being killed by GoS ground troops or aerial attacks.

When we'd ask if they were able to maintain their fields and harvest crops, they all cited examples of the fields being burned just before harvest by incendiary bombs or raiders targeting the food supply. For subsistence farmers, this was devastating. In addition, herds were targeted, wells destroyed, and villages burned. For those taking refuge in Tobanya (a town nearby), many were from further north and were now occupying homes among the rocks left by others who had fled in earlier waves towards Yida. Many women were alone, having seen their husbands off to war. After a while, it was senseless

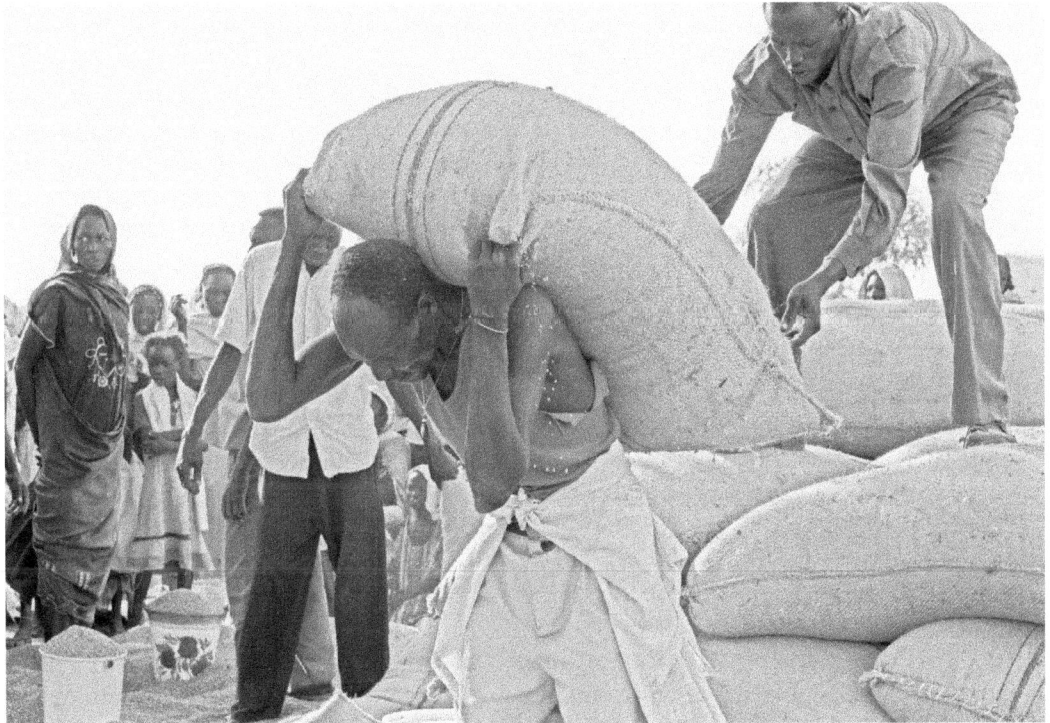

Unloading grain during one of the many humanitarian efforts on the behalf of IDPs and refugees from the Nuba Mountains (John C. Jefferson).

asking questions as the answers were all too common and painful. A well-orchestrated plan for destruction, both of crops and the Nuba people, was underway. We couldn't stop it, but we could undermine it with a bag of grain, some salt and sugar, a prayer to God, and a story for the world outside to hear.

Despite everything, I have to say that the Nuba (region) was far more beautiful and tranquil than I ever expected, though the threat of war loomed ominously and everywhere there were signs of it. In contradistinction to the beauty and seeming tranquility of the Nuba Mountains, "fox holes" to escape bombardment were outside just about every *tukul*.

After successfully making it into the Nuba Mountains against not a few odds just a few short months after my wakeup call about what was happening there, I tried to garner some level of satisfaction of what we had accomplished. After all, we had been able to get 1,000 lbs of grain, along with some sugar and salt, into an area not only extremely difficult place to reach but which was currently a war zone. We had also made an unlikely coalition work, and collected key information on real events in real time. But this was only the beginning.

A Second Trip into the Nuba Mountains, Spring 2013

My next trip to the Nuba Mountains took us to a very remote area called Kao Nyaro, of which little was known, even by a lot of Nuba from outside of the particular area. The Kao Nyaro people had been suffering greatly for at least a year before we got there. Tellingly, just as we were preparing for our team's third trip (Sam Totten had made a second one by himself in December 2012), NRRDO had requested help in getting food into the area.

Crowded in the front cab of a Land Cruiser pickup and bouncing along a deeply rutted dirt road in 100 plus degree heat isn't exactly most people's idea of a good time, unless of course you have planned, prayed and plotted for a few months in the hope of being in just such a situation. It also beats being in the back of said vehicle with a couple of drums of fuel, a ton of luggage and supplies, and a host of well-armed soldiers with live rounds of ammunition. After having faced a high level of scrutiny from the local authorities in Melut (in South Sudan)—both the local police and military personal questioned us about where we wanted to go and why due to the fact that an active civil war was being fought—dealings with unscrupulous merchants who raised prices hourly, the threat of a deluge of rain, reluctant truck owners who inflated their rates once they heard where we wanted to go, and a host of other obstacles, it was actually a great relief to finally be on the road and heading toward the destination ENG had been told was an area of great need. A sense of destiny had taken hold over the doubt, dissonance, and fear so prevalent during the planning stages back in the States. Though rough, the road proved to be in relatively good shape and we made excellent time as we drove north looking for the last city on the road, leaving Malakal before we headed toward the South Sudan/Sudan border.

With the last purchase of food we made, the tense moments of walking around the aforementioned city with over $15,000 in a backpack (as prices were being negotiated, renegotiated, and negotiated again, for the sorghum, hiring local males to load and unload the food coming in, and fuel for the vehicles) were behind us. Also behind us was the uncertainty as to whether we would even get this far: first, there was the torrential downpour portending a potentially, and most unwelcome, early rainy season (in the end, fortunately, the rain did not last long); second, there was the emergency evacuation of one of the team members who fell ill with an unknown malady; and third, there were a series of security meetings we had to endure until the authorities were convinced that our mission was worth the risk of letting us venture beyond the city limits.

The weather had been hot and the air dry, but soon the sun went down and the trip resumed under the cover of darkness. We bumped along into the night without incident, though I mused how easy it would be to get ambushed driving along a road of deeply rutted, dried mud, encased by walls of dense brush and tall spiny trees on either side. Our driver, Ahmad, seemed to know just when the bumpy road would turn into a launching pad and would press on the brakes and slow down just enough to make it seem like we hit an obnoxious speed bump, thus preventing the guys riding in the truck's bed from being shot out like projectiles, or sending the heads of those of us in the cab smashing into the roof of the truck. At one point, we came to a sudden halt, and the rebel soldiers jumped out quickly to check rustling in the bush. After a few tense moments, with the occasional shout coming from the thick of the brush, I saw a donkey come into focus surrounded by three soldiers who were going through the contents it was carrying. No owner was in sight. My first instinct was to feel sorry for the mystery owner. His milk, a small amount of food, and probably his most precious possession (or at least, most valuable)—that being the donkey—was now in the hands of these men; the same ones to whom I was more or less counting on to protect my life. How were they going to handle this situation, I wondered? Were they going to act like soldiers of fortune or bandits? Or were they going to behave more like guardians of the realm? As I pondered this matter and the incident faded behind us in the cloud of dust made by our Land Cruiser, Ahmad explained through George (who had now squeezed into the cab of the truck with me) as the interpreter, that the man with the donkey was an "Arab" herder, or more accurately a Baggara. With this brief explanation, I still found myself feeling sorry for the guy, who had just gotten shaken down by the rebels, as if he were a homeless man on a street in New York City having had his shopping cart emptied and turned over by a bunch of gang bangers. That sentiment, however, changed in light of new information Ahmad shared while we bounced along the dusty bush road.

In South Kordofan State, as in other parts of Sudan, Khartoum (in other words, the GoS) has used such semi-nomadic herders to disrupt or end the lives of the indigenous Africans or Nubans. In many cases in the relatively recent past, such herders, armed and dangerous, and, with the GoS' imprimatur, raided villages, captured children for the slave trade, destroyed crops, and displaced Christian, animist, and moderate Muslim farmers and herders and then encouraged loyal, Islamized Sudanese to settle on the newly "acquired" land. Part of the problem is that instead of the GoS seeing the Nuba civilians as people who were caught in the middle of the new war, it (the government) equated the elderly, the women and children as part and parcel of the rebelling faction. This perspective lent itself to making targets of the Nuba civilians. Furthermore, and conveniently, it justified allowing the Baggara to grab the Nuba land and villages, after they (the Baggara) had helped GoS troops drive the Nuba out of the region. In this context, it became a little clearer to me why the soldiers handled the situation the way they did. Likewise, my initial and naïve response to the situation—and misguided sympathies for the owner of the donkey—are emblematic of the danger of relying on partial information to complex situations. This is neither to say all Baggara are bad nor the SPLA rebels are always right in how they handle situations, but it taught me a good lesson about the danger of prejudging situations, one which I hoped I would not have to learn over and over again as the journey continued.

Making Deliveries in the Kao Nyaro

The Kao Nyaro region is hotter and drier than that of the region in Sudan due north of the Yida Refugee Camp, from whence we first ventured into the Nuba Mountains. It is also much more remote, and thus the people, being more isolated, did not have the benefit of what little support the the GoS had offered residents of northern South Kordofan, prior to the war. Likewise, the Kao Nyaro people also lacked contact with NGOs, which provide all sorts of valuable services.

The region is named after the people who are spread out over a large area bordered by "mountains" or large hills that rise up from flat lands to the south leading back down to the Nile Valley and the town of Kodok, where we began our journey northward. Whether it was true they had been completely isolated or not I cannot say; but there were no signs of NGO activity in 2013, and almost no development. (There were a few old buildings probably dating back to the Colonial Era, but that was it.) When we first arrived in the area, we were told we were the first "white" (non–African) people to show up there in years.

The tradeoff for having to deal with the extremely tough trek into the area was the satisfaction in finally arriving at our destination (i.e., the compound where we stayed at the edge of a village, after having spent over thirteen hours en route over hot, dusty "roads"). A bucket shower and a ring of beds laid out around the interior of the compound (mosquitoes not being an issue in the dry season) was the perfect conclusion to what had been a torrid day and body aching ride over rutted, rocky, dusty roads.

I really didn't know what to expect on this trip. We had had so little prior contact with the people inside the region, it was hard to get a read on how to actually reach the place, much less have a good sense of the conditions we were likely to encounter. We had had to negotiate with local suppliers in Upper Nile State in order to purchase the grain we wished to haul up to the Nuba, which was no mean feat given prices kept rising as the news of *kawajas* or "white people" interested in purchasing grain spread. Our NRRDO partners had procured a truck large enough to carry over fifteen tons of grain at a time in order to help us shuttle the combined 60 tons we had co-purchased with NRRDO to deliver to the Kao Nyaro. Because this was the first time in a long time anyone had ventured there on a humanitarian mission to deliver food, no one had any idea whether or not what the amount we were hauling up would be enough. We also feared we might face the specter of such severe need that our delivery might result in food riots and/or the people taking their frustration out on us, which had actually happened to another group attempting to deliver aid in another region within the conflict zone of Sudan.

Fortunately, for us, even though the people's condition was extremely dire in Kao Nyaro, what I experienced of the people was contrary to all of the aforementioned speculations. The people had no stores of food, and had been reduced to eating roots, grasses and insects, which they showed me as they crowded around when the food distribution started.

Ultimately, we were able to deliver a large portion of the 60 tons of grain purchased by the combined forces of ENG and NRRDO and to see to it that more or less equal amounts were distributed and stored in Kao, Nyaro and Werni, the three main villages of the region. Throughout the three main villages we heard the stories of how Nuba civilians were being bombed and attacked by their own government in a futile attempt to drive them from their land. They were, justly angry at being deprived of their basic human rights of liberty and freedom, and were upset that their children were being denied a basic education and health care. Their clothes were worn and tattered and their abodes ramshackle, but their spirits were strong.

Any trepidation about being in such a place or around the people in Kao Nyaro vanished as we went from area to area. Just about everywhere we went, we met people who captivated us with their stories of survival and determination to remain in their ancestral homeland. One case in particular rattled me. A little boy stood boldly in front of me after being jostled and pushed to the front of a crowd gathering in front of my Nikon and proceeded to allow me to interview him. He was dignified, but disheveled, with lighter skin than most, and a dusty Afro to match his baggy shorts and bareness from the waist up. He wavered a bit as he tried to hold his head up and speak directly to me through an interpreter (the adults around him coached him, as Sudanese elders are wont to do). He also had one half shut eye and dried snot under his nose, but he possessed as much charisma as Martin Luther King, Jr., delivering one of his famous speeches. The contrast between the young boy's appearance and his delivery, squinting in the setting sun with beads of sweat forming lightly on his dusty brow, as he responded to my two main questions—"What do you want the world to know about you and the Nuba people?" and "What do you want to tell the world?"—was so great it bordered on the comical. Upon reflection, it was a rather adult-like question for a boy who appeared to be only six or seven years old, but, then again, in this part of Sudan, with rampant malnutrition and disease, one can't assume age and physical stature always correspond. After recording his little monologue, one of the men I was traveling with told me the boy had directed his remarks to Sudanese President Omar al-Bashir and the Antonovs. I chuckled to myself, musing that here was this defiant young boy, who didn't even own a shirt, standing up to a ruthless dictator in a war zone and unflinchingly telling some American with a camera what he thought of the situation. This, I thought, is the spirit of the Nuba. This is why the Nuba will never be completely under the domination of an oppressive regime without first putting up the fiercest fight anyone could possibly muster.

I later found out the boy was an orphan who had been taken in by some relatives after he found his way to their village. The next time I saw him in the village center, with its shuttered shops and deserted markets, I had the driver stop the vehicle and I jumped out. I removed the shirt I was wearing and handed it to him. Everyone around me chuckled as I handed the boy the t-shirt and pulled my button-down on to cover up my "ghostly white" flesh. With some coaching of the elders, he put the shirt on, then stood at attention and delivered a brief thank you address. I was torn between laughing and tearing up. Sometimes Sudan stories get punctuated by memorable events, driven by the unlikeliest of people and circumstances. I went to Kao Nyaro to come to the aid of a people in a hopeless situation, and found myself overwhelmed with admiration, respect and appreciation to be among them.

Several women in the village of Kao were especially forceful in their opinions of the war and their plight. The stories, translated by George Tutu for us, were about atrocities committed against them and their families by the GoS. One woman kept silent until she was prodded to speak, and when she did it seemed like a teakettle had gone off as she recounted how she and others were driven from their villages along the plains up into the hills and mountains. Like a professional mime, using her hands, she indicated how planes would come from overhead, drop their deadly payloads, and leave a wave of devastation in their wake: burning crops, screaming children, and hundreds fleeing in search of safety. Each story she related was confirmed by the other women via the nodding of heads and verbal affirmations in their mother tongue (Kao).

When it was time to say goodbye to the people in each village, the mood would always shift to friendly parting words and blessings with smiles and waves. The Nuba had been listened to and heard by people willing to risk their lives to help them, and who promised to take their stories and share them with the larger world. The question, of course, was: Would the world listen and then act?

The Turning of the Tide

Leaving the Kao Nyaro was an exercise in exhilaration. We could now tell the world about the Kao Nyaro, who have largely been ignored by the rest of the world (including the international community), and what they've been subjected to at the hands of the GoS, not to mention their ongoing suffering. From the very beginning, the goal of the End Nuba Genocide project was to not only expose what was happening to the Nuba, but to help reverse the effects of starvation, malnutrition and lack of access to medicines.

Though our contribution was relatively small, we brought hope, truth, light and some sustenance, while at the same time paving the way for others outside of the Nuba to know and, hopefully, eventually act on what they now know. No longer were the Nuba a forgotten people, because now, a small group of people and churches located thousands of miles away from

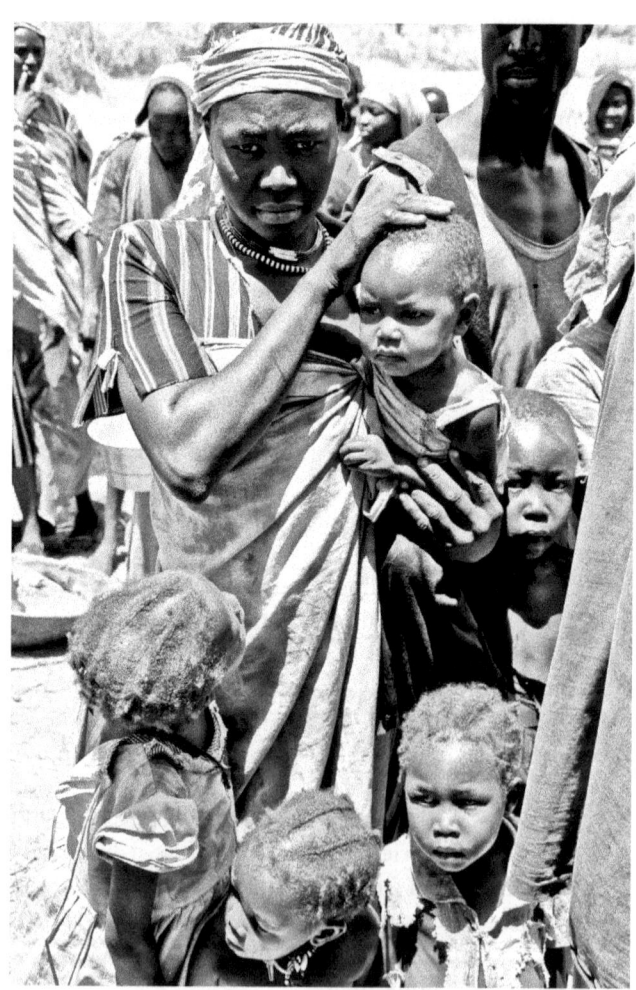

A family in the Kao Nyaro living the barest of existences as a result of being targeted by the SAF (John C. Jefferson).

the Nuba Mountains were taking action, making noise, and joining forces to do what nations and the humanitarian community were failing to do.

Return to Kodok

During my first trip to one of the more remote regions in the Nuba Mountains, we had discovered that there were hundreds, if not thousands, of refugees in Kodok, a city in southern Sudan. Because we were anxious to get out to Kao Nyaro, we had spent very little time in Kodok and thus did not get an opportunity to visit the refugee camp located there. As ENG mulled over our options in regard to returning to the Nuba, we started to hear reports of a new conflict erupting in South Sudan. It was December 2013.

The horrific and internecine fighting and vicious killing of both fighters and innocent civilians in South Sudan very much impacted plans to return to the Nuba Mountains. Basically, the Nuba civilians were caught in between two vicious wars. Still, ENG decided to proceed with its efforts, and thus it was in this context, in January of 2014, that the ENG group started to explore options for a resupply mission to people we knew were in desperate straits in Kao Nyaro.

It isn't easy to get into a war zone, or, for that matter, out, but when one who is intent on getting in *and* knows enough crazy people, things can happen. Or so it seemed in March of 2014 when, still reeling from the outbreak of civil war in South Sudan in December, those working to help the Nuba people were trying to continue their efforts. I was scheduled to return to the Nuba as my partners in End Nuba Genocide and I had raised sufficient funds to undertake a resupply mission, but short of commissioning a private plane to Upper Nile State, there seemed to be no way for us to get in this time around. Vicious battles were raging all across South Sudan and commercial flights to cities along the Nile, such as Malakal, had been shut down. With larger humanitarian aid organizations focused on their own missions in South Sudan—and, in many cases, focused on the evacuation of their personnel from the extremely dangerous situation— we were swimming against the tide in trying to get to our ultimate destination, Kodok, where the refugees who we wished to help were located. At one and the same time, the cost to hire a charter flight loomed in the neighborhood of $25,000 USD, an amount close to the entire budget allocated for the resupply effort. Reaching out to anyone I knew who might be going to the region, one option remained viable, and that was the potential participation of Dr. Allan Kelley of MedTeams WorldWide (MTWW). As mentioned earlier, my first trip to Sudan in 2004 was with Dr. Kelly, and I knew he was willing to take risks many others would not. Luckily, I discovered that he was on his way to Melut, South Sudan, with a team of fellow humanitarians, and right away I was hoping he might have space on his charter plane. Melut (which is upriver from Kodok) would put me in striking distance of the refugee camp in Kodok.

It wasn't until about seven days before actual departure from the States that I ended up with a confirmed seat to and from Melut (up until then it was only one-way for reasons I no longer remember, but I was willing to take that and figure out the rest when I got there). I was able to get my visa in less than 48 hours from the South Sudan Embassy in Washington, D.C., a reasonably priced last-minute fare to Nairobi, and initial logistical intel from the field, courtesy of partners at Empower One, a faith-based organization dedicated to working with the people of North and South Sudan. The timetable was tight as I had to pull off the mission within the timeframe set by MTWW (which was limited to six days on the ground), plus navigate an additional 70 plus kilometer barge trip in order to transport the food to the refugee camp. This was all in addition to procuring said foodstuffs in the midst of an outbreak of civil war in South Sudan.

After spending two days in Melut sourcing food and supplies, with help from two pastors referred to me by another contact with the South Sudan Baptist Church, finding a way to change a few thousand U.S. dollars to South Sudanese pounds, and locating a boat willing to go the "wrong way" down the Nile (not just against the flow of the water, but against the flow of refugees fleeing fighting further south), I was ready to insert both food and some medicine into the Kodok camp (which lies south of Melut along the Nile, but is still in Upper Nile State, South Sudan). The thought of failure, with so many people having contributed funds, the total of which was in excess of $20,000.00, was not even a possibility as far as I was concerned. (Some 25 individuals donated to my fundraising page on the Operation Broken Silence web site, and five different churches, scores of online donors through a "Mommy Bloggers" network and other faith based organizations all kicked in money for the effort.)

The price of the transport more than doubled as the boatmen started to realize they'd have to carry 150 90kg bags of grain and four passengers up river in a very short time frame. Even getting permission from the local military commander to take the boat up river from Melut was risky. After all, if he had said no, what would I have done? (Before even attempting to get permission for the trip, I had been told repeatedly that I would not be able to go up river to Kodok under the current circumstances, i.e., fighting in the area, and, in fact, I was only granted permission after a lengthy meeting with Medical Teams WorldWide personnel, plus the interjection of a rebel commander who issued some very bold statements to our entire group about his ability to control security in his area. Interestingly, when I approached him after the meeting and asked if it was truly safe to travel to Kodok, his actual words to me were: "Sure, it is safe, it is all safe, go wherever you like." Rousing laughter erupted from all those gathered within hearing distance at his words.)

Despite all the obstacles, I found myself floating down the Nile five days after I had left the San Francisco airport en route to Sudan. While we were told the trip from Melut to Kodok would take about four hours, we arrived over seven hours later. It was dark, and the air was heavy with something like hot, steamy fog. The mosquitoes were as thick as the humidity, and as I stood on the dirt rampart in the pitch black I wondered where I would sleeping that night.

As flashlights flickered and my companions, two South Sudanese pastors, debated in Arabic about what to do next, the headlights of a jeep appeared. A stern looking SPLA sergeant got out of the jeep along with several rebels accompanying him, and cautiously approached us. He immediately appreciated the complexity surrounding the arrival of this "foreign dignitary" in a very unstable area in the middle of the night, and immediately took us to a compound where my companions and I were able to get showers and bed down under mosquito nets.

I had 24 hours to complete my mission, but with the food at the dock and my back resting on a nice comfortable mattress, I was suddenly feeling a lot better about the prospects of completing this mission.

The refugee camp, I discovered, had been in existence for at least a year, but was yet to be registered by any UN organization. In fact, the refugees were being encouraged to migrate to Yida, hundreds of miles from their home and pretty much inaccessible by land.

By the end of the afternoon the next day, we had the grain loaded and we headed out for the camp. I now had only a couple of hours to get back to the river and negotiate a return trip. Arriving in the camp, I saw hundreds of Nuba streaming out of makeshift *tukuls* with blue and white UNHCR tarps covering the tops of them. We had, I now discovered, actually passed right by the camp as we floated down the Nile the night before with the 110 bags of sorghum on board. If I had known that—or if someone had told me—I could have insisted that we dock right next to the camp and unload the sacks. Instead, it took another whole day of waiting for a truck to transport the food from the town of Kodok to the camp, a scant four to five miles away.

That said, upon delivering the food I was warmly greeted by the Nuba, some of whom I had seen the previous year in Kao Nyaro. (I was actually being accompanied by two men I ran into in the market place in Melut, whom I had first met in Kao.)

We immediately went about distributing grain. I also made a point of interviewing several of the leaders and women in the camp, asking what they had been going through as a result of the war in their country. They told me stories about their homes and fields being bombed and how they fled from their villages out of fear of being killed. They also told me of their struggle in the camp, despite help from the local Shillouk community. More specifically, they spoke about how they were bereft of almost all basic necessities, such as food, shelter and water. Since they had not yet learned to fish in the river, most had been reduced to foraging for food.

I saw many sick children, often with signature indications of malnutrition. Disturbingly, the medical tent (i.e., the clinic) was almost bare when it came to supplies. I was even more pleased that I had thought of bringing along four boxes of Plumpynut (a nutritive paste) to donate to the clinic.

Of course, different people under different circumstances often have vastly different images and/or an understanding as to what a "refugee camp" is: some envision UN flags flapping in the breeze and/or row after row after row of UN tents, cooking fires, people lugging water, etc., all spread over a vast landscape. That is not the Kodok refugee camp. Picture a dirt road going through what used to be flat, open land, with insufficient soil composition to be used for subsistence farming, and in a torridly hot region with a lack of shade due to a paucity of trees. At first, the only clean water source was located in the town of Kodok, a walk of some 4.5 kilometers. If it weren't for the fact that 3,000 people were living in an area more suited for a clan of less than 50, it wouldn't be so bad. Indeed, the Shillouk hosts were more than gracious to allow the Nuba to settle on the spit of land they (the Nuba) were now calling "home," but without any recognition of it as an official refugee camp there was little in the way of assistance that refugees generally receive. Add to that the harsh conditions in northern South Sudan with exposure to malaria, measles, cholera, typhoid and even polio, and one is facing a bleak existence. Frequent shortfalls in food availability was worsened by the onset of the civil war in South Sudan (meaning that transport of food to the people in the camp was often virtually impossible due to the vicious fighting on the ground all across South Sudan). That, in turn, only increased the prospect of the outbreak of opportunistic diseases, especially among children and the elderly.

As I looked around the camp upon our arrival, I saw the refugees' "homes" were the barest of shelters. Their possessions were equally bare; generally a bed, a few cooking implements, and a fire pit. It was apparent that the children wore what was on their backs until it wore out, and then went naked until someone came along with clothing. Runny noses and ears were common, and bright white streams of fluid stood out on their dark skin in stark contrast to the raw, red areas of exposed flesh from endless irritation due to constant rubbing and scratching. Though the natural color of the children's hair should have been black, many had the red hair characteristic of protein malnutrition.

Some of the kids in the camp had swollen bellies from worms (many of the younger ones) as well. Fortunately, I had brought along enough deworming medicine for a couple hundred kids, and I instructed the sheik at the time how to treat the worse cases.

One boy in particular really touched me. He walked up slowly and extended his hand, which seemed to emerge from a tattered, dirty, green, ill-fitting smock. Then he raised it and touched his eye, which at first had a little white pus in the corner, but almost immediately erupted with thick fluid. I instinctively pulled at the sleeve of his smock and then raised both hands palms out while smiling to show I meant him no harm and got his point very clearly. I was swearing inside that I'd do all I could to get eye and ear drops, along with more deworming meds and anti-malarials back to the camp as soon as possible. (As fate would have it, when I returned to Melut, there was a Médecins Sans Frontières (MSF) doctor who I was able to give a full report to right before I left for the States. She had actually been to Kodok and the refugee camp once, but informed me that MSF had left the area when the fighting started and that she hadn't been back since. She promised to redouble her efforts to try to get back there again.)

My encounters were all during the dry season, so being in the low lying camp during the seasonal rains would have meant even more sickness and suffering. Just the thought of that was heartbreaking. One young man in particular, Mukhtar, would be particularly bad off. You see, he literally crawled around on his hands and his knees. I'm not sure of the cause of his disfigurement, but he was practically paralyzed from the waist down and though his arms were strong enough to lift his body weight, his hands were partially atrophied—to such an extent, in fact, it is dubious as to whether he could have even held a pencil in them. His knees were frozen with his legs bent at roughly a 90-degree angle. So, he moved around by supporting himself on the palms of his hands and his knees, with his feet flying behind him. He didn't have a wheelchair or another way to get around. I'm not sure how he even managed to get from his village to the refugee camp, and I could hardly imagine the challenges he had already faced, let alone those that would bare down on him in the future. But like all the young Nubans, he was there, beating the odds and asking for books, pencils and instructors to help pave the way to a better future for his people. Just as astonishing was the fact that his English, though limited, was very clear, and his comprehension strong. It moved me beyond words that he spoke of his keen desire for education, and his ardent wish to return to his home someday.

Planting of the Seeds of GNAC (Greater Nuba Action Coalition)

Upon returning to the States from this last mission, I became increasingly convinced that such missions of mercy would not ultimately improve the lives of the Nuba people. My thinking turned toward a more holistic approach, a broader coalition, and a foundation built not on meeting the exigent needs, but built upon a long term vision comprised of eternal truths: Christ and His church.

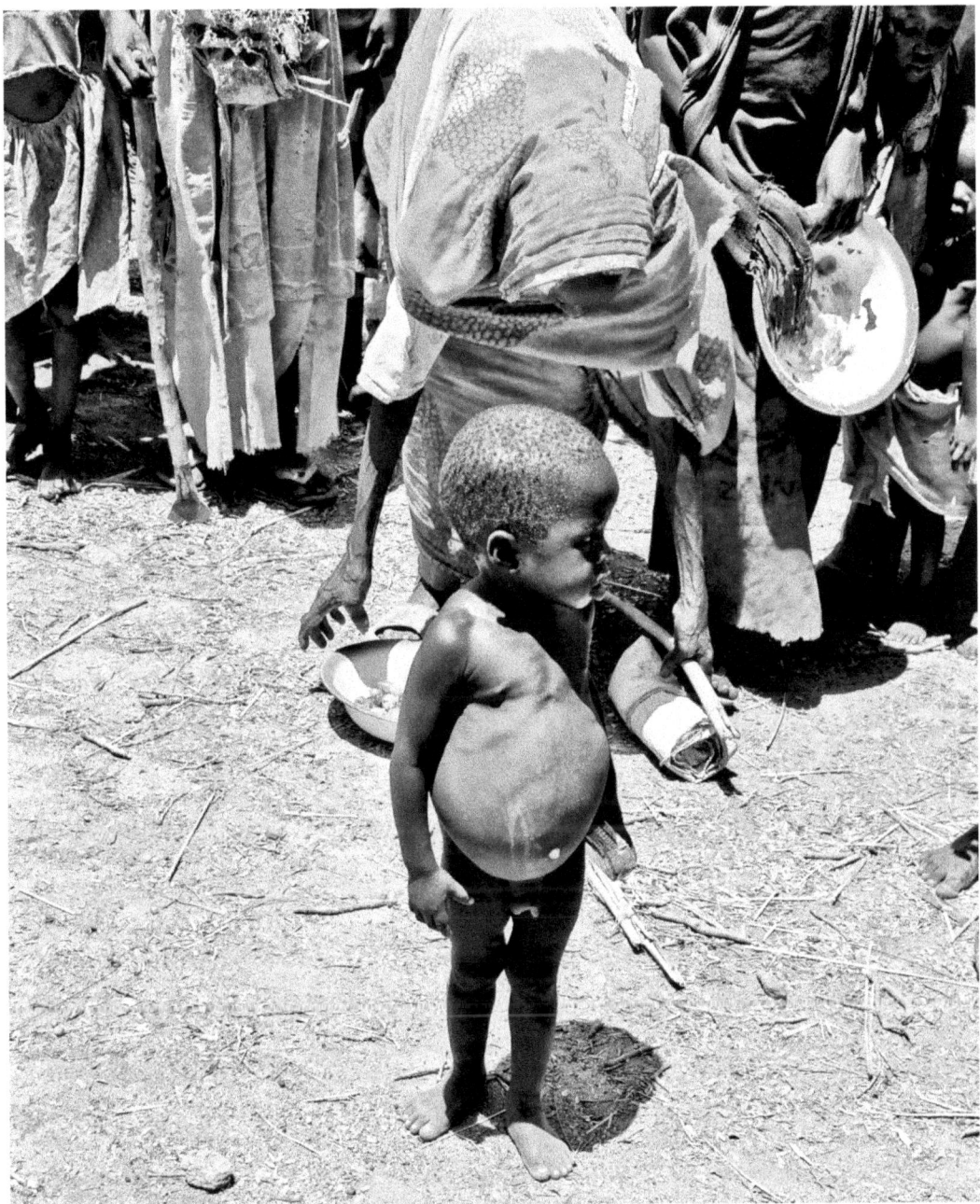

Boy in Kao Nyaro with swollen belly due to hunger, or worms, but does it really matter which it is? (John C. Jefferson)

In the intervening years since I had first traveled to Sudan, I had become conversant with some of the many organizations operating in the region, many of which had also established themselves in South Sudan following the latter's independence. In addition, through my ENG connections, I discovered some extremely dedicated individuals and groups that were working tirelessly on the behalf of the Nuba. Providence led me to individuals such as John Becker of Vision 5:9 and AIM, Rob Moore of Frontiers, and others who may not want to be mentioned, but were ultimately instrumental in building a coalition that fit my vision. Of course, initially, I shared my vision with ENG, which readily assured me of its support. (By this time, Sam Totten had left ENG in order to go it alone as he continued to make mission after mission into the Nuba.) All of its remaining members were to eager to be a part of the new coalition, while also remaining faithful to the original vision and mission of ENG, as was I. Thus, the Greater Nuba Action Coalition (GNAC) was born, with the intent of directly involving the Nuba in the relief and spiritual work that was so apparently needed both in Kodok and other parts of the Nuba community inside and outside of Sudan.

Beginning of the Beginning

The *main idea* of GNAC was to bring together as many of the Nuba, along with as many of the people supporting and working with them, as possible. Almost immediately, it was apparent that it was imperative to reach out to the Nuba leaders directly. I had already decided that most of the coalition members would be faith-based NGOs and churches from both inside and outside of Sudan. The composition, I also decided, should also include laypersons, such as myself, who for one reason or another, were dedicated to aiding the plight of the Nuba. So I began looking for various business professionals, academics, journalists, doctors, and independent missionaries to join the effort. Finally, with backing from my home church, most of the original ENG members, and my new missionary contacts, a series of brainstorming and planning sessions morphed into the aforementioned coalition, which led directly to the planning of a conference and humanitarian mission planned for the fall of 2015. Much like the period after the inception of ENG, a whirlwind of human planning and the seeking divine guidance led to miraculous results in a short amount of time.

Forty church leaders and missionaries meeting together in a room for two days isn't necessarily a miraculous an event—not unless they are from a closed country (herein, "closed" means "not open to the Gospel or evangelism"), and are marked men and women who have all seen their own and others' homes and farms destroyed, friends and fellow believers tortured or killed, been forced to change their names to hide their identity, and/or been forced to flee the country of their birth. Furthermore, when the focus of the gathering is the spiritual and physical empowerment of a people facing overwhelming opposition to their very existence, it can be a very powerful event. This is what people like Joseph, Paul, Jamilla, Ibrahim, Mohammed, Tabitha, Grace and others experienced during the first GNAC conference, which preceded my next attempt to reach the Nuba people with the hand of friendship and the love of God.

The aforementioned conference was held in Yei, South Sudan, over a period of three days in a relatively bucolic setting as compared to the previous ENG missions to the north. The fact that we were able to fly directly into Yei from Entebbe (Uganda) meant we were able to get to the Episcopal Church of the Sudan conference center and relax within an hour of our arrival versus the two days it normally takes to get to our destination in the Nuba. It also meant more time with the Nubans themselves, in a safe environment, something currently unknown in Sudan. As a result, it was also my first chance *to really, closely and personally, engage* with the Nuba people over an extended amount of time.

Getting to know them, their thoughts, dreams and desires for freedom and empowerment was empowering for me.

Most of the pastors present did not need a translator to communicate in what was their third language, English. Their beliefs, their passion, and their hopes came through loud and clear. Over and over again, I heard their desire to reignite the faith of their people and bring them hope, not only via the Gospel, but through providing them with education, food, medicine, and the other basic elements of life delineated in the Universal Declaration of Human Rights.

GNAC made good on the promise of not only addressing spiritual needs throughout the conference, but also turning the dialogue into action by establishing plans for the first GNAC coalition relief mission immediately following this unprecedented gathering in Yei. The target would again be Kao Nyaro, just a few months after my last mission to the Kodok refugee camp and just over a year after my first trip there with ENG.

First GNAC Conference and Mission-Failure, Then Success

As previously mentioned, the outbreak of civil war in South Sudan in December 2013 vastly complicated ENG's efforts to get aid to the Nuba, since much of the fighting was (and continues to be) going on in the Upper Nile State and areas close to the border with the North. The fighting had been going on for almost a year when we set out again—this time in late November of 2014—to engage the Nuba of Kao Nyaro in their homeland. Timed on the heels of the rainy season, we were hoping for ideal conditions as we attempted to reach Kao Nyaro and all the people who had been cut off for the better part of the last few months by the impassable routes in and out of the region due to the heavy rains. Knowing their situation was dire to begin with, getting the fifteen odd tons of grain in as soon as possible was a top priority for us.

Though this was the first trip involving the newly created GNAC group, there was a lot of institutional knowledge from the previous missions with ENG and other partners, who were part of this new configuration. One of the benefits to having the new coalition was the addition of new folks to the usual skeleton crew of two U.S.-based ENG members: a South Sudanese pastor, a representative of the Nuba government, a Nuba evangelist, a photographer, and a missionary from Europe.

Most of the $15,000 raised to cover the cost of the mission came from an individual grant, along with monies raised from long-time supporters of ENG and other coalition partners. Unfortunately, we arrived in Kodok to find the worst news possible. There was flooding on the road leading to the north and it was only with great difficulty that we were able to negotiate the "rental" of two tractors (one of which broke down along the way) at the precipitously high cost of $1,000 each to take us in since there was concern about all other vehicles getting bogged down and stuck until the rains subsided or someone came along to pull them out of the viscous muck. And, actually, there were no other vehicles available. We also kept hearing more and more stories of a "big lake" covering the entire access route to the border. Due to the fact that we'd have to ride at least to the "lake" on tractors, it was decided that only two of our team would travel north (George Tutu and I were the logical candidates having been there before), and the remainder of the team (Pastor John, my wife Dawn, and a European missionary, Tristen) would work

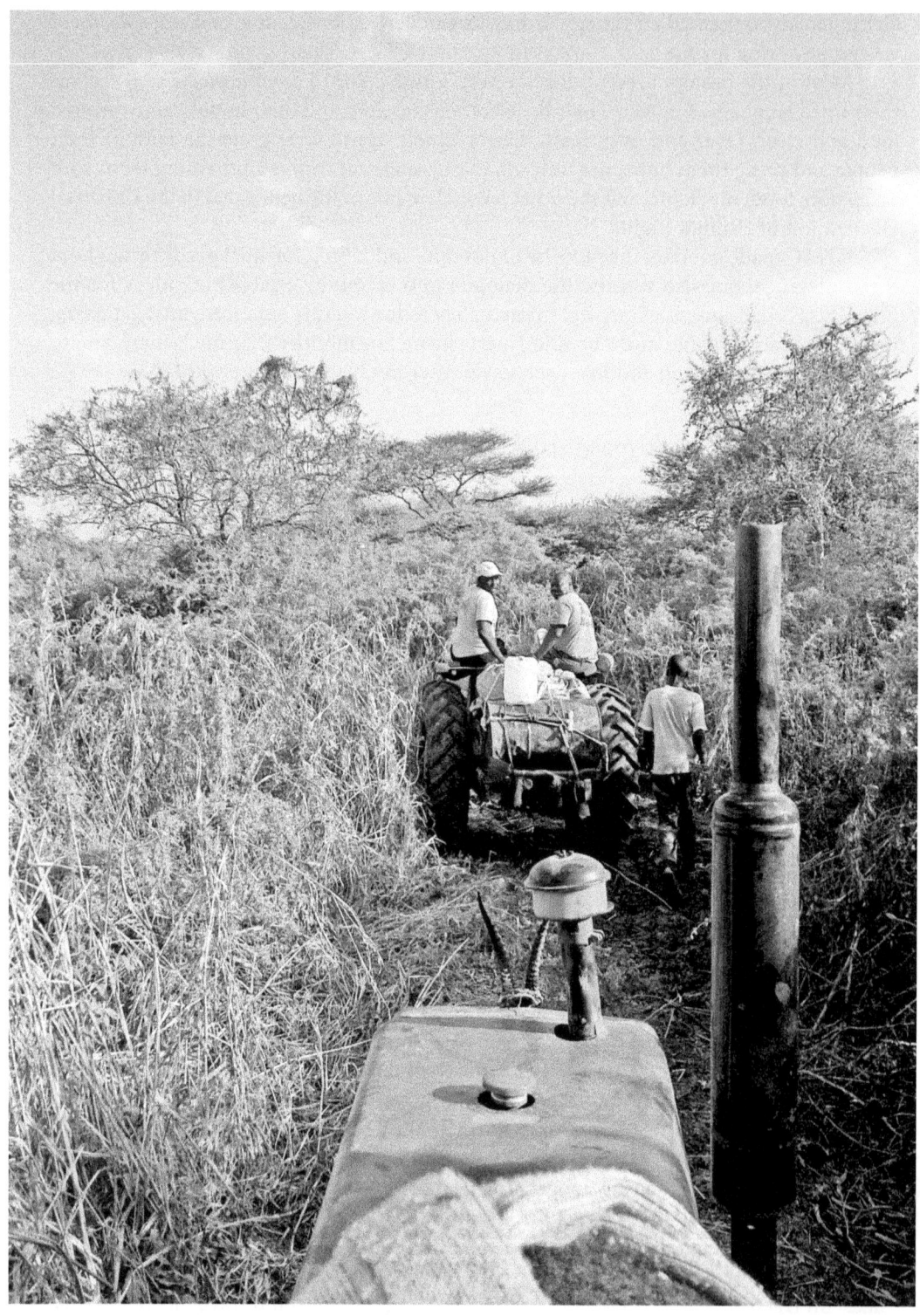

The bush road less traveled is sometimes the only way to get into a war zone (John C. Jefferson).

with the refugees from Nuba and the IDPs in South Sudan (as a result of the ongoing civil war). As usual, time was working against us as we had scheduled a charter out of Kodok seven days after our arrival, which would have been ample time to accomplish our mission had there not been complications due to road conditions and vehicle availability.

George and I began the journey across the muddy expanse that used to be a road—and would be again during the dry season. The way was difficult to say the least, and we were forced to bed down on the side of the "road" for the first night—cold, muddy, damp and hungry. I thought about the children on the road ahead, the old and infirm, who all had to live in these conditions all the time, not just during a two week mission. Not just that, but that many had had to take this same route under duress, leaving homes and possibly family members to face an uncertain future in South Sudan, not knowing how they would provide for themselves once they had arrived.

The food we purchased, along with medicines and supplies, eventually made it all the way to Kao Nyaro, but George and I only made it to the border of South Sudan/Sudan before time ran out on us, and we had to return to "base camp" to connect with the rest of the team we left behind. We actually missed our rendezvous with the rebel soldiers coming to meet us from the north by only a few hours, so they are the ones who ended up transporting and delivering the food and supplies we had purchased and staged. That said, the time spent getting supplies to the border was memorable and set the stage for our return a few months later, making us all that more determined to make it all the way to our destination. Ultimately, we spent a day and a night in the bush, basically arriving at the border too late to cross and thus we had to turn back. We ended up walking the last half-day in order to get to Kodok after the second tractor got stuck on the return journey.

A Future and a Hope

By spring of 2015, only four months after our aborted trip to the Kao Nyaro, I was once again on a flight to Nairobi. A young Nuba man, James Kuti (name changed), who attended the 2014 GNAC conference, was now part of our team, along with another man from the States, Chris Ward, who had been part of Dr. Alan Kelley's mission to South Sudan in April of 2014, when I made the trip to the Kodok refugee camp from Melut via the Nile. Hearing about my solo trip up the Nile and as well as my experience at the refugee camp inspired Chris to go back home and raise funds for a mission to the Nuba, making him the newest member of the ENG coalition. (Think of ENG as a GNAC partner.) As for James, he impressed me as a Nuban intent on changing the destiny of his people—not only through his own education and self-development, but via his willingness to work with others. He was not afraid of the perils of traveling back to a country from which he had fled from as a youth, nor the inherent risk in traveling in light aircraft over war zones, large overloaded trucks over unpaved bush roads, or walking unarmed through villages that had been raided and ransacked over and over again for decades.

On this particular mission, we were able to deliver over 40 tons of grain, school and medical supplies, print Bibles, audio Bibles, *and* make several presentations about the Gospel, all in the course of a few days. It was monumental in terms of the impact, and a step up from anything we had done in the past as a coalition, either as ENG or as

GNAC. This was due in part to the ability to leverage the human and material resources of several organizations and coalitions, i.e., funds were donated by various organizations, individuals brought Arabic Bibles and audio recordings of the Bible in Arabic played on solar powered Mp3 devices, food was procured ahead of time by working with a pastor in Kodok, medicines were acquired by the NRRDO Health Secretary, and lots of prayers were sent from churches all across the U.S., Canada and beyond. The very idea of GNAC is that the whole is always greater than the sum of the parts, a truth in this case born out by the results.

James, Chris and I, along with others on our mission team made up of Sudanese and South Sudanese, had a lot of time to talk during our travel, which was invaluable for getting to know one another's stories, insights, and hopes and dreams. As for Pastor John, he worked with the Nuba in the refugee camps, and in his role with Empower One he was becoming a well-known entity among them. He was graciously working with the Nuba even though he was a Dinka and had his own war stricken people with which to concern himself. Two other members of our team, Musa and Mustafa, both of whom are Nuba, were excited at the prospect of seeing their "estranged" brethren, the people of Kao and Nyaro, who had been separated for so long from their brethren to the west in the Nuba Mountains as a result of the presence of warring militias and incredibly difficult terrain. This was a team of tremendous experience, love for God, and dedication to the Nuba and the spread of goodwill and the Good News.

Conclusion

Where my sojourns in the land of the suffering strong will take me next only God knows. What I do know is that I remain dedicated to helping the Nuba, both to grow in Christ and to help ease their physical and emotional suffering as the current war takes its daily toll on so many innocents.

Notes

1. SPLA stands for Sudan People's Liberation Army, the main rebel faction that fought against the government of Sudan up until the Conditional Peace Agreement of 2005. The most recent iteration is the SPLA–N or North to differentiate itself from the relatively independent South Sudanese regular armed forces.
2. Meals Ready to Eat.
3. Nicholas Kristof (2012). "If Only Our Leaders Had Mariam's Guts." *New York Times*, Opinion Section, June 6.

Doctoring in the Nuba Mountains During Wartime

JOHN P. SUTTER, M.D.

When anyone asks me how I ended up working in the Nuba Mountains in Sudan, I tell them by way of a little bit of luck and a lot of inspiration. Riding on Amtrak from New York City to Washington, D.C., a year prior to my heading to the Nuba Mountains, I had a chance encounter with a former colleague of mine riding the same train, Dr. Kate Sugarman. I had previously worked with Kate at a community health center, Unity Healthcare, in Washington, D.C. She knew of my interest in global health and tropical medicine, and during the course of our conversation she mentioned Sister DeDe Byrne. She went on to relate that Sister DeDe was a Catholic nun and a physician who had served overseas in Afghanistan as a surgeon in the U.S. Army. She also mentioned that Sister DeDe had done voluntary work in some place called the Nuba Mountains in Sudan, at a place called the Mother of Mercy Hospital. Up to that point I had neither heard of the Nuba Mountains nor Mother of Mercy. Neither had I, at that point, met Sister DeDe; but when I did, her life and her commitments became a real inspiration.

Sister DeDe is a colonel in the United States Army, a dedicated nun who runs the Little Workers of the Sacred Heart convent, in Washington, D.C., where she cares for the elderly sisters residing there, and is double boarded (i.e., certified) in family medicine and general surgery.

Upon my return to Washington, D.C., I called Sister DeDe, and we arranged to have lunch at The Little Workers of the Sacred Heart with her and the other sisters. In part, we ended talking about the fact that we had both grown up in the Arlington and Falls Church area of Virginia as well as about our mutual friends and contacts, but mostly we discussed our prior international medical work. I shared with her that my specialty is family practice, and that over the years I had done medical work in Malawi twice, both times as a medical student; Tibet, also as a med student; South Sudan, twice, both times as an attending resident; and Mindana, Philippines, twice, again as an attending resident. I informed her that the various trips lasted between four and eight weeks; that, at times, I assisted with surgery, during others I primarily handled anesthesia; and during all of the trips I provided both inpatient and outpatient medical care.

I told her I was especially interested in her work in Nuba. She went on to describe a very remote and highly functional mission hospital capable of treating a wide array of patients. Sister DeDe described Mother of Mercy hospital as the perfect place for a doctor like her and Dr. Catena to practice, and for someone like myself to work at, too; and not only that, but I'd also learn a tremendous amount as well just by working with Dr. Catena.

Because of her broad skill set as a general surgeon and a family practice physician, she is one of the few physicians capable of handling the workload at Mother of Mercy Hospital, and one of the few trusted physicians that can relieve Dr. Tom Catena, the only surgeon at the only fully functioning hospital in the Nuba Mountains.

I have tremendous respect for doctors like Sister DeDe and Dr. Catena who go "all in!" They've trained and sacrificed for a very long time to be able to take care of everyone.

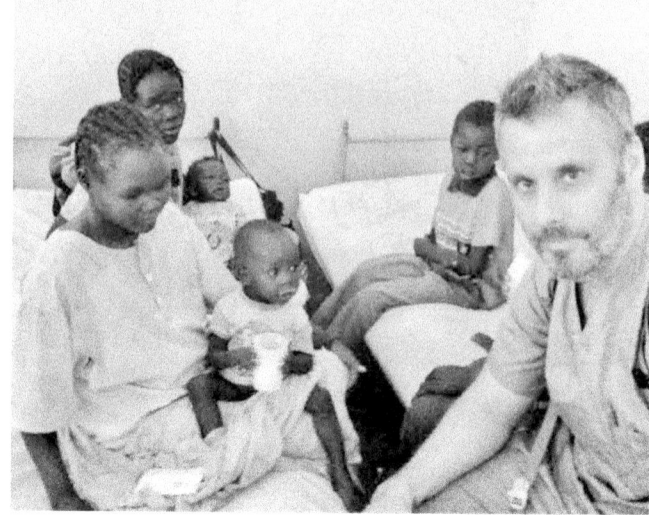

Many children come to Mother of Mercy Hospital for treatment of malnutrition. The child here seems concerned that I might take his nutrition supplement, and is holding on to it tightly (Tom Catena, M.D.).

"John, you have to go to Nuba!" she said.

I think she had sized me up, and thought I'd really enjoy it and that I could be of some help to Dr. Catena and his patients.

Over the next few weeks we met and talked, and as we did I envisioned a scale weighing the risks and the rewards. The chance to work in Nuba was a very unique and special opportunity Working there, I'd have the opportunity to help people that were in dire need of medical attention in an area that most (doctors, among others) do not have the opportunity to experience, among a relatively untouched native and ancient population. Plus, all that I heard about Dr. Catena was both intriguing and encouraging, and I mused, "What an opportunity to be able to work with him."

On the other side of the scale, there was the war in the Nuba between the Government of Sudan and the Sudanese People's Liberation Army-North. No matter the incredible opportunity, it involved all the risks of going to a war zone in a remote corner of the world.

Eventually, about a year later or so, I contacted Dr. Catena and we exchanged numerous emails in which he filled me in about the war, the aerial bombings in the region, the roads (dirt, rutted, and rough to travel over), the topography, and so on and so forth. In spite of all this intel gathering, my journey to the Nuba and work at Mother of Mercy came down to a "lets roll the dice" moment, and I just went. My time there spanned about two month's time, from November 2012 to January 2013.

While my particular journey to the Nuba Mountains at the time seemed special, it is the very same way almost everyone gets to Nuba these days. That is, it involved multiple flights and multiple connections from the United States to Nairobi, Kenya, onto to Juba (the capital of the Republic of South Sudan), another flight to the Yida Refugee Camp in South Sudan, right along the South Sudan/Sudan border. Luckily, for me, Bishop Macram of the Diocese of El Abeid, who is the Bishop who built Mother of Mercy Hospital and whose office in Nairobi runs the logistical supply operation to and from Mother of Mercy, and Sharon, his assistant, had a small plane flying from Juba to Yida to pick up amputees, all of whom were victims of the current war in the Nuba. So, I was able to hop that flight from Juba to Yida.

In Africa, there are three ways to arrive for a flight. You can get there on time, but because Murphy's Law is sometimes at work, the plane will have left early. You can go late, and miss the flight, because the plane has left more or less on time. Or, you can go many hours before the flight and wait and wait and wait. I chose the latter, and got to the airstrip in Juba just before sunrise. I ended up waiting and waiting; in fact, I was there for about three hours before anyone else even got to the small cargo terminal.

"Put your bags on the scale," the airport clerk ordered me. No problem, both within the weight limit. Then the clerk looked at me and motioned towards the scale and said, "Now you get on the scale." Keep in mind, I spent the previous two weeks working at a hospital in Chagoria, Kenya, where I unfortunately succumbed to a raging case of gastroenteritis and lost a significant amount of weight. In spite of my recent weight loss, this clerk wisely knew that the Cessna 208 we were flying on, while a proven African bush plane, could only handle a determined amount of weight—and there was supposed to be absolutely no wiggle room. Sizing me up, he knew that my current weight was—in comparison to the weight which was clearly spelled out next to my name on the passenger list—absurdly incorrect (and this was true even after my having lost a good number of pounds during my illness); and thus, in dark red ink, he crossed the number out on the passenger list and wrote in a few more kilograms. Luckily, I still got on the flight, and the change in my newly recorded weight did not preclude others or their cargo from getting on the flight as well.

Taking off, with just two other passengers on board, the pilot mentioned we were stopping in Old Fangak prior to Yida.

"Old Fangak! Jill Seaman!" I exclaimed.

The other two passengers were Nuer, and they were returning to Old Fangak. I immediately struck up a discussion with them reminiscing about my time there in December 2005 working with Dr. Jill Seaman. I had gone on a medical trip there as a second year resident for the express purpose of working with Dr. Seaman in Old Fangak.

Approaching the dirt "runway" in Old Fangak (really just a field), I immediately recognized the bone yard of planes, many more than when I had been there, that didn't make the take offs or landings over the years, all scattered along the tree line. On a piece of paper, I hastily scribbled: "Hi Jill, hope all is going well in Old Fangak!—John." I handed the note to one of my fellow two passengers and asked him if he would kindly deliver the message to Jill—and, also, to give her and the others in Old Fangak my regards.

As we were about to take off again, this time en route to Yida, I was reminded of the harshness of life in Old Fangak. Especially the flies!

One fly managed to get into the cabin of the plane, and that's all it took—one stinging bite of an Old Fangak horsefly—to remind me of the millions that awaited anyone who arrived in Old Fangak. I'll never forget those flies!

As we approached Yida, we circled around in preparation for the landing. Yida, from the air, appeared as any other sprawling refugee camp: a massive number of tents, people milling about, a central open market area, another bone yard runway strip littered with shattered white planes and Russian made helicopters, and smoke rising from small cooking fires.

Upon the final approach, the pilot and I finished up our conversation, and as we did, he said, "You're going to Gidel? You know, they're bombing there."

Before I had a chance to respond, he began telling me about the pilot who flew the last plane out of Kauda in June 2011. When the war started, the pilot was in Kauda (a main town in the heart of the Nuba Mountains) with his plane on the airstrip (which is, essentially another field). He was up there on a routine supply run for the hospital (Mother of Mercy) in Gidel, when all of a sudden the Sudanese Armed Forces (SAF) began bombing the airstrip. The war—unannounced and without warning—had just begun. He ran to the plane and took off, luckily and skillfully avoiding any hits.

That was the last civilian plane in Kauda from June 2011 to present; and ever since then, all supplies, people and food heading to Gidel have had to be driven in overland from Yida, a good nine to ten hour trip over rough, dusty, bumpy dirt roads.

We landed in Yida around 12 p.m. I was immediately met by a thin man in a well-worn and dusty polyester three-piece suit, Mr. Ali. He sternly looked at me, almost accusatory for being late (were we late?), and said, "OK, we go." I hopped in the Toyota Land Cruiser, and he and I started our drive to Gidel.

Ali and the vehicle handled the drive over dirt roads, paths, dry creek beds, and seemingly no roads at all, quite well. He knew a little English, I knew no Arabic, so the ride was mostly without conversation. We passed multiple checkpoints along the way, usually consisting of two posts made from tree branches with nothing but a sliver of rope across the road—more of a marker, really. At each checkpoint we had a short conversation with a few guys with Kalashnikovs and continued toward our destination.

About five hours into the journey, we came upon a place called Abu Leila. Ali pulled to a stop. There were more people gathered there than any other place we had passed thus far. There were a few lorries (long haul trucks) transporting as many people as they could cram into the bed, along with many Nuba refugees traveling by foot to Yida. There were a few makeshift stands where locals sold typical fare: batteries, soap, fruit, and so forth, and a rather large tukul served as a restaurant.

As we got out of the vehicle, Ali motioned to me and said, "We'll go here and eat and take a rest." The tukul was dark and shaded inside, which was a nice relief from the sun. Ali and I sat down on some cheap plastic stools and ate rice and goat in a circle with about ten others.

We were having a nice meal, with relaxing conversation, when all of a sudden all conversation stopped and the expressions on everyone's face in the tukul changed to one of concern. Immediately, everyone jumped up and rushed outside, and as we did one man in uniform pointed up to seemingly nothing in the sky and pronounced: "There!"

Adjusting my eyes toward the distant and clear, bright blue sky, I saw the Antonov to which he was pointing. Then, the sound. Throughout the course of my life I've heard the sound of prop planes in the distance without even taking notice, really—that faint whurrr that almost peacefully approaches and then dissipates. And that's exactly what I heard as I stood there, staring at the Antonov, except this time there was nothing peaceful about it.

Ali and I looked at each other, and almost telepathically did a risk assessment and made a decision in about three seconds, and with a nod, we got into our vehicle and drove like hell. Now, a white Toyota Land Cruiser with a plume of rising dust trail behind it must make for a delicious target for a SAF bomber.

Driving and bouncing across the mountainous desert landscape, sun setting behind us, with our heads out the window looking every direction we could in the sky, we kept calling out "There! There it is!"

The plane made multiple passes, but still seemed at a high altitude, which I estimated to be about 15,000 feet. Finally, Ali had enough and veered off the dirt road and pulled under a scrawny tree. We got out, and watched the plane. Circling above like a shark, then becoming clearer and obviously lower and closer, it dropped its bombs, which hit a hillside a safe distance from us. "Relief" is hardly adequate to describe what I felt.

Ali looked at me and said, "They're done."

With that, we reentered the vehicle, and continued on our way.

Gradually, the sun set, which provided me with a false sense of security, for I assumed the SAF wouldn't attack at night. Ali then told me that they bomb all the time, and my brief moment of solace vanished.

Driving through the night, without headlights, we used my headlamp intermittently to attempt to ascertain particularly sharp dips and/or large rocks, but for the most part we basically drove blind.

In the darkness I smelled the smoke of burning timbers. This smell permeates the developing world, where most cook over an open flame. This time, however, the smoke was thick and choking and intensified as we drove onward. When I was in Old Fangak I learned that the Nuer often burn the fields during the dry season for agricultural reasons, and I thought that that was what I was encountering on this journey. I was wrong; these fields in the Nuba Mountains were not set afire for agricultural purposes, but resulted from the bombardments. Destroying crops and homes and schools and any other remnant of life are the goals of the SAF. In complete darkness, rounding a hillside then ascending toward the top, through thick smoke, I saw a ridge-line of fire in the not too far distance, then another line of fire, then another. Driving though this smoke and fire, a cliché-like but apropos thought came into my head, I couldn't help but think we were driving through hell.

Six hours later (eleven in total), we arrived in the middle of the night at Mother of Mercy Hospital. What we had just completed was, I was informed, a typical ride from Yida to the hospital in Gidel.

Ali dropped me off at the physician housing compound, but there was nobody around, so I walked over to the hospital. Approaching the office, I heard this booming voice, speaking English, that at first I thought was scolding someone. Listening more intently, I could tell it was, in fact, someone having a nice conversation with family about Thanksgiving. ("Oh yeah," I mused. "Today is Thanksgiving!") I poked my head into the office, and saw that it was Dr. Tom Catena on Skype with his family. Once he was off Skype I introduced myself saying, "Hi Tom, it's me John." He looked puzzled, then it connected, "Oh, John!!!" My trip had been arranged so quickly he wasn't notified that I was going to be there *that day*, and so my arrival was somewhat unexpected. We talked for a while, but it was late, and we agreed to continue our discussion at 7 a.m. during hospital rounds.

Going to sleep that night I wondered about family and loved ones celebrating Thanksgiving back home, then I remembered, "Shit, today's my birthday."

Prior to heading to the Nuba, I had just finished up three years of locums work in rural southwest Bethel, Alaska. Again, by way of luck and inspiration, I landed work there on the recommendation of Dr. Jill Seaman. Dr. Seaman works the dry season in

Old Fangak, South Sudan, and in the rainy season (when the mud is waist deep and nothing moves in South Sudan), she works in Bethel, Alaska. She, like Sister DeDe, once told me "John, you have to work in Bethel." If someone as inspiring as Jill Seaman tells you to do something, you should do it.

In 2010, I had just finished a four-year U.S. government scholarship commitment working at an inner city community health center, and as a result I had no debt left over from my schooling, and a life wide open in front of me. Seemingly out of nowhere at that time, almost five years since I worked with her in Old Fangak, I received an email from Dr. Seaman: "John, what are you going to do now? You should go to Bethel!" I hadn't talked with Dr. Seaman in years, how'd she know I had finished my scholarship commitment? Dr. Seaman described the work in Bethel as "the closest you'll get to the African Bush without leaving the U.S."

So off to Bethel I went. What a wonderful experience it was; indeed, I miss it still. Bethel is a 25-bed critical access hospital in the tundra of southwestern Alaska, and *it is* the closest thing one can get to working in the bush. The hospital serves a subsistence-living Yupik population of 28,000, in an area about the size of Wyoming. The small group of doctors in Bethel handle everything, including obstetrics, pediatrics, emergency, medevacs—and they do it well. It was one of the better healthcare systems I've ever encountered. I was really able to hone my skills in Bethel, and was excited to bring this to the Nuba.

Early the next morning I met Dr. Tom for breakfast, consisting of a dense flat roll with peanut butter and instant coffee. That was, in fact, to be our breakfast everyday—which did wonders for my leftover gastroenteritis from Chagoria.

Rounds, every day, consisted of seeing every patient in obstetrics, labor and delivery, pediatrics, the women's ward, and the men's ward—all 300-plus of them. The usual "suspects" were all there, including: malaria, malnutrition, diarrhea/dehydration, pneumonia, tuberculosis, leprosy, and all the worms you could handle. Scattered throughout were the victims of war trauma, mostly women and children with disfigured and missing limbs. After rounds was surgery, followed by seeing 100 plus patients in the

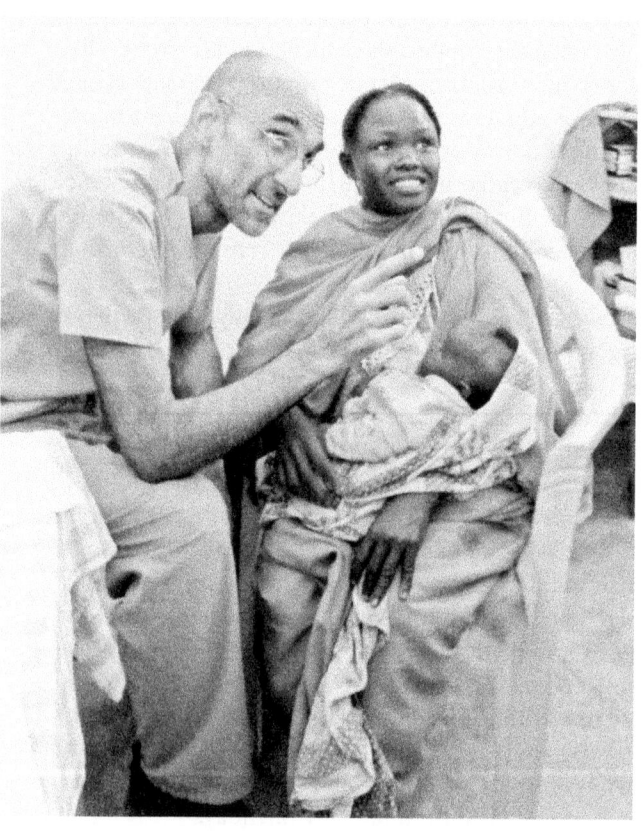

Dr. Catena giving directions, with humor and loving firmness, to staff regarding patient care (John P. Sutter, M.D.).

outpatient clinic. All of that was followed by night calls, handling any emergent patient that presents him/herself after the sun goes down. Do this 365 days a year, year after year, and you're superhuman—or, Dr. Tom Catena.

In the moment, you don't really think about the suffering in front of you. There are patients to be attended to, there are assessments and treatments and medicines to be given, and surgeries to undertake—all must be done, constantly, all the time. Sometimes afterwards, however, when it is quiet or during a rest it all hits you—and every once in a while it smacks you right in the face right in the moment. For example, there was a newborn baby, about two weeks old, which showed up at the hospital with its momma, with a rapid staccato cough. Pertussis. Cute little baby. We put the baby on antibiotics, but the cough persisted over several days. One day, the coughing stopped ... followed by the piercing cries, wailing and screaming of the baby's mother and the other women who had cared for the baby.

Another case involved an elderly man, a tough old guy, who had a bowel intussusception that was successfully resected. Day after day, he rested in bed, with his friends and family around him, fully alert, seemingly doing well. Then one day, he sat up abruptly and started shouting, gasping for air ... *fully aware that he was breathing his last breaths.* It was too late to give him sedatives or morphine or anything else that would afford him some peace. He, wide-eyed, and in panic, rocked violently back and forth in his hospital bed screaming—all the while his relatives holding his shoulders so as to minimize his thrashing—and then, struggling to even get out his last few screams, he was gone.

And then there was Vivienne. Most days during hospital rounds there was this eight-year-old girl with bright eyes and a vibrant smile who would greet us as we passed her bedside. Dr. Tom would joke with her and she'd smile even brighter and laugh. Thus,

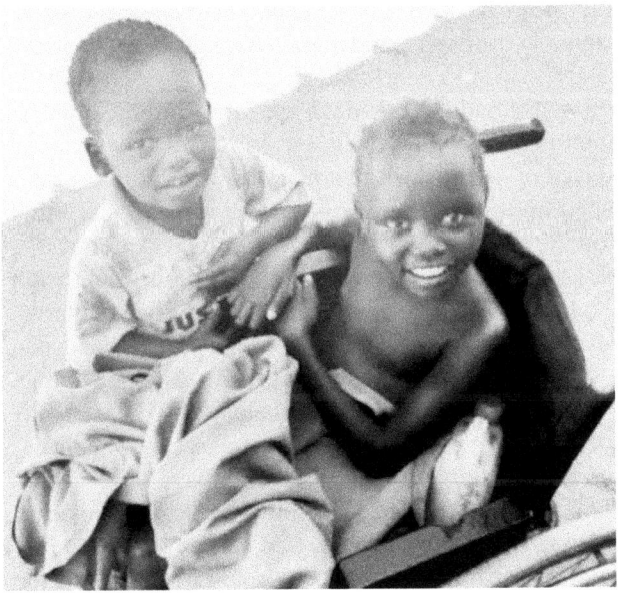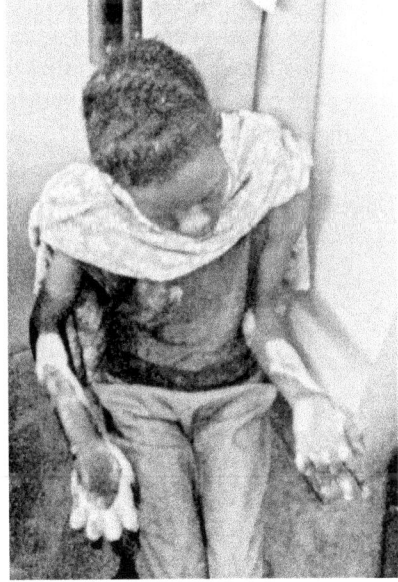

Left: Here is a photo of Vivienne (right) and her brother. Vivienne was unfortunately paralyzed from the mid-chest down, a traumatic victim of an Antonov attack. Note that she is seated in a wheelchair. *Right:* This photograph of Vivienne was taken during morning rounds on the children's ward (John P. Sutter, M.D.).

each day, in the middle of rounds with the sickest and most destitute there would be a moment of joy and hope. Vivienne and her brother were orphans. Vivienne had been cut down by an Antonov and paralyzed from the mid waist down. She and her brother lived at the hospital and were taken care of by the staff. Some days, however, our hospital rounds didn't encounter this joy; rather, Vivienne would lie under her covers on her bed, smelling of incontinent urine—a consequence of her traumatic spinal lesion—seemingly overwhelmed with her lot in life at that particular moment, maybe realizing that each day forward, as she grew older, life was only going to prove more and more difficult.

In preparation for writing this personal essay for inclusion in this book, I pulled out the journal I kept while in Gidel, only to realize that most of what I wrote therein is boring and technical and mainly contains diagnoses and treatment regimens we made in Gidel. But, I did, in fact, discover that it also contains one other thing: a list of the bombardments we experienced. One bombardment, in particular, stood out; it was on Christmas day, when the SAF bombed nearby Kauda.

Kauda is a town about ten miles from Gidel, and when the bombs fell that Christmas morning the sound was deafening and the shockwaves shook those thick stone hospital walls as well as my innards. It hit me that the bombs of the Antonovs dropped that morning were much more powerful than the ones dropped near me on my journey to Gidel. I also realized that we probably should consider digging some more foxholes. (Prior to that, I had developed a series of irrational safety plans in my head, more or less along the line of: "Where will I duck if the bombs fall?" We had one foxhole at the time, but it was in the housing compound, not at the hospital. I looked around at the thick stonewalls of the hospital, and thought, "Maybe these would provide some protection from a bomb." After the aforementioned bombing of Kauda, I quickly made a new assessment of the situation.)

One morning at breakfast with Dr. Tom, he said: "Did you hear the plane last night? It was buzzing around all night, and finally dropped some bombs near Heiban. We may have some patients from that today."

I commented that I hadn't heard it, as I had slept through the night and the bombings. Dr. Tom continued, "Yeah, sometimes I sleep on the floor." I immediately formed an image of the floor of the room I stayed in, covered with fat hairy spiders and the occasional scorpion, and realized it created quite the quagmire—"Do I dive head first into scorpions and spiders, or do I sleep on the bed and take my chances with the Antonovs?"

With all the bombings, and stress of the day-to-day work I sat in bed one night and briefly pondered, "What am I doing here?" First, I like to blame my parents, particularly my mother, who instilled an over developed sense of empathy in me, especially focused on those with an unlucky lot in life. Growing up herself, she was very involved in helping South Asian refugees who resettled in our neighborhood. I tagged along with her during such endeavors, and saw—first hand, at an early age—what some people go through just to survive and get through life. This made quite an impact. Second, I've always had a longing to see everything, not to miss out, and to explore. This selfish search for the next best adventure, along with an upbringing focused on service, had led me to that point in my medical career: lying on the floor swatting spiders and scorpions, hoping not to get bombed.

While Mother of Mercy Hospital is in an extremely remote—and some may even consider it to be an exotic—locale, the day-in and day-out functions of the hospital require work. A lot of work. And the fact is, while we did take care of trauma victims of

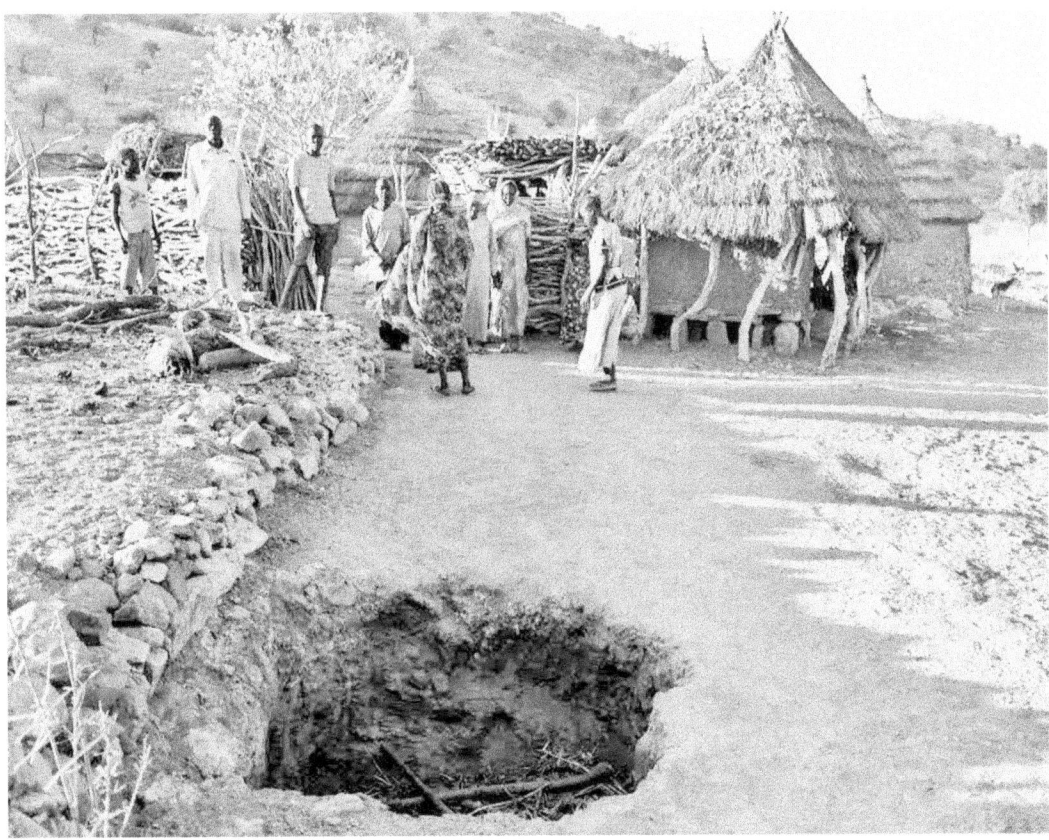

Most villagers have dug holes in which to seek shelter during aerial bombings (John P. Sutter, M.D.).

the war, there were just as many—and really more—very sick Nuba who required healthcare, and they all came to Mother of Mercy Hospital.

My work consisted of seeing patients on the wards with Dr. Tom every morning, assisting in the operating room (OR), sharing night call, and seeing patients in outpatient.

I estimate about fifty percent of the patients I saw were sick children. The three most common childhood maladies I attended to were: malaria, pneumonia, and diarrhea/dehydration. Many of these required admission to the hospital for more intensive care. The second most common patient was the pre-natal/obstetric patient, including many first trimester bleeders and missed pregnancies who required dilation and curettage. Without these treatments, almost surely all of these patients would have died.

There was a real problem with dog bites when I was there, and unfortunately a rabies outbreak as well. There are a lot of stray dogs in Nuba, and they breed like ... well they breed like wild stray dogs. In vain, we tried to get a good history to see if we could find the dog that had bitten the patient in order to place it in quarantine, but the bite story was always the same:

"Where were you, and what happened?"

"I was walking in the market, and there was a dog, and when I walked by it bit me."

"Where's the dog?"

"It ran away."

We received some rabies vaccine from MSF (Médecins Sans Frontières or Doctors without Borders), and provided the post bite vaccine series for most but unfortunately not all. Rationing rabies vaccine is no fun.

Tuberculosis patients were started on 4-drug therapy and sent to the "TB Village" for their entire treatment time (9–12 months). Leprosy patients were treated for twelve months, but stayed in the hospital for the entire course. There was one elderly woman I saw every day during rounds. She was missing her distal fingers and thumbs on both hands due to leprosy, and she lived at the hospital, at least until her twelve months were up.

One day in clinic a young woman, who had been carried in by her relatives, was limp, with a bloody frothy cough in acute respratory distress. Her lungs were full of fluid, and she was hypoxic. No Code Blue, no ICU, no prolonged intubation/ventilator care at Mother of Mercy, so time was of the essence. She had delivered a healthy baby three weeks prior, and we thought her symptoms were consistent with peripartum cardiomyopathy, and with IV diuretics and steroids she ended up surviving.

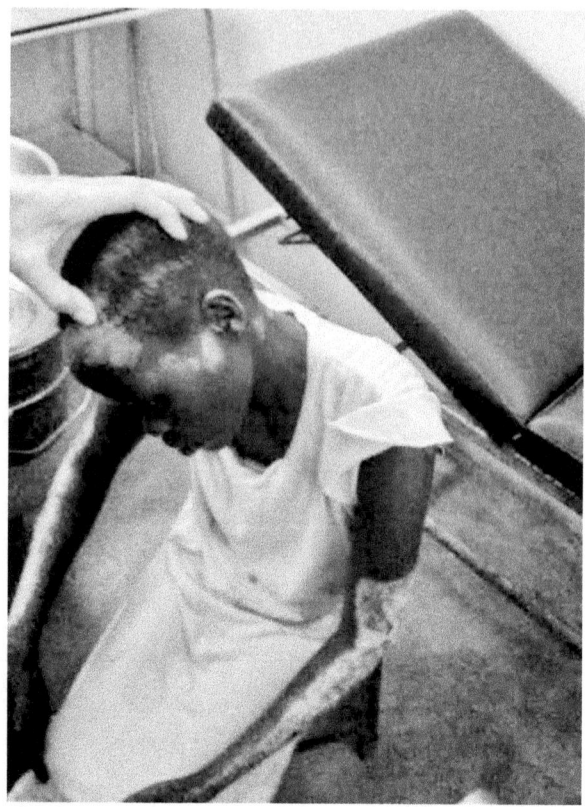

This photo was taken during daily wound care of a young girl who was scalded during an Antonov attack. Notice the scars on her forearms and forehead—you can picture her covering herself with her arms as the bomb exploded and burned those areas (John P. Sutter, M.D.).

And, as mentioned, we, of course, took care of casualties of the war as well. One morning a truck sped into the hospital compound and dropped off four war casualties, all of them with shot up limbs. They had some ingenious tourniquets (made out of grass/plant structure sewn together to create a tight seal and provided ample pressure to stop arterial bleeds). I triaged the four: two required immediate surgery, the other two were stable and could wait. We took two to the OR that day for above the knee amputations. Dr. Catena performed the surgery, I assisted.

I'll always remember a patient that day who was one of the more stable ones, and as a result waited for treatment. He was an elderly SPLA–N soldier, looked to be about 65 years old, who was shot in the foot. He was calm, just laid on the gurney with his arms folded behind his head resting. I talked with him briefly, and he reported he'd been fighting off and on for most of his life. Later that day after the other amputations, we debrided and cleaned and dressed his foot wound. He was stable, but the wound was bad. I'm pretty sure that he eventually lost his foot. During the debridement, which took out

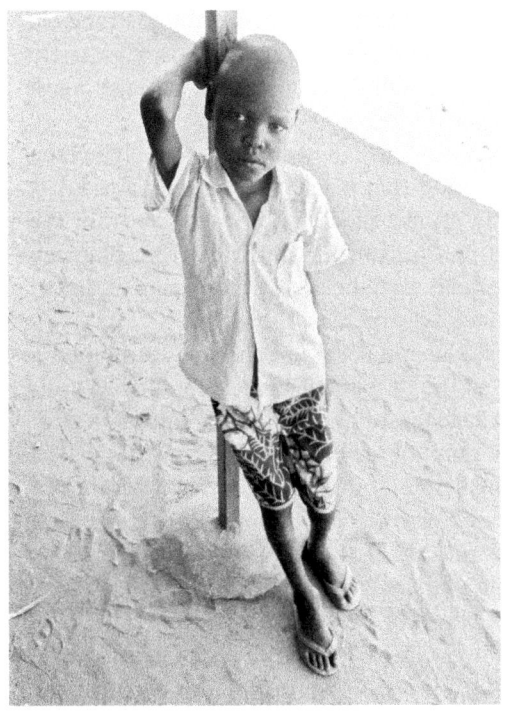 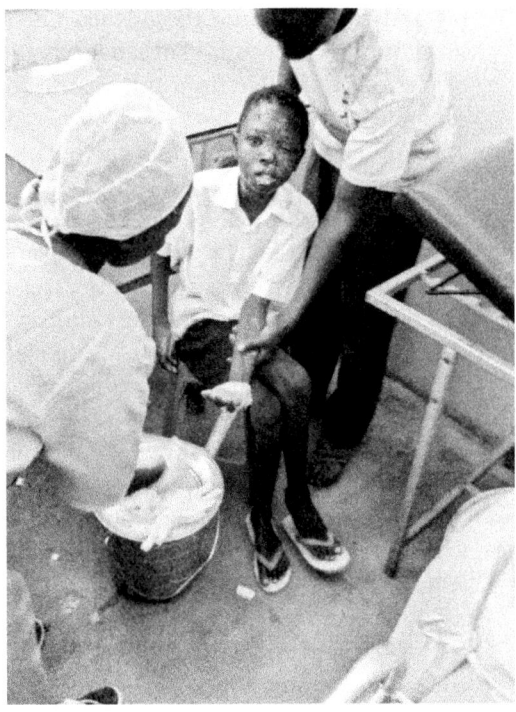

Left: This is a photograph of a boy who was emaciated and had tuberculosis. After just six weeks of treatment, one can see how he's on the road to recovery. *Right:* This young boy happened upon a land mine. Not knowing what it was, he and his brother threw rocks at it and it unfortunately detonated, leaving him wounded and scarred, along with some vision loss (both John P. Sutter, M.D.).

pieces of bone, with questionably effective anesthesia, he just laid there with his arms behind his head as calm as could be. He was one tough old man.

One day during rounds I took a brief respite and sat down with a group of nurses—all of whom were Nuba—who were eating their breakfast. They were eating a pasty dark brown gruel of sorghum, and they invited me to join them. It was a bit bland, but appealing. As we ate, we had a discussion about life in Nuba and in the United States. Curious about what we ate in the United States, they asked me to bring them food from America on any of my subsequent trips to Gidel. More specifically, they asked me to bring them a pig. Apparently, a few months earlier someone got ahold of a

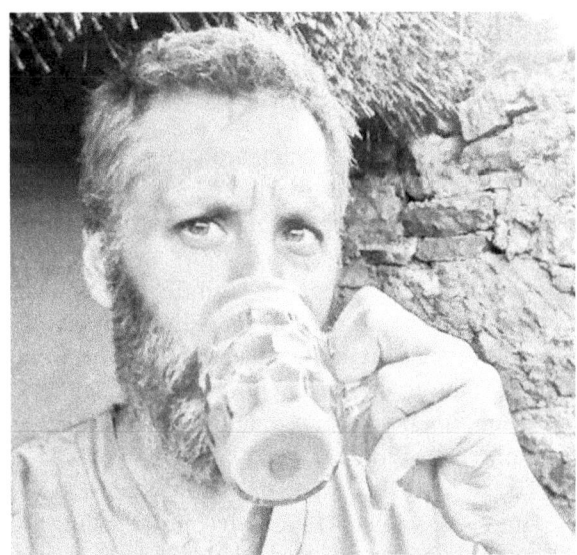

The Nuba have a mild special home brew that is delicious. Here I try some during a visit to a nearby village (John P. Sutter, M.D.).

pig and cooked it, and these Nuba nurses were just thrilled with this unique magical meal of pork they had. I subsequently blew their minds describing to them the variety of products available from this wonderful beast, including: bacon, ham, sausage, maw, scrapple, and spam.

Although they are strong and healthy, in part because they don't eat pork, the Nuba are vulnerable if their food source is destroyed, and that is what is happening today—and has been throughout the current war. The grind of facing daily assaults from the bombs dropped by the Antonovs have, overtime, prevented the Nuba from planting sorghum; or, even worse, in many cases their fields have been outright bombed, burnt and destroyed. As a result, many continue to face ever-increasing hunger.

As my weeks working at Mother of Mercy hospital passed along, I developed a friendship with the translator assigned to me in the outpatient clinic, Khamis. Khamis is a young man about 30 years old who was a teacher, but had left teaching as most of the schools in the Nuba have been shuttered because of the bombings. Khamis, it just so happened, had been shot in the foot and was operated on by Dr. Catena at Mother of Mercy. He now walks with a limp, and had an oozing festering osteomyelitis in his foot, which resulted in daily debates over whether the foot should be amputated or not. Khamis taught me much about the Nuba, particularly its soldiers. When asked about the fighting, Khamis would crack a smile and say "they like the fight."

Nuba boys are brought up with the sport of wrestling, a brutal but respectable athletic endeavor combining grappling and pummeling. I have to wonder if this spirit of the fight, along with surviving in a tight knit culture and community in a harsh landscape for thousands of years, lends itself to a population of soldiers that not only are able and willing to fight, but in some degree are eager to meet the enemy combatants of the dictator who is killing their families and destroying their culture.

The one thing the SAF has, however, which the Nuba are defenseless against, is the air assault by the Antonovs. Imagine an old school bus with wings, with all the seats pulled out, filled with kegs of nails, metal shards, and gunpowder, dropped indiscriminately from 15,000 feet on schools, farms, villages, and people below. If this goes on long enough (and thus far, it has gone on since June 2011), over time the Nuba children quit going to school, the people fear tending their farms, and the Nuba are often relegated to the life of NGO-dependence in a refugee camp. Ultimately, there is the very real possibility that the Nuba culture will be lost. While this current crisis may not meet the criteria of a physical genocide, if this smoldering war continues then, in the end, it could result in cultural genocide.

While the Nuba have no defense against the Antonov, they do pretty well on the ground. Khamis described an ill-equipped SPLA–N force which patiently planned well-coordinated attacks against the SAF and were, remarkably, often successful. The Nuba are fighting on their own turf and have the will to fight. The SAF, on the other hand, seem to rely on marauding opportunistic contracted barbarians, as well as a generalized conscripted force.

Khamis described one battle where the SAF hired taxi drivers in Khartoum to transport SAF soldiers to the Nuba border, telling them they would be paid handsomely to take the soldiers to a barracks near the border. Instead of dropping the soldiers off at a SAF military barracks, the taxis drivers were directed to the front lines of an ongoing battle, and subsequently came under heavy fire from the SLPA-N. Khamis described how the taxi drivers, and their SAF passengers, fled in complete fright at the sight of the SPLA–N.

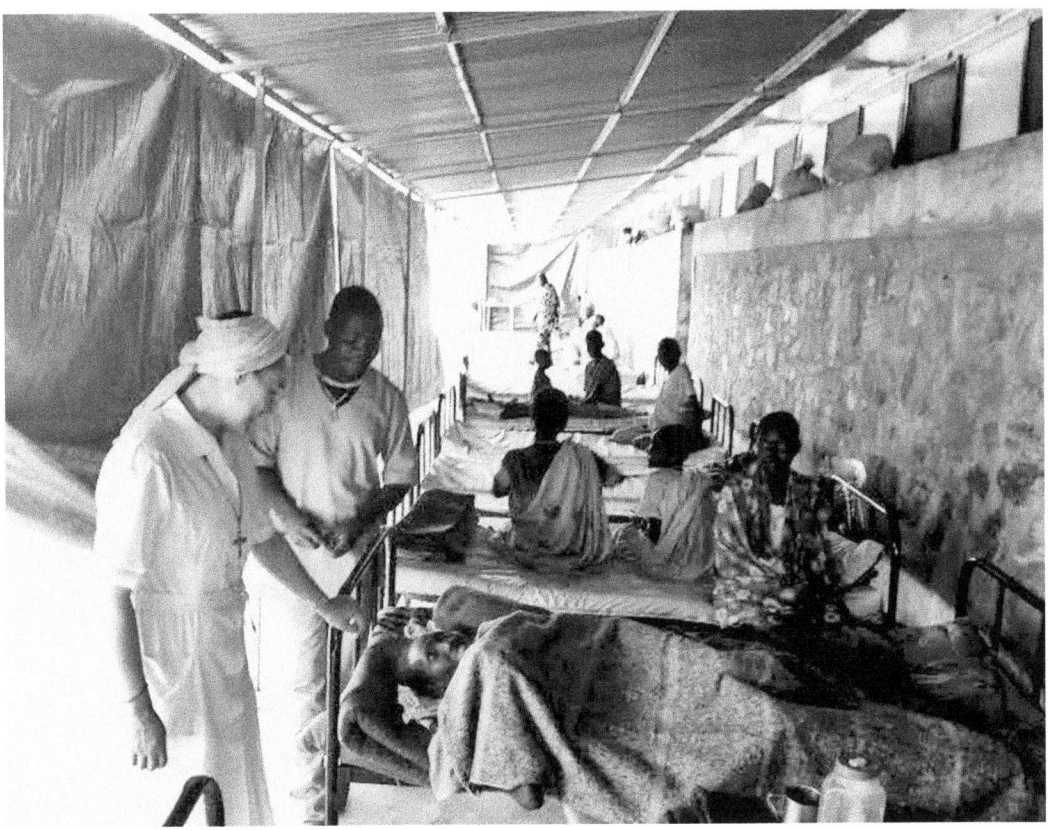

A photograph of the overflow area (outside) of the hospital. Here Camboni Missionary Sister Rosia (foreground) and a Nuba Nurse attend to patients (John P. Sutter, M.D.).

Thus far, though, the ground war has gone back and forth, with no significant movement of battle lines by either side, while the Antonovs continue to drop their bombs. It is the prolonged exposure to the threat from the sky that will eventually do the Nuba in (or, at least the Nuba civilians) if the war is not stopped.

During my time in Gidel, more foxholes were dug, and the bombs continued, but life weirdly enough became routine: wake up, have breakfast, go to work, see patients, eat dinner, socialize a bit, try to get some sleep, check your shoes for scorpions, listen for the planes above—day-after-day. As the abnormal became the new normal, the day-to-day routine lent itself to developing friendships, with Dr. Tom, the Catholic Sisters and the Nuba staff. All are tremendous people, and because of them Mother of Mercy was a terrific place to work in spite of the hardships and sadness of the injuries and maladies faced by the patients. The Nuba have a great sense of humor, and it was just a lot of fun joking around with them. It is no wonder that my last day there was filled with heartfelt good-byes.

The ride back to Yida was actually uneventful. It wasn't just myself and Ali this time in the vehicle, but various hospital staff, all of whom were heading to Yida and then onwards for school and training. That made the eleven-hour spine-shattering ride enjoyable, with lots of jokes and good conversation. And this time, there were no Antonovs flying overhead or bombing the region through which we traveled.

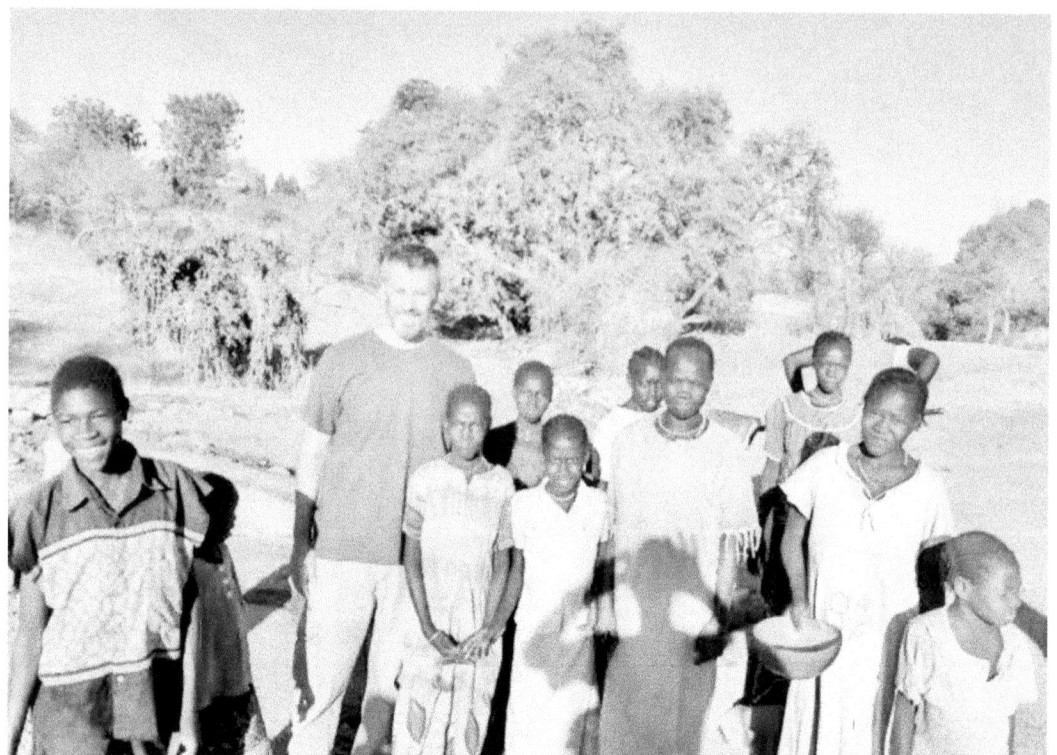

On the way back from a visit to a nearby village, we stopped by the local well (Tom Catena, M.D.).

I spent a night in Yida, explored the refugee camp a bit with a Nuba friend, then tucked myself into a tent, only to be awoken soon after by the scuffling sound and appearance of hundreds, if not thousands, of rats that emerge after sunset to scour the squalor of the refugee camp. Their appearance kind of made me yearn for the scorpions and spiders in Gidel.

There were many nuns and priests in the compound where I spent the night in Yida as they were on their way to Kenya for the annual diosocean meeting with Bishop Macram. That morning we all made our way to the makeshift, dirt airstrip in Yida to board the Hawker 748 to Lokichoggio in Kenya. As the crew unloaded the cargo of hospital supplies they had just flown in to Yida, I noticed people hauling 50-gallon steel drums and placing them next to the plane. As the last bit of cargo was unloaded, the crew started loading the 50-gallon drums onto the plane. When I inquired what the barrels were, I was informed that they were empty barrels of jet-A fuel and that they were being transported back to Loki. At that point I thought, "The Antonovs didn't get me but it looks like the Hawker might!"

As I boarded the plane with about twenty sisters and priests, I immediately met the familiar smell of vaporized gasoline. It reminded me of when I used to transport lawnmowers in my station wagon as a teenager and the gas would drip out and the whole car would smell like a Molotov cocktail. As I sat down across from Sister Rosia, she looked at me and we glanced at the stacks of unsecured steel drums behind us, and we both started our prayers, as our pressurized tube of highly flammable fumes ascended into the air. I racked my brain, flipping back and forth between, "Are those barrels going to expand or contract as we gain altitude?" and "What about the pressure in the cabin?" In the end it didn't matter. The fumes in the drums either expanded or contracted and began "popping." Just a few pings at first, but as we gained altitude it crescendoed into the sound of popcorn being microwaved. And it did it again on the descent into Loki. Looking around in the cabin at all the priests and nuns, I mused, "Well, if it's going to happen, I can't think of a better lot of folks to go down in flames with." And, added to that, I thought, "At least nobody is smoking."

So, why did I go to the Nuba and work in Mother of Mercy, and why will I go back?" Honestly, the answer is bound to sound rather selfish. The short and totally honest answer is: The longing for adventure, to see the world, and to challenge myself. This challenge, though, is tempered with the desire to use the skills I developed as a physician for what they were meant for. In the United States, so much time as a physician is wasted on tasks unrelated to delivering care to patients. At Mother of Mercy Hospital, all resources are limited and nothing is wasted. All decisions and actions are necessary and important, and the actions save lives. That is a very satisfying way to practice medicine.

There was also the desire to do something outside of myself, as it were, for the betterment of others. To engage in service to others. My parents taught me this, and it was reinforced with my Christian upbringing. But really, my small adventure and small contribution pale in comparison to those that are up in the Nuba working day-in and day-out, month after month for years on end. What is an adventure—and now a story for me—is daily life for those such as the drivers that dodge the Antonovs to bring supplies to the hospital as well as for Dr. Tom, the sisters and the Nuba staff, who risk everything, every day, to serve the victims of war and disease.

The Nuba are good people, and it is odd how their plight is, for the most part, ignored, especially by the West. It is a shame that no one has stepped up to stop the bombers from carrying out their daily bombing missions.

The Nuba I met have values and traits that mirror what we strive for in the West—tolerance (Muslims and Christians living together without issue in Nuba), a fair rule of law, respect for women and children, an appreciation for education, and an emphasis on the preservation of the family unit. I'm lucky to have been able to work with them, and once again, I'm inspired.

Medical Missions to the Nuba War Zone

CORRY CHAPMAN, M.D.

I've been to the Nuba Mountains three times. I traveled there in my capacity as a physician.

Every time I have gone, it was rough. And I got homesick. I couldn't wait to get out. But then, after getting back home, I realized each experience had been one of the most real of my life. It was eye-opening, and that's true for numerous reasons: the starkness of life there, devoid of comfort and devoid of the pettiness of First World living; the great appreciation for small things, like the act of drinking a cold Coke out of the lab refrigerator at Mother of Mercy Hospital deep in the Nuba Mountains after weeks of sweltering in the heat; the hospitality of the Nuba people; the Milky Way at night. Yes, all the Eat, Pray, Love clichés. But most of all I went back for Tom. Dr. Tom, as he's known in the Nuba Mountains. Dr. Tom Catena. He's my friend, and I love him.

The last time I went, the region was at war with the government in Khartoum. That was a new development. I understood it to be more dangerous than it had been in the past, but I didn't realize how bad it was until I got there. The upshot is, after that last time, with the bombing and death, I don't think I can go back any time soon.[1] I can't get myself killed. That wouldn't be fair to my kids. Plus, I'm scared now. The bombing and death I saw last time scared me.

Backing up a bit. It took me ten years to get a college degree, in history. During that time I worked multiple jobs in different areas, including construction, retail and clerical. I was a computer software designer when I decided to go to medical school. I started at Georgetown University Medical School when I was 33, a lot older than most of the other students.

My undergraduate training in history was comprehensive in terms of learning about the human experience. Medicine, in my opinion, is hands-on liberal arts combined with science; thus it encompasses all learning: math, physics, philosophy, art, religion, etc. It was a good fit for me, as I'd always been a restless person who couldn't choose one particular career.

I chose medicine because I wanted to combine a humanist career with job security. Growing up, my family struggled financially, so having a job where I would always be employed was important. It took years to decide on medicine, however, since I had a variety of other interests. At different times in my life I thought about being an artist, a writer, a teacher and a journalist.

In med school I liked all the specialties, but was focused on doing international work. Family Medicine seemed the best specialty for that, as it incorporated internal medicine, pediatrics and OB/Gyn, with some surgical training as well. Perfect for working in countries where one can encounter all kinds of emergencies and problems in the very young to the very old.

In residency I wanted to be an international doctor. I planned to work somewhere in Africa, maybe South America. Sweat it out in a jungle clinic, get malaria, deliver babies and stock my arsenal with stories to impress friends and family back home.[2]

One of my residency preceptors was Dr. Deirdre Byrne, a nun and medical missionary. She had worked in some rough places, including Afghanistan, Haiti and Kenya. In 2008 she invited me to go with her to a Catholic hospital that had just opened in a remote area of Sudan called the Nuba Mountains. The Nuban people were returning there after decades of civil war, to a devastated region without roads, electricity or health care.

Dr. Byrne told me about Tom Catena, the only doctor they had been able to recruit for the hospital. He was an American physician who had only ever worked in Africa. He didn't have a wife or kids. He was a devout Catholic. A plane had dropped him off in Nuba a few months back, along with a year's worth of supplies—beds, generators, medicine, food—and a mandate to get the hospital running.

Before we could leave for Sudan, Dr. Byrne got called back to Afghanistan, so I went alone. It took five days of flying, driving and delays to get there. A prop plane left me on a grassy airstrip near a village not on Google Maps. Next came a ninety-minute drive through muddy creek beds that served as roads during the rainy season.

Though the hospital had been open only a few months, it was already swamped with patients. Herds of them filled the courtyard. Women wrapped head to toe in brightly-colored cloaks and scarves despite the heat, sitting in any shade they could find, with children in their laps, while men of all ages squatted nearby, their bare feet as gnarled as tree roots.

I wandered into the hospital, a high-ceilinged, green-walled warehouse crammed with beds and patients. IVs dripped quinine from wooden poles into patients with malaria. Nurses mopped the concrete floors and changed urine-soaked sheets. Patients coughed and spat, babies wailed, the injured and post-operative moaned. In the middle of a group of nurses gathered around a patient's bed stood a tall, gaunt man, his shaved head tanned by the Sudanese sun. In a baritone voice he murmured orders to the staff as he flipped through the patient's "chart," loose bundle of handwritten notes and graphs. His overgrown, bushy black eyebrows and prominent nose made Catena's face instantly unforgettable, while his intense, deep-set eyes took in the chaos around him with a mixture of amusement and sadness that would lean more towards haunted as I saw him several times over the next few years.

On the bed in front of him lay a twenty-something woman with uterine cancer. She'd had vaginal bleeding for weeks. Catena had tried chemotherapy, using some of the few cancer drugs he had on hand, but the bleeding wouldn't stop. A vaginal exam showed a protruding mass halfway up the canal. Her belly was swollen as though she were pregnant, but putting hands on the bumpy, irregular mass beneath her skin elicited groans of pain and more bleeding. She was bleeding to death. Catena wanted to transfuse her but none of the Nuba—including her own family—would donate blood. A superstition about exchanging blood was just one of the many frustrating obstacles to care that Catena would encounter in a region of the world that—medically speaking, at least—seemed barely out of the Stone Age.

On that day and for many days after I followed Catena in the routine he began in 2008 and which continues to this day. He is a poor sleeper and usually awakens long before dawn. After brief prayer at the nearby chapel, he begins rounds on hundreds of patients, first children, then women, then men. Case after case, decision after decision, for up to 400 people a day. Medication orders, dressing changes, whether to discharge, whether to give up.

Once hospital rounds are over, usually in the early afternoon, Catena operates. Depending on the number of cases, their complexity, and whether any trauma patients show up, he can be in the operating room for many hours. After operating he usually sees patients in the outpatient clinic, which for most of the day is staffed by what are essentially medical residents who refill medications and refer any complicated patients to Catena; thus, many times during the day, while he is on rounds or even in the OR, Catena must stop what he is doing and consult over whether a patient should be admitted to the hospital or is an urgent case. Catena usually stays in the outpatient clinic until the last of the patients have been evaluated. His workday ends long after dusk.

Clinic is followed by a dinner of lentils and possibly meat, then administrative tasks and checking email via the Internet connection provided by solar power and satellite. Then bed. Then do it again. And again. For years.

It didn't take long for me to realize I could never do what Catena does. I don't have the faith. Neither Catena's faith nor the faith of the nuns and priests I met who work with him every day as well, taking care of the sick and powerless, for years on end with no publicity, no fanfare, no expectation of reward. Missionaries who had spent five years in the Congo, then three years in India, now possibly two or more years in Sudan. Women and men in their 60s or even 70s sweating, cleaning up filth, risking death from disease or violence for no pay, the work not a stepping-stone to better things but rather the only thing they would ever do, until they became too old to do it or died doing it.

Every single time I went to Sudan I couldn't wait to leave. I spent a month with Catena in 2008, another month in 2010 and still another in 2014. I saw many patients with illnesses and injuries that medical students in the U.S. only read about, everything from advanced leprosy to fulminant rabies to rare cancer in its most advanced stage. I saw children die of tetanus, starvation and burns. Dead neonates wedged in the birth canal. Then, in 2014, I saw war.

Sudan split into two countries in 2011. The Nuba Mountains were ceded to Northern Sudan, much to the dismay of the Nuba people, who had only ever been persecuted by the government in Khartoum and keenly desired to go with those who formed The Republic of South Sudan. A small rebel army took up arms to defend the region. Violence erupted. Planes came and bombs started falling. Catena's role changed almost overnight, from that of humanitarian doctor helping the Nubans rebuild to war zone surgeon, running what is essentially now a MASH hospital. Most of his staff evacuated after the first bombs fell. Instead of daily goiter and prostate surgeries, he has been called to the OR night and day for amputations, shrapnel wounds to the head and abdomen, and to tend to women and children mutilated by bullets and bombs.

While it may sound odd, I saw my job at Mother of Mercy as being company for Tom. I was not essential. The place runs well without me. I'm not a specialist, like an ophthalmologist or ENT [Ears, Nose, Throat] doctor, so my visit wasn't critical. I assisted Tom somewhat in the operating room. I also saw countless patients during the day in the outpatient clinic, triaging and admitting the sickest. In that regard I'm was a help, but Tom has other staff who do what I can do.

Most of my time there was spent following Tom around, keeping him company. Joking and talking, bringing him some much-needed American sensitivity. He is pretty isolated out there, surrounded by a culture he is not part of and likely never can be. He loves the Nuba people, but interaction and communication is not easy. He's a foreigner. I think most of the time he just carries around in his head all his intensity, worry, fear and determination, like a red hot boiler keeping him going, vented daily with prayer but without any real release until he can sit down with an American and let it out over drinks. I love when we see each other after a few years. Lots of stories to tell, frustrations to release, horrors to relate. Our graveyard senses of humor match perfectly.

My last trip to see him, in February 2014, was my last until the war stops. As I said, I don't have Catena's faith and what I experienced there was too dangerous to go back.

First of all, we could no longer fly directly up to Kauda, which is only a dozen miles or so from Gidel, where Mother of Mercy is located. Rather, we flew to the border of South Sudan and Sudan, to the Yida refugee camp, which itself is a sprawling ghetto of displaced people. Then we had to drive an entire day through the state of South Kordofan in Sudan to get to the Nuba region. We were stopped at numerous checkpoints by the Nuba—that is, the "rebel" army. At one checkpoint they told us a bomber had recently passed overhead, and that we might have to take cover. I'll never forget the queasy feeling I got then—worse than just fear—imagining the bomber suddenly appearing and me scrambling for a hiding place somewhere in the dry, yellow dust; the bomb falling, shrapnel ripping me apart. What I felt was the first whiff of panic. Thankfully, though, I didn't see any bombers while driving to and away from Nuba.

What I did see during my stay there were the casualties from the bombing of a nearby village. That experience is spelled out in a good amount of detail below. I had seen injury and death before, but never in such a catastrophic way. It's grotesque what exploding metal does to the body. Arms and legs ripped off, faces destroyed, intestines hanging out, blood, pain and death. The minute I saw it, I was afraid and wanted to go home. I realized there was no law, no safety, no civilization [when it came to the actions of the Government of Sudan]. And that there was no reason I wouldn't be shredded by the next bomber. My sense of myself as a special person, a doctor working hard to help people, was gone. The banality of the chaos and violence terrified me. I wanted to get out.

Bombers flew over or near the hospital after that almost every day. One day they came so close that I almost jumped in a foxhole. The sound of the airplane engine terrified me. "Get me the fuck out of here," I thought, again and again.

Catena looked thinner and more tired than ever. Patients filled the hospital and the hospital grounds, with beds outside under awnings or in tents. Children missing limbs hobbled on crutches after playmates. Wounded soldiers, women and kids were everywhere.[3]

Foxholes had been dug all over the hospital grounds. Whenever a bomber flew overhead, staff and patients scurried to them. The nearest large town, Kauda, had been bombed regularly, its airstrip destroyed. Almost every day I heard the faraway rumble of munitions. The hospital had not yet been directly targeted, although Catena expected at some point it would be. Possibly only Catena's worldwide notoriety prevented the Sudanese government from killing everyone there.

On February 13, 2014, near Um Dullu, a village close to the hospital, impoverished Nubans combed the region looking for slivers of gold. If wildly successful, a forager might find $20 of gold after a week of work. An impromptu market had sprung up nearby. Women and children sold tea and snacks out of straw lean-tos. The jets came around noon. It's unclear whether they bombed or strafed the crowds. One survivor ran to a foxhole and jumped in on top of people already hidden there. *Just before his legs* were torn apart, he realized everyone else in the hole was dead.

Later that day coming into the hospital I heard screams. Blood-soaked casualties writhed on stretchers lining the main hallway. A woman close to me moaned and lifted her arm. It had been blasted open at the elbow.

Catena pushed past me, already on his way to the operating room. Inside, a young soldier on a stretcher gasped for breath. We cut off his clothes and Catena pointed to a small hole in his right chest—his only wound.

"Got to put in a chest tube," Catena muttered. He grabbed a kit off the shelf. The kit flopped open, its protective seal and the tube inside gnawed to bits by a rat.

"Shit!" he yelled. He rifled through the chest tube kits; almost all of them had been destroyed.

Meanwhile the dying man screamed, sat up, fell back. Lying there, he screamed again, in English: "Why? Why?"

Finally Catena found an intact kit. He opened it and grabbed a scalpel, made a large incision in the man's side and inserted the tube, hooked the tube to a vacuum bottle. We waited for blood to pour out. Nothing happened.

The man stopped screaming. He breathed slowly, longer pauses between each breath. His head rolled to the side, eyes open, fixed.

"He's gone," Catena said.

Quickly the staff replaced him with another victim, then another. We cut the clothes off the woman with the blasted arm. A single loop of intestine protruded from her abdomen, full of stool. Her left knee was blown open as well. She stared at us, awake, in shock, moaning. She would go to the OR first. The woman after her, older, had also had one of her arms mostly amputated by shrapnel. She didn't moan or scream. As I began to cut off her clothes, she stopped me and helped me take them off so I wouldn't ruin them.

Another woman, pregnant, had a shrapnel wound to the face. A crater passed from her jaw up into her sinuses. Catena was able to insert his finger all the way through to her nostrils, and pluck out bits of bone while she submitted quietly, whimpering. She had had no pain medicine. The bone surrounding the bottom of her eye was gone. Her lips were shredded.

In the OR, Catena found shrapnel and multiple areas of injured bowel inside his first patient. He resected one section and rejoined the bowel; in other areas he sutured to stop bleeding. After the lengthy laparotomy, he amputated her right leg. He predicted her left arm might have to come off as well, but the pulse in her wrist was strong. He would monitor her for now. As she awoke he noticed her mangled fingers, two of them barely attached. With a pair of surgical scissors he quickly snipped them off.

Next he amputated the arm of the second woman. By the time he finished it was nearing midnight. The other injured could wait until tomorrow; many of them would need amputations but there were no further chest or abdominal injuries to attend to.

We walked out of the hospital in a daze. "Come on," he said. "Let's get some chocolate." He led me to small office where a freezer hummed, used to store lab samples and vaccines. Hidden under the supplies were five chocolate bars, unbelievably rare and precious. We grabbed all of them and headed back to the OR, where Catena treated me and his operative staff to cold candy.

Over the next two weeks the casualties of Um Dullu healed. Several more amputations were required. The woman who lost her leg did indeed lose her arm as well.

Watching Catena change the bandage on a stump of one young girl, I asked him: "Can you imagine what that's like? One day you're ok and the next shrapnel takes off your arm?"

"Yeah," he said. "You never know when it's your time."

For Catena, everything is in God's hands, including himself. Every day he tries to do God's work, essentially to live according to Christ's mission: "Inasmuch as you do to the least of my brothers, you do to me." Murder doesn't demoralize him; terrorism won't break his spirit.

Six years of long days helping the powerless has taken its toll but evidently not shaken his faith. Not just faith but love motivates him as well. Catena loves the Nuba Mountains and its people. He wants them to be able to live in peace in a region free of persecution, with more than one hospital and one doctor for the sick. That's his dream. It's an unlikely dream but he's giving his life for it.

Notes

1. I'll definitely go back if the war concludes. Despite how harsh it is, the Nuba is stunningly beautiful and populated by people you'll meet nowhere else on earth. Seeing the Milky Way every night, living simply, making such a huge difference in people's lives—those are some of the reasons. The main reason though is Tom. As long as he's there, I'll go back. He's an inspiration and he's my friend. There's nobody like him.

2. I was given time in my Family Medicine residency to do rotations abroad, which I eagerly pursued. That is how I ended up in Sudan with Tom. I also worked in Haiti. But despite my idealism, I discovered that the grueling, hard and thankless work of international medicine was too much for me. It's dangerous. You can die. It's often boring, frustrating and bleak. There are incredible moments as well, good moments, but the work is not for the weak or unsure. It also helps to have faith. Especially when you're facing death. Or when you're facing extreme suffering, suffering that seems meaningless. So I abandoned the international doctor dream and stayed in the U.S. I had kids I needed to raise and a family who I didn't want to say goodbye to. Plus the money was good, even if the work was not professionally satisfying.

3. On rare occasions Tom will leave the hospital and visit the village right outside the gates. It's called Gidel. There are makeshift, ramshackle shops and "cafes" there. I walked out of the hospital with him a few times, and every person who walked by greeted him. They love him there. Invariably we would be asked to come into a café and offered chicory coffee and food. The Nubans are generous, kind, low-key and love to laugh. They are also very guarded, given the constant persecution in their history. I've had much less interaction than I would have liked. That is largely due to the fact that I don't speak Arabic. Now that Tom speaks it rather well, he has had an opportunity get to know everybody. As I said, the Nuba love him, and he loves them back.

Sowing Seeds of Peace
My Life at Mother of Mercy Hospital

MARGARET CAMARCA

I would like to make an appeal to those in possession of greater resources, to public authorities, and to all people of good will who are working for social justice: never tire of working for a more just world, marked by a greater solidarity. —Pope Francis, Rio de Janeiro, July 25, 2013

In the summer of 1988 I had recently graduated from Virginia Tech University with a biology degree and was headed to Texas to serve as a volunteer for a year at a residential treatment center for abused and neglected children. Before I left, my mother gave me a hand-embroidered needlepoint graced with the following poignant words of Ralph Waldo Emerson: "All are needed by each one, nothing is fair or good alone." Although now faded, I keep the needlepoint in my bedside table and often reflect on its profound implications.

I was raised in a Christian home with four sisters and four brothers in Northern Virginia. My parents were devout Catholics with quiet faiths who exemplified the importance of family, service and forgiveness. My mother was a humble, hardworking woman who, more than anyone else, shaped how I came to understand the world around me. She was from a poor family in Washington, D.C., married at 35 and proceeded to have nine children. She did not have a college education, she did not win any awards for service, she did not start any humanitarian movements, she simply lived an honest life dedicated to serving others. Her life was the classic example of doing small things with great love, always seeing Christ in whomever she met. She was jovial, kind-hearted, and never did I experience her having a "bad day," although I am sure she had many. After sustaining a brain injury later in life she was unable to care for herself and was bed bound in her home for her final three years of life. She died surrounded by her loving children one year prior to my departure to Sudan.

Early on in my catechism classes I was taught that we are all parts of one body, all children of God, sharing one sacred humanity. Decades would pass before I came to a mature understanding of this teaching.

Throughout my life I have been greatly encouraged by stories and examples of people who not only talk of "love for their fellow man" but live it out, often in ways that are seemingly deleterious to themselves. Thus, for example, during my young adulthood I was influenced by Sister Angela Murdaugh, a Franciscan Sister of Mary and midwife, who started Holy Family Birth Center, a birthing center which cares for impoverished migrants of the Rio Grande Valley; by Dr. James Ronan, who helped found Mercy Health Clinic, a clinic for the uninsured in Montgomery County, MD; and, Dr. Buzz and Melissa Auvil, who co-founded "Hope for Kabingo," a program addressing a variety of needs in an impoverished area of southern Uganda. I was fortunate to work alongside these models of self-sacrificing love, be it briefly or for an extended period of time. One dominant theme throughout their good works was a heartfelt understanding of the inherent dignity of all human life; a dignity that stems from the belief that we are all made in the image and likeness of God.

And then there was a close friend of mine who was living in an area of conflict in what is now the Republic of South Sudan. A war had been raging with the north since the country's president, Omar al-Bashir, assumed power in a coup d'etat in 1989. I visited her in 2003, specifically to bring her medical supplies that she needed: dressing supplies and medicine. During that trip I was introduced to Bishop Macram Max Gassis of the Diocese of El Obeid. At the time, the Bishop was planning to visit an impoverished region of his diocese, the Nuba Mountains, to meet with the local people and discuss his desire to build a hospital in the region. I was struck by the Bishop's ability to "dream big" in such a harsh and remote area scarred by war. In 2008 his dream came true with the opening of The Mother of Mercy Hospital.

Although I financially supported Mother of Mercy over the years, there was always an underlying yearning to do more. With a renewal of fighting in 2011 between the Government of Sudan and the Sudanese People's Liberation Army-North (SPLA-N), most non-governmental organizations (NGO) left the Nuba Mountains and almost all assistance vanished.

Concerned about the plight of the Nuba people, I followed the events that were unfolding in the region, that resulted in my watching a video about the ongoing war. As I viewed the latter, I was both sickened to see the Nuba people literally being starved to death due to the aerial bombardments and the "scorched earth" policy of the government of Sudan (GoS), *and* the largely silent response of the international community. Outraged by the situation, a U.S.–based Christian organization, among others, gathered truckloads of food and delivered it themselves. I remember thinking good for them and good for all those serving at the Mother of Mercy Hospital. Although saddened by the atrocities in the Nuba Mountains and greatly inspired by those serving in the area, I still wasn't motivated enough to act. I was too comfortable in my own life, but things were to dramatically change a year later.

In July of 2013, I went on a two-week mission trip to a little village in southern Uganda. Upon my return I was telling a friend of my experiences there and she commented that it sounded like something I might like to do full time. I told her, "Yes, someday." She responded by asking me, "What's stopping you from doing it now?" When she said those words, it was as if Jesus himself was speaking. *What was stopping me?* I was single, no dependents, healthy, financially stable and the list went on and on. Upon reflection, the answer was, "Nothing was stopping me." And with that realization, the very next week I submitted an application to the Catholic Medical Mission Board (CMMB) indicating my interest to serve as a volunteer at Mother Mercy of Hospital. That November I found myself at Mother of Mercy Hospital in Gidel in the heart of the Nuba Mountains. The hospital workers welcomed me with songs, jewelry, food gifts, and a bird with clipped wings, instantly making me feel at home.

Up until that time I had, for the last several decades, been working as a clinical nurse and as a study manager in the medical research world. The Mother of Mercy hospital, though, needed a pharmacist. And so, I became a pharmacist. There was nothing glamorous about this role. You could often find me sweating, covered in dirt unpacking medication that had just made the long, arduous, dusty journey from South Sudan. My nursing care was limited to children coming into the pharmacy wanting their wounds to be dressed and giving shots to the outpatient department (OPD) patients.

The position, nonetheless, was a perfect fit for me. I was able to support the employees, care for and visit with patients, organize the pharmacy and most importantly be touched by the villagers' stories. I feel privileged to share some of these stories with you.

Although the Nuba have known war for decades, they are a resilient, gracious and gentle community. My transition to life in Gidel was easy. The villagers smile and greet anyone who passes by, even small children come up to say hello ("kaafe") and shake one's hand. There are over fifty different tribes in South Kordofan who, variously, hold Christian, Islamic and traditional religious beliefs. They get along well. Mixed marriages are not uncommon. When you are invited to someone's *tukul* (hut), expect to stay for hours, to meet and be greeted by extended family members and friends, and be waited on by many in the household.

Soon after my arrival in the Nuba Mountains, war broke out in the Republic of South Sudan. The warring factions in the Republic of South Sudan are predominantly between two major tribes (the Dinka and Nuer). It was not surprising that this new country, composed of people who have known nothing but war for decades, was experiencing major growing pains. The fighting there unfortunately affected hospital logistics as the hospital's chain of supplies has to go through the South Sudan to get to Gidel. Truckloads of sorghum were stolen, supplies were indefinitely stranded in Juba, and a clinical officer was also unable to get through making the hospital's hectic outpatient department even busier.

Initially, my daily work consisted of assisting the hospital's pharmacy store manager, Joseph. Joseph's story was like many there. As a result of the Second Sudanese Civil War (1983–2005), his family members have been separated from each other for years with little communication. Joseph's education was constantly interrupted by the war so he was unable to complete primary school. He has, though, a great thirst for learning, is conversational and a smile was never far from his face. I loved working with him.

The hospital pharmacy was well stocked with a variety of antibiotics, cardiovascular, diabetic, gastrointestinal and pain medications. I supplied drugs to OPD, dispensing pharmacy and medical supplies to the ward staffs weekly. Approximately 150 to 200 patients (who have either spent the night on the hospital grounds or walked for an hour or more to get there) are seen each day in the OPD by two to three clinical officers or seen by the hospital's one doctor, "Dr. Tom" Catena.

As with the OPD personnel, the ward staffs are incredibly busy. Apart from common illnesses such as malaria and pneumonia, they also attend to the tragic victims of the conflict. The hospital was built for 80 patients but due to the lack of healthcare facilities in the area, it houses 350 or more in- patients at any one time. Beds line the corridors making dressing changes, IV insertions, patient privacy very difficult. Family members often sleep under the bed of their sick relatives.

I remember one pediatric patient, Manair, who lost his right arm and leg to shrapnel. He would hop around the office on his leg, or skooch along the floor on his buttocks

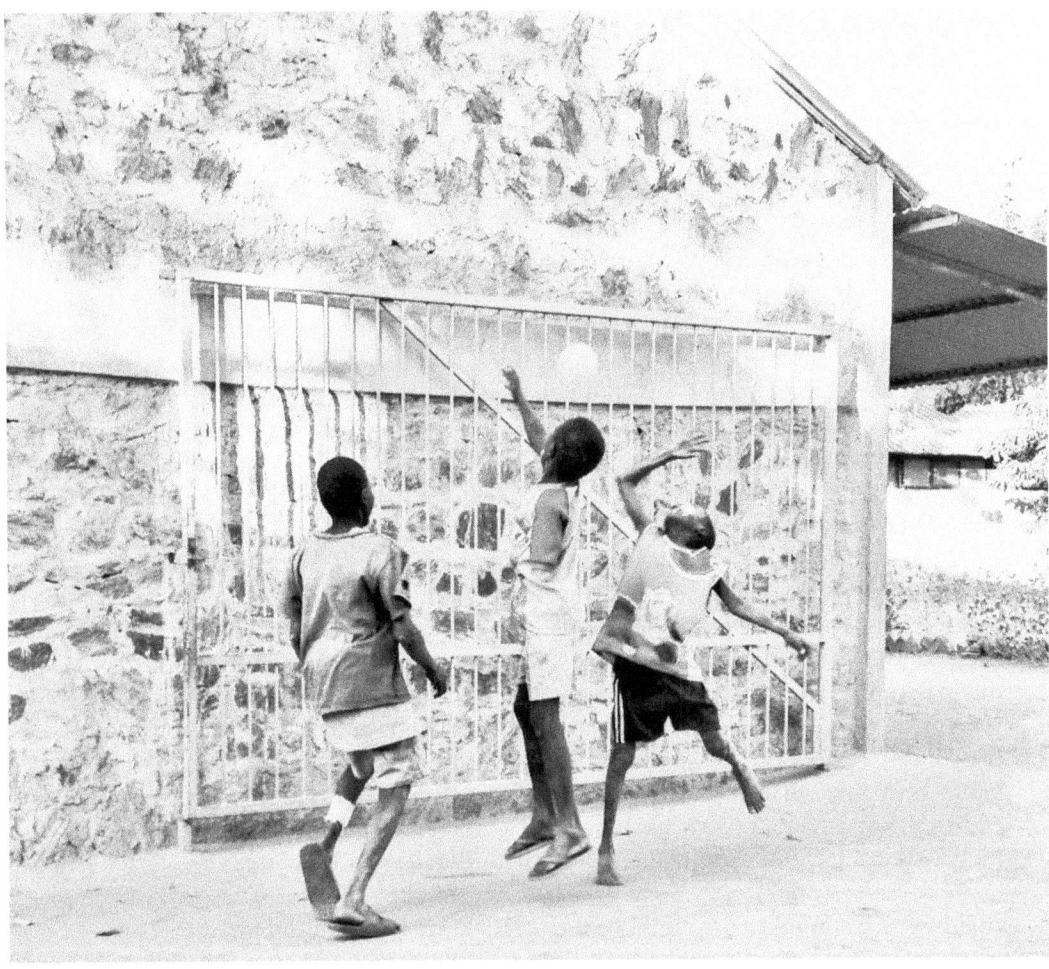

The middle boy was the first child I met while at the hospital who was maimed by a bombing (photograph by Margaret Camarca).

when he needed to move quickly. The morning that the doctor informed him that he was being discharged Manair asked the hospital matron to convince the doctor to let him stay. He was frightened to return home, especially now that he could not run when the bombers appeared in the sky.

How do you explain to a child that there is no safe place? During my first year in Gidel, Antonov planes flew overhead weekly, threatening relentlessly to drop their bombs. Nighttime provided no relief. The heat was stifling in the Nuba Mountains so oftentimes I slept under the stars. Fighter jets passed by throughout the night, where they were headed I had no idea, perhaps they were on training excursions. No matter, their appearance contributed to one of the constants in the Nuba Mountains: the complete and utter disruption of work and social activities.

I was blessed to share in the life and prayers of a religious order stationed there (the Comboni Sisters),[1] and to witness them serving in small and large ways. The sisters were from Uganda, the Congo, Sudan and Mexico. Although they carried heavy crosses, they were always quick with a smile, story, and welcomed one to their compound. I liked spending time at their compound, as many things went on, apart from the hospital activity, that you would never know about unless you saw it yourself. For instance, while in the States (this was prior to my going to the Nuba) I watched a video about a boy, Daniel, who lost his arms to a bomb blast years before. I remember being horrified when his uncle told a reporter that the "boy wasn't of much use anymore." Daniel went back home to live with his uncle but word got around that he wasn't being fed. The Sisters sent a driver to find him. He returned to the hospital half dead. I met Daniel at the sisters' compound, where he had been nursed back to life. The sisters built a little tukul for Daniel and his friends, enrolling all the boys at the parish school.

The issues at the hospital were many and varied. Just caring for the patients and staff present many unique challenges for the administration, but there are countless others as well. One example was a boy named Kuku. A shy boy of about eleven years. Dirty with matted hair, he was always alone. I never saw him with a parent, sibling or friend. As it so happened, Kuku was interested in everything I did. Before long, I started giving him small jobs like moving boxes from the warehouse to the pharmacy and helping me deliver supplies to the wards. He loved "working" and never asked for anything in return, but I paid him in toys, mangos or candy for his labor. I finally asked the hospital matron, Sister Angelina, if she knew why he was in the hospital. After some investigation we realized he wasn't a patient or co-patient, just a boy who lived an hour away who decided to make the hospital his home. He slept, we discovered, on the ground outside the male ward. He was not well cared for by his mother and had been on his own for years. Due to the lack of development and infrastructure, there are no "social service" networks in Nuba. Sister Angelina spent a long time talking to Kuku telling him the hospital was no place to live. Ultimately, she had him bathed and gave him some new clothes and told Kuku he had to go back home. He agreed to go and went. However, Kuku returned two days later stating he was going to the hospital's "school." He started going home (or somewhere) each night and stopping by the office each day to show me he could write his numbers. Eventually, the parish church took Kuku in.

The hospital school was the brainchild of the Comboni Sisters. At Mother of Mercy, hospital patients with tuberculosis (TB) and the children and siblings of TB patients stay six months or more for their TB treatment. Normally, the caring physician would send TB patients home, if stable, after a couple weeks of treatment and have health care workers go to their households with a DOT (directly observed therapy) program, where a healthcare worker physically watches the patient take his/her TB medications. Originally Mother of Mercy administered a DOT program, but the TB treatment failure and relapse rate was high. Patients were scattered all over the region and it became impossible to manage the program. TB patients and their families now stay in tents at the hospital for the full treatment course. Although the living situation is not ideal, the treatment success rate has improved. The hospital school was started to help these children keep up with their studies, but it has had its challenges. One of the many challenges was the fact that a good number of village children not associated with the hospital, like Kuku, attended it due to a lack of schools in the area. Unfortunately, the hospital eventually was forced to close the school due to a measles epidemic.

While I was in the Nuba Mountains my niece turned ten years old, and for her birthday she and her friends made gift boxes of stickers, markers, paint and bracelets for the village girls. I enjoyed handing them out as the village girls remarked that they had never seen such "wonderful things." This is true as there is currently no place to purchase such items. Today, during the war, anything not grown locally is considered contraband as the GoS allows no business transactions. It is no wonder that the Nuba frequently pepper their talk with "before the war…" They are usually referring to that little window of peace between 2005 and 2011 when war was no longer a constant in their lives. (The Second Sudanese Civil War lasted from 1983 to 2005, and resulted in some two million dead.) Trade was common between the north and the South Kordofan state during that short window of peace, and the markets were full. Clothing, shoes and consumables were readily available. A little market even sprang up just outside the hospital's gate. Business was particularly good there because people visited the hospital from all over (even as far as Khartoum) and would patronize the shops. In fact, Joseph, our pharmacist, ran a little café that did quite well. While I was in the Nuba, Joseph and I visited his café, which had fallen into ruins. When peace returns he dreams of restoring the café and buying a little refrigerator for sodas. He even mentioned having Internet access! Currently the only real market is about a 20-minute walk from the hospital. Items that can be produced in the area (sorghum, limes, goats, local beds) are sold there, along with other small items smuggled in from the north, such as packages of dried milk.

In early May 2014 I started receiving urgent emails from friends and family back home. They had seen ominous news reports about bombings of Mother of Mercy. May 1st and 2nd marked the first time the hospital was directly targeted by the GoS. A drone was seen days prior, taking pictures of our compound no doubt. That morning the parish priest, Father Francis, was saying an outdoor mass at St. Joseph's Secondary School. He was celebrating the feast day of St. Joseph the Worker (May 1st). That was the only service he never completed. I was in the pharmacy watching medications tumble from the pharmacy shelves, wondering what could have caused such a deafening explosion. Within a split second Joseph appeared at the pharmacy door yelling at me to take cover, we were under attack.

I remember the incident like it was yesterday. In particular I remember everyone (staff, students, patients, visitors) frantically packing up their belongings to find safer surroundings. As the planes flew overhead, patients begged Sister Angelina to unlock the hospital's back gate so they could quickly exit. Right after she did so, a bomb dropped near her and she was forced to take cover in an open field.

I ran towards a foxhole behind the OPD, tripping on a short wire fence I didn't see. I jumped into the foxhole brimming with eight other patients. An elderly patient's leg was wounded and bleeding due to her fall. We attended to her as best we could while we awaited the jet's return. The first bomb dropped behind the TB village causing no damage. As I heard the jet's piercing engines once again, I got down as low as possible, in a curled position (not wanting to lose a limb) and I covered my ears. I prayed God would protect us from harm. The next bomb was closer, hitting immediately behind our housing compound's fence. The fence was destroyed, trees were singed and shredded, windows were blown out and doors were thrown off their hinges. Roofs buckled from the bomb's concussion force.

Afterwards, hospital workers, the police, reporters and others walked the grounds for hours taking pictures and surveying the damage. People recounted their stories of what transpired that morning over and over again. The next day brought an eerie quietude. Most of the patients had completely fled but a few were staying in the rocky cliffs just beyond the small market outside the grounds of the hospital. By 10 a.m. the Antonov planes returned. I ran to a foxhole by the pharmacy, lying low and making room for

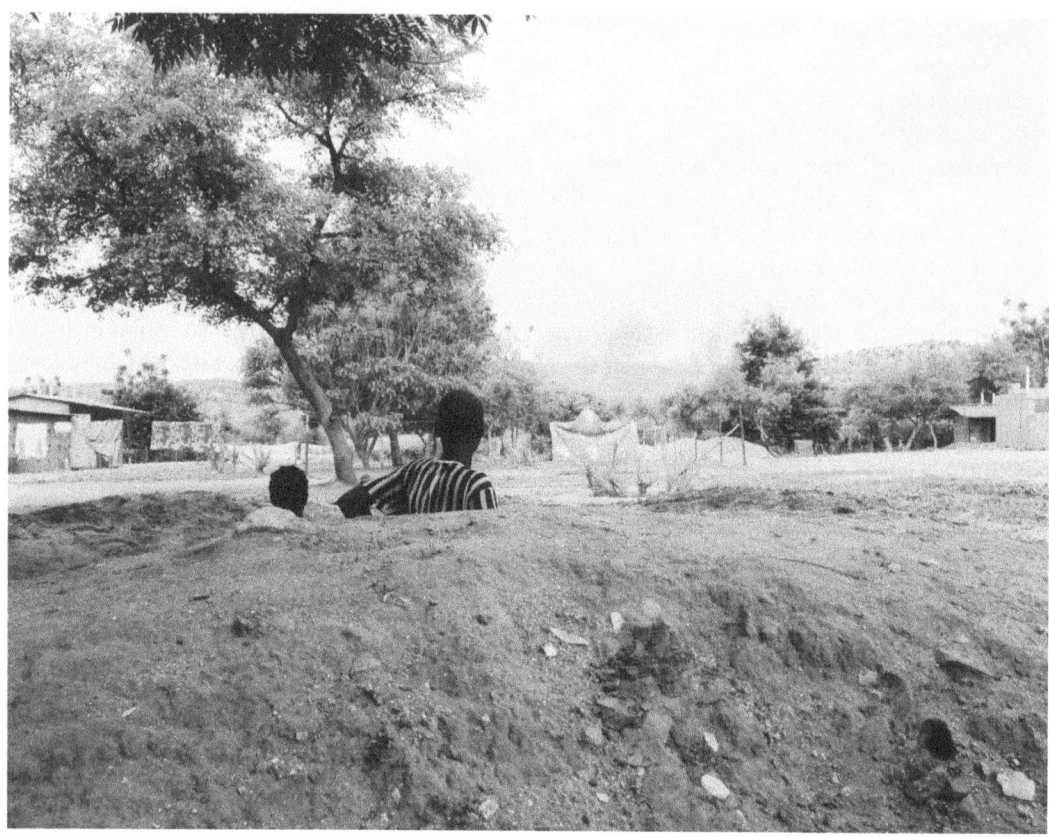

In a foxhole watching a bomb explode just outside the hospital compound on May 2, 2014 (photograph by Margaret Camarca).

others. We all laid stone still and quiet anticipating the KABOOM and rattling of the earth once again. Moments later I saw smoke rising in the distance, just beyond the river that borders the hospital's compound. Miraculously eight bombs were dropped that second day with little damage being done. One man hiding inside the trunk of a majestic baobab tree was injured as shrapnel flew through an unprotected hole penetrating his ankle but there were no other casualties.

Some Nuba were afraid we'd leave but everyone's resolve was that if a structure remained and patients still wanted to be seen, the hospital was open for business. The Nuba civilians had done nothing to deserve such treatment, and the bombings were such a blatant war crime it made staying easier. I felt blessed by God for the opportunity to serve there and I wanted to continue doing so.

When Antonovs pass overhead you have some time to prepare, unlike when the jets attack, so Antonovs are a bit less frightening. I know it sounds strange but you could often find us laughing in the foxholes. This was a mixture of nervousness and a sound awareness of the absurdity of the situation. While in the holes we would brush the dirt off each other, straighten out our clothes, put the shoes that slipped off while jumping in back on and clear the area of leaves, ants and sticks so we could lay down if need be. I purposely carried bubbles and other toys in my pockets so I could distract and play with the children while in the holes. When the planes passed directly overhead we would quiet down considerably and I would start praying. Once the planes disappeared we would assist each other out of the foxholes which, for us shorter folks, was no easy task and often led to more laughter. I usually experienced a tempered feeling of lightheartedness once I emerged. I don't know why. Perhaps this was due to a feeling that we had "cheated death" once again or just plain gratefulness that no one was hurt although the anxiety of wondering exactly where the bombs dropped lingered.

Not a few ask why I remained at Mother of Mercy Hospital after the hospital bombings. My reasoning was simple: I was completely confident that I was living the life God had prepared for me. This instilled in me an overwhelming sense of peace. By nature I am not a courageous person, nor am I one to seek adventure. Although the sound of the bombs and rumbling of the earth were frightening, I still slept soundly at night. The Nuba are very brave, which rubs off on you. From the beginning I understood that the region was not safe. In 2003 I visited the memorial site of fourteen children and one teacher from Holy Cross Primary School in Kauda who had died during a bombing in 2000. During this visit, I met a schoolgirl who had been maimed in the attack. I understood that President al-Bashir wanted to eradicate the region of the Nuba people and I was aware that all of us caring for the sick were considered criminals by the Khartoum government. Ultimately, I understood that my life was in the hands of God, so nothing else mattered. I witnessed firsthand the dedication of others in the region making exceedingly greater and more dangerous sacrifices than mine and I wanted to continue supporting them and the villagers. Soon after the targeted bombings one of the nurses, Kucha, entered the pharmacy crying. She was frightened, exhausted and wondering if the war would ever end. She told me how she had survived the 2000 bombing at Holy Cross Primary School. My mind immediately flashed back to the memorial site and the maimed schoolgirl I had met years before. Kucha and the other villagers have been living this nightmare their entire lives. I, on the other hand, had been living a secure life of plenty for decades. Clearly, the time had not come for me to leave.

We didn't experience any further direct attacks from the government but a feeling of vulnerability was the new norm for weeks afterwards. Over a month passed before I stopped jumping at the sound of every thunderbolt or large passing truck. The hospital's foxholes were made deeper, from three to four feet deep to five to six. The local police also instructed the market's venders to dig holes in front of their shops. It is assumed, and largely proven true, that as long as one can reach a trench in time, one will remain safe as the shrapnel flies a foot or more off the ground. Children are often the victims of these attacks because they don't appreciate the critical need to get as low down to the ground as possible.

I was not surprised by how the Nuba marked the one-year anniversary of the bombing. They threw a party, a big one. The students at the secondary school invited us to join in their "St. Joseph the Worker" celebration. The day was festive with lots of speeches, songs, dancing, acting (playlets) and food. As Father Francis rose to give his speech in front of the assembly he did an impromptu reenactment of his fright-filled reaction from that fateful morning of one year prior. The students started to laugh—in fact, not simply laugh but roar. I thank God for His protection on that day and for the witness of the villagers who carry on despite constant adversity, an adversity far beyond anything I have ever experienced.

The almost constant aerial and ground attacks against the civilians of the Nuba Mountains during both the Second Sudanese Civil War (1983–2005) and the current war

(June 2011–present) has sorely, and negatively, impacted the operation of schools. As a result, many young Nubans have been hard-pressed to attain a high school diploma, let alone a university degree. Most of the villagers one meets who have finished secondary school were educated, as least in part, in Kakuma (a large refugee camp in Kenya). The diocese's schools had to close in 2011 with the renewed fighting. They opened up again, despite the conflict, in 2013.

Soon after the targeted bombings Fred, St. Joseph's schoolmaster, coordinated a volleyball match between the hospital workers and the secondary school students for some R & R and stress relief. Fred thanked the players for a good game and encouraged them and the visitors not to lose hope in a more peaceful future. After the match, Fred asked if I could teach biology as one of his teachers returned to Kenya after the bombings. I couldn't refuse.

In early 2014, the hospital started experiencing yet another calamity. A newly emerging measles outbreak placed an enormous strain on an already overburdened hospital and caused the closure of the few operational schools in the area. Measles mimic many other respiratory diseases and several days can pass before the pathognomonic rash appears. Ward patients admitted with one diagnosis were found during the doctor's morning rounds to also have measles, having been infected by an unidentified case. As the epidemic grew the hospital was forced to erect isolation tents to handle the staggering number of cases. Prior to the current war, the hospital's Tuberculosis (TB) control program and Expanded Programme for Immunizations were supported by the GoS's Ministry of Health. TB drugs and vaccines provided by the World Health Organization were also readily available. With the renewal of fighting and blockade of all international and governmental aid to the rebel-controlled area of South Kordofan, diseases that had long been controlled were reemerging. Despite the lack of any governmental assistance though, the hospital limited the measles's mortality rate to less than 5 percent and continued the TB control efforts with self-purchased drugs.

I fondly remember one TB success story. Owal was a five-year-old Dinka boy who had been transferred from the Yida Refugee Camp in the Unity State of South Sudan to Mother of Mercy in the Nuba Mountains. Upon arrival at the hospital, Owal was lethargic and extremely emaciated with purulent sores on his hips and buttocks. Although treated at the refugee camp and at other hospitals in South Sudan, he was not getting better. His father had heard of Mother of Mercy and opted to take the risk of transferring his son to Gidel.

Owal was immediately started on a trial of TB medications. As he proceeded to get better, Owal would stop by the pharmacy often to make paper airplanes or show me his latest tractor made out of dirt. Bittersweet was the moment when he informed me of his pending discharge. After nine long months and several surgeries, his osteomyelitis was finally healed. Had it not been for Mother of Mercy, Owal would have surely died, thus adding to the large and growing number of senseless and preventable deaths in the Nuba Mountains.

The end of each rainy season marks the start of the GoS's bombing campaign in South Kordofan. As part of its scorched earth policy, the government attempts to prevent the villagers from harvesting their crops. On Thursday, October 16, 2014, for example, numerous bombs were dropped in Heiban resulting in the murder of six girls, three of whom were sisters. One of the girls arrived at Mother of Mercy without any sign of external damage except for a nose bleed. Be that as it may, she perished shortly thereafter due to a cerebral hemorrhage. A fourth sister suffered several corneal lacerations but survived the traumatizing incident.

A few days later more bombs were dropped near us, this time south of Gidel. Two casualties were brought in, one of whom hemorrhaged to death from a massive leg wound; the other barely survived a major abdominal surgery.

The villagers, although frightened, maintain extraordinary hope. One such example is a woman from our cleaning crew named Hawa. She invited me to her home for dinner the day of the 2nd bombing. She sent her daughter, Bibiana, to accompany me to her (Hawa's) tukul. Hawa has ten children, four of whom were in school and able to translate for us. Her children played outside as we ate. Another cleaner, Hanan, stopped by with her children and both husbands joined us once their day of harvesting was complete. My animated hosts thoroughly enjoyed themselves throughout dinner. As I listened to them laugh, I couldn't help but be struck by the contrast of their joy and the war around us. I stayed past sunset. Hawa's girls walked me back home singing the entire way. I had a flashlight and asked if they needed it for their return trip. They said no, they had the light of the moon.

The dry season allows for movement from the Yida refugee camp once again. During the year's end hospital workers and teachers leave for their long holidays but visiting doctors (some of whom are specialists) and others arrive to fill in the gaps. For weeks beforehand villagers from all over start appearing in anticipation of the visitors' services. Among the services provided are vesico-vaginal fistula (VVF) surgeries, cataract surgeries and the fitting of orthopedic limbs. A VVF repair is a specialized gynecological surgery. Prior to moving to Africa I hadn't heard of VVFs, but the condition is well known in countries with poor obstetric care. Usually caused by prolonged labors, small holes are made between the bladder and vagina. The seepage of urine is constant. The condition is emotionally debilitating so I was happy to see the women get them repaired.

Despite all the challenges, the hospital continues to function at full capacity, conduct formal training courses for new workers, send Nuba staff for additional medical training outside the country and expand its role in the community by supporting community outreach clinics. Plans were even in the works to add additional outreach clinics and start an HIV counseling and testing program.

January of 2015 was relatively quiet until mid-month. The government's ground forces started shelling near Mendi, a location of one of the hospital's outreach clinics, and as they did so, the inhabitants of Mendi fled. A GoS victory in this region would've likely resulted in an emboldened military attempt to overtake Kauda, the SPLA–North's defacto political "capital."

This period was the closest any GoS forces had come to the hospital since the conflict began in 2011. One of my former secondary school students, Bibiana, was in Kauda when a bombed dropped on January 13th. Bibiana is an orphan and was staying in an abandoned government school with her little sisters and grandmother. She was alone when a jet dropped its bomb near her dwelling. She arrived at the hospital two days later with shrapnel imbedded in her thighs and ankle. I visited her in the hospital and asked her if the incident kept her up at night. She said no; a typical, courageous Nuba response. Her greatest difficulty was being separated from her younger sisters. After a week of shelling the government troops were turned back and a tenuous calm returned once again.

I was able to visit my U.S. home in February 2015, and then returned to Gidel the following month. My journey back included four days in Nairobi, four days in Juba, one night in the Yida refugee camp followed by an eight hour truck drive due north to Gidel. The Yida refugee camp is home to some 70,000 Nuba, and was started by Samaritan's Purse (a ministry of Billy Graham's son, Franklin) in 2011 when war broke out in the Nuba Mountains. I was amazed to see how well the Nuba adapt to whatever situation confronts them. A refugee camp is no place to live, but homes and small makeshift schools are being built, church services are being held and commerce was occurring.

Despite the harvesters' best efforts, life can be precarious in Nuba. Inadequate rainfall results in food shortages causing everything in the markets to become extremely expensive. Normally various NGOs can fill in the gap until the next rainy season, but it is far from easy there since the government uses food as a weapon of war. Due to the early and weak rains of 2014 the subsequent year's harvest was poor. Hundreds of villagers arrived at Saint Peter and Paul's Church compound searching for food. Sister Angelina created a "work for food program." Those requesting food cleaned inside and outside the hospital complex, and I must say, the grounds never looked so good.

The fighting in April 2015 proved to be more intense than the earlier years. Most of the fighting took place, along the front, several hours away. My coworker in the pharmacy, Alfonde, lost his brother in one of the battles. When I went to give Alfonde my condolences he quietly responded saying it was the price of freedom. Yes, a costly and all too elusive freedom. In toto, Mother of Mercy received over 70 causalities during this period.

I was happy to receive some educational supplies from the U.S. my second year in Nuba. I brought them to a local school called Kumo Faulk. The school had been supported by Save the Children but along with all of the other NGOs up in the Nuba, it pulled out in June 2011 shortly after the current war broke out. In spite of being left with no support, Angelu, the headmaster, carried on. He has 300 primary school children attending class in the morning and an adult education class in the evening. The villagers pay him small quantities of food for his service. The children sit on wooden logs in makeshift classrooms with no chalkboard or easel and few, if any, exercise books. While at the school I recognized one of the students (Makki) who had been a long-term patient at the hospital. I remembered being surprised after giving Makki a notebook while in the hospital and seeing that he could write his letters and numbers. Most village children spend their days caring for siblings, tending the family's goats and cows and fetching water. Makki was one of the few fortunate ones being educated.

Angelu assembled the students to dance and sing for me in thanksgiving for the school supplies I had given them. They were extremely grateful despite the paucity of supplies I provided. I enjoyed meeting people like Angelu while in the Nuba Mountains. His devotion to duty in the face of abysmal odds reminded me that learning, inspiration and good example do not necessarily need material goods to be passed on.

Life is fragile in South Kordofan, which seems to foster this sense of devotion and duty to one another. One of the most striking characteristics of Nuba life for me was the Nuba's sense of community. The impetus to welcome and care for each other is strong especially when another is suffering. While passing through the pediatric ward one day I met a child name Tia. Tia's mother, Hawa, was in Yida when Tia fell into a fire while cooking dinner. Although his situation was dire, I was a bit shocked at the news of his death as I had visited Tia and his mother the day before. Severe burns, especially on children, are difficult to overcome in the hospital's primitive environment. Despite the staffs' best efforts, flies often penetrate the cages burn victims sleep under and lay eggs in their wounds or the skin grafts performed by the doctor get infected and fail. Moreover, the additional nutritional requirements the child needs for wound healing oftentimes just can't be met.

Although Tia was from a village far away, his mother did not mourn alone. The hospital has a small mortuary and crematorium. I searched for Hawa to give her some items for her long, lonely journey home and found her sitting with others outside the mortuary. Women staying at the hospital, unknown to Hawa, stopped by to grieve with her. Heroically and through a stream of tears, Hawa thanked the head nurse and told him how much she appreciated the care of her son. Tia's was a very sad case but I know, and am thankful, that he didn't die in obscurity. As my sister reminded me at the time of his death, God knows and loves each and every human being that has ever lived. No one, however poor, obscure or lost is concealed from His sight.

I befriended another courageous mother named Jerusalem after she stopped by the pharmacy asking

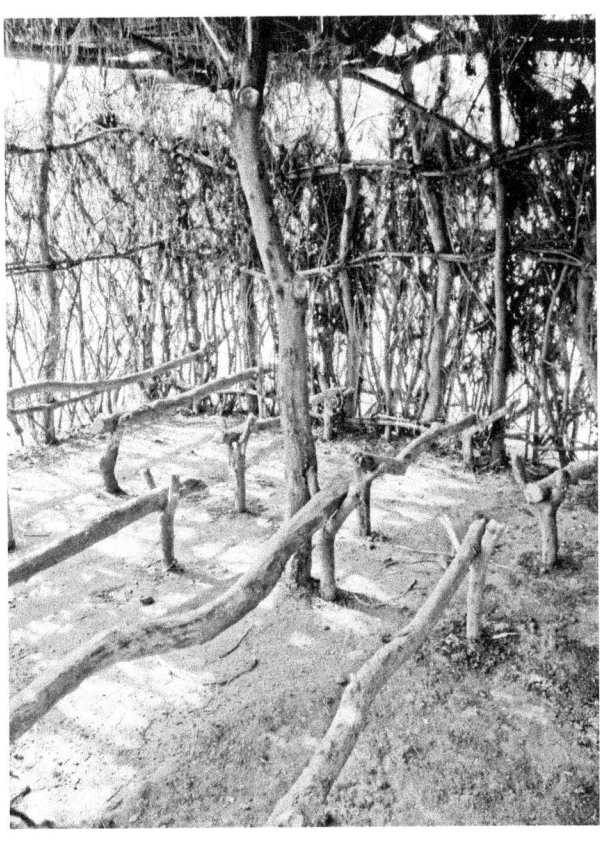

Typical Nuba "bush" classroom (photograph by Margaret Camarca).

if I had any diapers. I did, but only adult size, which she was grateful for. As with many women in the Nuba Mountains, Jerusalem is a determined mother of four doing her best to survive in dreadful circumstances. She is from a village close to the front lines. In 2012 Jerusalem left her village for the Yida refugee camp searching for a safer environment. She arrived during the rainy season. A generous stranger took her and the family in until she was able to build her own shelter. As Jerusalem was trying to establish her new life, her three-year-old daughter, Christina, fell sick. Christina stopped eating and started having loose, bloody, stools. Jerusalem repeatedly brought Christina to the camp's Medicins Sans Frontieres (MSF) hospital but her condition did not improve. Jerusalem then took Christina to a fee-for-service "private clinic" in the refugee camp where six injections were administered in Christina's buttocks.

Christina improved and was doing well for several months when her mother noticed some painful swellings over her buttocks and a foul smelling discharge emanating from her vagina. She brought Christina back to the MSF hospital where she was admitted for two weeks and then discharged. Unfortunately, while at home Christina's condition deteriorated. Not only did she begin to lose weight and have a vaginal discharge but she then also developed multiple fistulas (tunneled openings) which were oozing pus on her buttock. The MSF staff transferred Christina to another hospital located an hour's drive outside the camp. Physicians at this hospital operated on Christina immediately and discharged her seven days later. Within a month the symptoms reoccurred so Jerusalem took Christina back once again to the MSF hospital. A MSF physician gave Jerusalem the disheartening news that his hospital was not equipped to handle Christina's medical condition and offered to fly Christina to a hospital in Juba.

At her wits end, Jerusalem opted instead to take matters into her own hands. Jerusalem had attended the teacher's training college in Kauda years before, and was therefore aware of Mother of Mercy. She scraped together 200 Sudanese pounds ($40), packed up her children and headed to Gidel. Within days of arrival Dr. Tom performed surgery, giving Christina a colostomy. He also started her on TB medications along with other antibiotics and put her in the hospital's feeding program. Six months later, Christina was flourishing. She grew beyond the 50 percent weight range for her age and height, her vaginal discharge disappeared and her fistulas resolved. Jerusalem attributed Christina's medical issues to the shots she paid for years previously at the "private clinic" in the refugee camp. Dr. Tom was not so sure. Either way she stopped blaming herself and looked forward to restarting life in her family home.

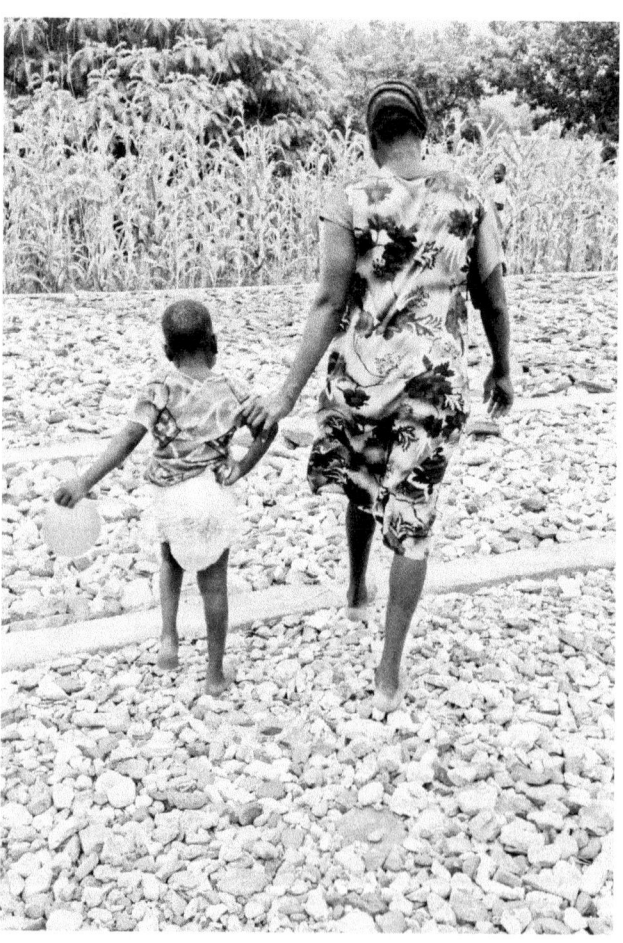

Jerusalem and Christina off to pick the hospital's maize shortly before Christina's discharge (photograph by Margaret Camarca).

For such an isolated place, I was always struck by how much went on in Gidel. In my second year there I attended an international nurses' day celebration, a primary school graduation ceremony, a wedding and a "radio station signal expansion" party. The hospital celebrated international nurses' day with a large parade through town, dancing, food and an awards ceremony. The hospital's administration awarded not only nurse training certificates but also "certificates of merit" to those who had been with the hospital since its 2008 opening. Starting the hospital was extremely difficult. The local community did not want it as they were convinced the employees were spies of the Khartoum government. A year had to pass before the workers convinced the villagers otherwise.

Certificates are extremely important in Nuba. The villagers have no documentation of their lives, no birth certificates, no wedding records, no photographs and very few have educational diplomas so any type of certificate is a highly coveted possession. The

International Nurses' Day merit awardees included nurses but also cooks, cleaners, maintenance men and plant waterers. I suspect it was the first time most of them had been publicly acknowledged for anything. I loved the quasi-standing ovation one of the older women, Laila, received when handed her certificate. Laila scrubbed the latrines, by far the most odious of jobs at the hospital.

The rains were stronger and more consistent my second year in Nuba and by August of 2015 our patients were already eating the maize and okra they had planted on the hospital compound. Throughout the year our diet consisted mainly of rice and beans with chicken or goat periodically served. I looked forward to the months ahead when cucumber, tomato, pumpkin and sweet potatoes would be available once again.

I administered many diclofenac pain shots during this period as the planting season is tough on the villagers' backs. There is scant equipment to assist with the farming so essentially all work is done by hand.

I spent my final months in Gidel cleaning, organizing and removing expired drugs from the pharmacy in preparation for our next big drug shipment. I also started training one of the pharmacy technicians to take over my role as the pharmacy store manager. It was a bittersweet time. My work was winding down and I suspected I might never return. Serving in the Nuba Mountains had been my great pleasure and I was grateful to be able to give back a small fraction of what I had received in life. The villagers taught me much about courage and trust in God. I was inspired by their strength, humility and tenaciousness. I clearly experienced how very little we actually need in life to get by. A case in point: I enjoyed learning that the local blacksmiths collect pieces of metal from exploded bombs and fashion them into hoes and other household items to sell in the market. Nuba resourcefulness is truly unrivaled.

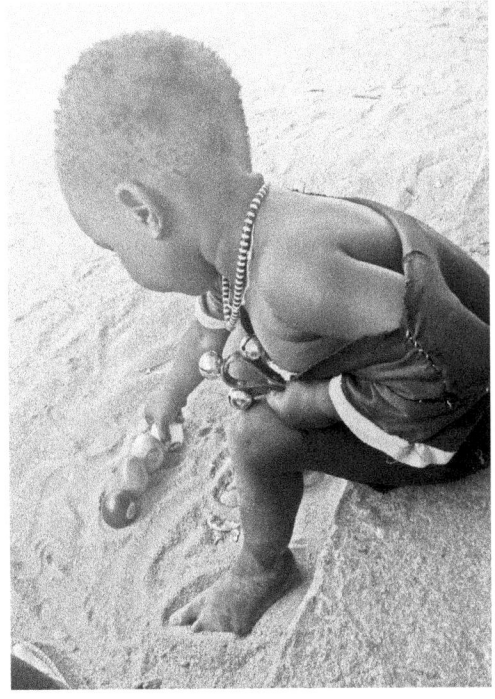

A pediatric patient playing with my shakers and completely oblivious to the war around him (photograph by Margaret Camarca).

Throughout my days in the Sudan I chronicled my life through a monthly "News from Nuba" letter that I sent to family and friends. I shared the daily joys, challenges, sorrows and successes I had experienced with the villagers. Some are curious as to what drove me to spend two years in the Nuba at Mother of Mercy. My commitment to stay was driven by a desire to live out God's will for my life. I believed my desire to work in Nuba was inspired by God who then ordered all things perfectly to allow me to undertake the journey. I felt even more confident about this resolution during my second year.

In my last letter to those back at home, I reminisced about the things I would miss most living in Nuba. I noted that I was going to miss many things, especially Nuba hospitality. Patients often walk for hours or days to get to the hospital. If they needed to rest along the way, the family could stop at any tukul and know the owner would happily accommodate them. Meals are a communal activity and villagers eat from one shared pot. Rare was the occasion, as I'd walk home from work, when I was not asked to join in a patient's meager dinner of maize, beans or sorghum. I still miss the constant "fadel, fadel" (i.e. "welcome, welcome") shouts from strangers.

I knew that I would also miss the children. Nuba children are given, at an early age, the responsibility of caring for their younger siblings. This creates strong familial bonds. I had lost count of how many American dollars I exchanged for Sudanese pounds so our workers could pay their siblings' (who are living abroad) school fees.

Nuba children are joyful and uninhibited even among strangers. Beyond natural curiosity, they have a great desire to help and to be part of your activity, if only to sit quietly and watch. I was going to miss the little helpers I had along the way.

And last but not least I was going to miss Nuba hope and joy. Despite living for decades under a brutal regime, the Nuba are quick to celebrate life. The villagers know they've been long abandoned by the international community, but are confident that God is with them. Although the distance between my life among the Nuba and my U.S. home is great, they will live eternally in my heart. Mother Teresa once said works of mercy are works of peace. Together, let us continue to sow these seeds of mercy throughout the world confident that they will eventually bear an enduring peace.

Note

1. Editor's Note: According to their website, Comboni Missionaries "are a world-wide group of more than 4,000 priests, brothers, sisters, and laity from diverse cultures who have dedicated our lives to following Christ's example and St. Daniel Comboni's missionary ideal of evangelization. St. Daniel Comboni was born in Italy in 1831. At an early age he felt a strong call to the priesthood and to take the Gospel to Africa. Today the Comboni Missionaries serve on five continents and 40 countries worldwide. [They] first worked in Europe and Africa, moving to North and South America in the 1930s, and expanding into Asia in the 1980s. In all the places 'we serve we share our deep faith in God through service to the poorest and most abandoned people throughout the world.'"

A Small Town Doctor Responds to the Needs of the Nuba

C. Louis Perrinjaquet, M.D.

Introduction

I'm a family physician but with a unique twist: nine months of the year I reside and work in Beckenridge, Colorado, ski town, and then for three months of the year I volunteer my services as a physician in remote underserved parts of the world. To date I've served in such places as Honduras, Langtang, Nepal, Darfur, Sudan, and the Nuba Mountains, Sudan.

By accident of birth, I was born healthy into a loving family. I grew up in a small farm town, Edgewood, Iowa ("The Town Between Two Counties"). My father ran the local feed and grain business.

My grandfather had immigrated from Switzerland when he was eight years old with his parents, an older brother and younger sister. His parents were too poor to feed the family so they literally "farmed out" the boys to work on the neighbor's farm for room and board until my great-grandfather had proven himself a hard enough worker to rent a farm himself. To rent a farm in those days meant that the landowner provided the land, while the renter provided all the labor. They split all expenses and profits 50/50.

Highway 13 ran through this little town of 800 people, mostly retired farmers or those working in the small businesses that supported farmers. Three churches and three taverns. It was a given in Edgewood that neighbors helped one another.

I can remember many times when someone's car broke down as they passed through town and they would end up at our kitchen table. If they didn't have the money to get back on the road, Dad would find some work around the feed mill or call one of the other local business men who could use a day laborer to help the fellow earn enough to cover the costs of getting his vehicle fixed. In the end, Dad would fill the guys car with gas to send him on his way.

My high school was tiny. There were 40 students in my class. I participated in a many activities: I was class president, student body president, and lead in the high school musical. I also participated in sports. All of this built my confidence leading me to believe that I could literally do whatever I wanted in life.

My high school science teacher, Mr. Johnson, suggested I consider becoming a doctor because I always liked a challenge, and it was a profession in which one would always continue to learn something new. I reasoned that if I could do anything why not pick a career where I could benefit others.

I always had a job at the family feed and grain business, "Perrinjaquet's Edgewood Feed Mill," which I knew I could fall back on if I didn't like medicine or didn't get accepted to medical school.

My parents are middle class folks, and fortunately, student loans were cheap in those days, so pitching in together we could afford my education. That, in turn, allowed me to pursue and enter a profession I love: medicine. It is a profession that pays me well enough that I have extra money with which to help others. By chance, I suppose, I have simple tastes that are easy to satisfy. It's rare that I feel a want for a material thing.

After my freshman year in college at Drake University in Des Moines, Iowa, I took a job as the night orderly in the Emergency Room at Mercy Hospital (also in Des Moines), and that solidified my commitment to medicine. I was fascinated by all the different ways people could get sick and by how much a doctor had to know in order to be able to help cure a person.

My major was Biology Pre-Med as an undergrad at Drake. My advisor, Dr. Bob Kodama, was a positive influence just by his encouragement and confidence in me. He actually re-typed my medical school application to get every letter typed in the middle of the blank, no erasures or white out to smudge the good impression he wanted me to give.

I can still remember my excitement when I got accepted to the University of Iowa Medical School. I shouted and danced and ran around my apartment like a crazy person. That excitement continued the next eight years of my education. It took me at least half way through my family practice residency to accept that I was no longer "becoming a doctor," but that I actually "was a doctor!" I chose family medicine as my specialty because, again, I wanted to learn more about everything. Family medicine also gave me a broader background as a generalist, which I figured would allow me to work in underserved areas of the United States and underdeveloped areas of the world where there were no specialists. So I was already thinking along those lines pretty early on.

Whether a patient has cancer or a cold, there is an emotional intimacy that a doctor and patient have very quickly. When someone is suffering and I have the knowledge to help relieve that suffering, we become friends quickly. Of course, there's a responsibility that comes with that knowledge, and also a huge reward. For me there's nothing more gratifying than the smile on the face of a grateful patient.

The Beginning: Volunteer Medical Missions

Over the years (beginning in the spring of 1999) I have made 20 trips to Honduras providing medical care and doing public health education in a dozen small communities along the Rio Patuca in the remote jungles near the Nicaraguan border. The people there, primarily subsistence farmers, are extremely poor. I have provided mass treatments for intestinal parasites and Vitamin A deficiencies. I have also provided safe delivery kits and prenatal vitamins for pregnant women, and birth control to those who did not want to get pregnant for a while. I also pulled a lot of really awful teeth, reliving a lot of pain. I got good at the anesthesia so people would line up for a free tooth extraction. I also provided toothbrushes, soap, bleach to sanitize drinking water and treated whatever acute problems a person happened to have the day we were passing through.

On one of my trips to Honduras, I read *The End of Poverty* by Jeffrey Sachs. Dr. Gerard Rudy, an American doctor working at a small mission in Ahuas, Honduras, recommend the book to me. At first I thought the idea of ending poverty was just fanciful dreaming. By the end of the book, though, I was convinced that poverty can be ended. We will always have relative wealth and poverty, but to end the extreme poverty of ⅙ of the global population—those living on less than $1.00. a day—is possible, and I believe it is the obligation of those of who us—the other ⅚ of the population—who were lucky enough to be born where we were into the families that we were, to work towards that and to see that it becomes a reality.

During the course of reading it, I learned of the extreme poverty of Sub-Saharan Africa, which actually made the subsistence farmers in the rainforests in Honduras appear well off. By sheer coincidence, at a social gathering not long after returning to Breckenridge, I ran into an acquaintance, Kendra, who had just returned from teaching epidemiology at the University of Khartoum. She knew the head of the medical school there, and a few emails later I was on my way to volunteer in medical clinics in the refugee camps in Darfur. That was in October 2007, over four years into the conflict in Darfur.

Darfur—October 2007

I was only in Darfur for a month, but I had never worked in a war zone before, never seen poverty on such a scale, never seen lines of people standing for hours all day long in the scorching sun waiting their turn to receive water, never been in an area where to get somewhere you had to weave your way through and around temporary brown grass shelters—as far as the eye could see—with blue or gray tarps serving for roofs. I was ready to come home when my month was up.

I had not really appreciated the gravity of the situation before I arrived. In fact, I had to go online for a little history: in 2003, two black African rebel movements in Darfur—the Sudan Liberation Army (SLA) and the Justice and Equality Movement (JEM)—took up arms against the Government of Sudan (GoS), complaining of disenfranchisement and marginalization, including the failure of the GoS to protect them, most of whom were farmers and thus sedentary people, from attacks by Arab nomads. Initially, the GoS simply ignored the complaints of the black Africans but when the rebel groups began attacking government facilities, the government carried out a scorched earth policy against the black Africans. Ultimately Sudanese forces and Janjaweed militia attacked hundreds of villages throughout Darfur. Over 400 villages were completely destroyed and millions of civilians were forced to flee their homes and estimated 300,000 to 400,000 Black Africans were killed.

I brought $12,000 worth of a new broad-spectrum antibiotic called Levaquin. Drug companies were more generous in those days, and through a local pharmaceutical representative I was able to get this donated by Janssen Pharmaceuticals, Inc. At $10 a pill or $100 for an IV dose this much medication actually fit in one duffle bag.

I was working with the Sudan Islamic Medical Association (SIMA)—in an IDP (internally displaced persons) camp. SIMA arranged for me to fly directly from Khartoum to a dirt landing strip in El Geneina in Western Darfur, near the border with Chad.

There were seven IDP camps in the area with a total of about 100,000 people who had fled from their homes as a result of the attacks by the Government of Sudan troops and the Janjaweed. The medical efforts were headed up by approximately 40 to 50 Sudanese doctors who variously worked under the auspices of ten to fifteen nongovernmental organizations (NGOs), such as Médecins Sans Frontières (Doctors Without Borders) from France, Save the Children, The International Red Cross/Red Crescent, and The International Rescue Committee.

While I was the only foreigner working with SIMA, most of the staff of the other NGOs were Arab, so it was very isolating being the only native English speaker.

The little hospital to which I was assigned was able to do amazing things with incredibly few resources. No electricity much of the time so no x-ray, oxygen, or lights. A shortage of medicine, bandages, sutures, and iodine to clean wounds was a regular occurrence. Most of the medical facilities consisted of grass mats for walls, a sand floor and a big blue tarp from the United Nations for a roof. That said, despite the primitive conditions, the care provided by both the Sudanese doctors and volunteers was quite good.

With only sand between the buildings, it was next to impossible to even roll a wheelchair or gurney outside the medical facilities. Because of that, patients were carried in an old fashioned canvas stretcher by two to four people. Inoculations were given without alcohol; instead, one simply rubbed the skin with a dry bit of cotton and gave the shot.

The clinic I spent the most time in had a lab technician equipped with a microscope to do blood slides for malaria and stool investigations for intestinal parasites. Having completed a Diploma in Tropical Medicine and Hygiene at the University of London and a Masters in Public Health from Harvard I had many more years of formal training than the young Sudanese doctors there, who were half my age. But I'd never worked in such a resource poor environment as this; in fact, I never really imagined the scale of what I was seeing there. Luckily the younger doctors were as eager to learn as I was, so together we taught each other a lot and did the best we could.

In the hospital there were wounded soldiers and civilians who were direct casualties of the ongoing war, but in reality everyone was an indirect casualty of war having been forced off their land, having witnessed or survived themselves beatings, rape, the trauma of seeing their families killed. We often found ourselves talking about the psychological stress that everyone, including the volunteers, was under and how essentially no programs were available to help people cope with their situation.

One night I watched a surgery being conducted under a single bare light bulb. Period! No EKG or oxygen monitors. The anesthetist didn't even have a stethoscope. I witnessed a C-section conducted with only the sunlight that seeped in through the window of the operating room.

I also spent some time at the Therapeutic Feeding Center. It had actually been built by Save the Children many years before the outbreak of the Darfur crisis, in response to previous food shortages before the conflict in Darfur.

The mothers themselves were malnourished and could provide no breast milk. On arrival the more severe patients were mere skeletons draped with loose brown skin that once covered muscle and fat. Too weak to even drink from a bottle, a feeding tube had to be inserted in their nose and on down to their stomachs in order to give precision formulas to save their lives.

At that time, the medical facilities were not overcrowded and had enough high calorie formulas to save all but the most severe cases, the latter of whom also suffered from pneumonia, typhoid, malaria or another infectious disease as a result of their weakened immune systems.

Understandably, it always lifted my spirits to see these beautiful tiny bodies getting stronger with the dedication of local nurses and the hope and love of their mothers who stayed with their children the entire time in order to give the required eight feedings per day.

The day after I arrived in Darfur, as I was shuffling through the sand streets of the local market looking at the bright red and green watermelons, colorful dresses of the girls and women, and beautiful dark almost blue-black faces, I was almost hit by a truck load of young men overflowing with large weapons and bandoliers of bullets. As I caught the eye of one of the men in the back of the truck, he seemed as startled to see me (a random white guy) as I was them.

The young Arab doctor, Mohammed, who had been assigned as my translator, explained to me that the men in the truck were from Chad and were hiding in Sudan, from which they planned attacks against their government. To my eye, they looked pretty much like the truckloads of Sudanese rebels who were fighting against their own government in Khartoum.

Mohammed went on to say, "Three hundred U.S. dollars buy you very, very nice machines guns which is available everywhere in the markets, and bullets is very cheaper.... It is common here that for not many money you can buy some guns, hire some guys, call you self some kind of army, kills a few peoples or just shoot some buildings and the government will have to negotiate with you and give you a government job."

With the exception of a woman's arm being amputated after she was bitten by a camel and had contracted gangrene, the surgical schedule was filled with cleaning damaged flesh away from gun shot wounds. I was told there was no active organized fighting going on in that particular area at the time, but there were guns everywhere—and they tended to go off.

Not being accustomed to hearing machinegun fire in the night, the first night I heard the staccato bursts I sat upright in bed and listened for clues as to what to do. The electricity and thus the fan had gone off at 9 p.m. It was stiflingly hot in our cement block guesthouse. The dry dusty air burned my nose. I never realized sand had a smell. The other doctor sharing my room snored straight threw the gunshots. I heard no shouting or running, so figured I was not in imminent danger and eventually dozed back off.

I never really got used to the sound of gunfire in spite of hearing it randomly through the night. Whether the bullets were aimed specifically at someone or just shot in the air out of boredom, they had to come down somewhere. (And, in fact, daytime hospital ward rounds revealed that the bullets did, indeed, find flesh.) I'm sure the refugees who had lost family and been driven from their homes by armed men were terrified by the sounds.

I spent most of my days helping out at in the IDP camps. The World Food Program (WFP) provided a minimal weekly ration of local grain, cooking oil and salt. The people's days were spent lining up for water, searching for firewood, cooking, caring for their children, planting, and/or looking for any work to help them and their families survive. The IDP's of West Darfur had been in El Geneina since the conflict began in 2004.

There were lots of weapons available in the camp, people from many different tribes all crowded together, no real security to speak of—no guards or peace keeping troops and often there were rumors of impending fighting between rival groups, so some days it just wasn't safe to enter the IDP camps. On one such day I met Dr. Khalid, a young man from the Nuba Mountains. As I was to learn, the Nuba is one of the most isolated areas in Africa, sandwiched between the world's largest desert, the Sahara and the world's largest swamp, the Sudd.

Having been educated by Christian missionaries, Khalid spoke English much better than my Arab translator. He so loved his beautiful homeland he made me promise that someday I would travel there to help his people.

At that particular point in time, the Nuba Mountains were actually enjoying a period of relative peace (from 2005 to June 2011). The Nuba were building schools, were cultivating again, and the there was even talk of a hospital being opened somewhere near Kauda in 2008. Khalid said he was the first person to be trained as a doctor from his area and knew how much work there was to do. As soon as he could complete a surgical internship in Khartoum he would be returning home.

In another coincidence a few years later, I just happened to approach a member of my church, Jim Gully, who I knew traveled extensively as he carried out development work, and asked him if he'd ever heard of the Nuba Mountains. He said that while working in Haiti he met a guy doing a safe water project who had told him about the Nuba Water Project. It just so happened that that fellow, Steve Riley, lived just down the mountain from me, in Denver. Not only that, but he still had contacts in Sudan. Long story short, before long I was on a plane to Juba.

From this point forward, I am going to take the liberty of quoting extensively from the diaries I kept during my several trips/missions to the Nuba Mountains. In doing so, I think the reader will glean a more "you are there"-like experience than if I attempted to recount what I witnessed, experienced, thought, and felt on each of the trips/missions.

At the same time, it should be understood I did not write these entries with the intent of publishing them, and thus I apologize for the "style" (i.e., truncated sentences, fragments, streams of consciousness, etc.).

Finally, some of these stories are graphic and even hard for me to write about, but I feel obligated to do so as a witness to what the Nuba people are living through. And I do so in the hope that somehow the stories will help to draw attention to the plight of the Nuba people and that that will result in help being extended to them. (I should note that I have submitted some of the following stories to a group of lawyers filing a case with the African Commission on Human and People's rights against the president of Sudan, Omar al-Bashir.)

Journal Entries from October 2011: Nuba Mountains, Sudan

Oct. 8—Juba. ... It's difficult to arrange a flight from Juba [South Sudan] into the Nuba Mountains because the Sudanese Armed Forces (SAF) keep finding out about flights and bombing the landing strip as the plane tries to land.

Oct. 9—We were able to fly to Kauda and arrange the hour-long ride in a Land Cruiser ride across the rough and arid terrain—down dirt roads and across dry riverbeds—to Mother of Mercy Hospital in Gidel.

Upon our arrival, I was greeted by Dr. Tom Catena, the director of Mother of Mercy and the only surgeon there. In fact, he is the only surgeon in the entire state of South Kordofan.

Dr. Tom, as everyone refers to him, gave me a tour of the hospital. Mother of Mercy was originally established back in 2008, during a time of peace.

The hospital was built to handle 200 patients. Tellingly, he now has over 400 patients. And astoundingly, he supervises the care of all of them.

I must say, I was not prepared for what I saw. Horrible! The wounds of civilians who have been hit by bomb fragments from the bombs dropped by Antonovs.

The Antonov is an Eastern European cargo plane used to fly thousands of feet above civilian areas. They are not precise military weapons. These are terrorist weapons. The Nuba try to reassure me saying, "The bombs hardly ever hit the people." Most of the people the bomb fragments do hit die, either on impact or after unimaginable suffering of having a limb blown off or their internal organs exposed with no medical care or medicine to ease their pain. I saw the "lucky ones" who survived the attacks and transported to this hospital. The wounds are horrific!

Oct. 10—At least one child dies of malnutrition every day, osteomyelitis (chronic draining infection of exposed bone)...

Oct. 12—Heard my 1st Antonov. Dr. Tom Catena pointed it out over sounds of fans, anesthesia machine, oxygen concentrator & people talking. "You hear that low rumbling sound?" Then back to surgery...

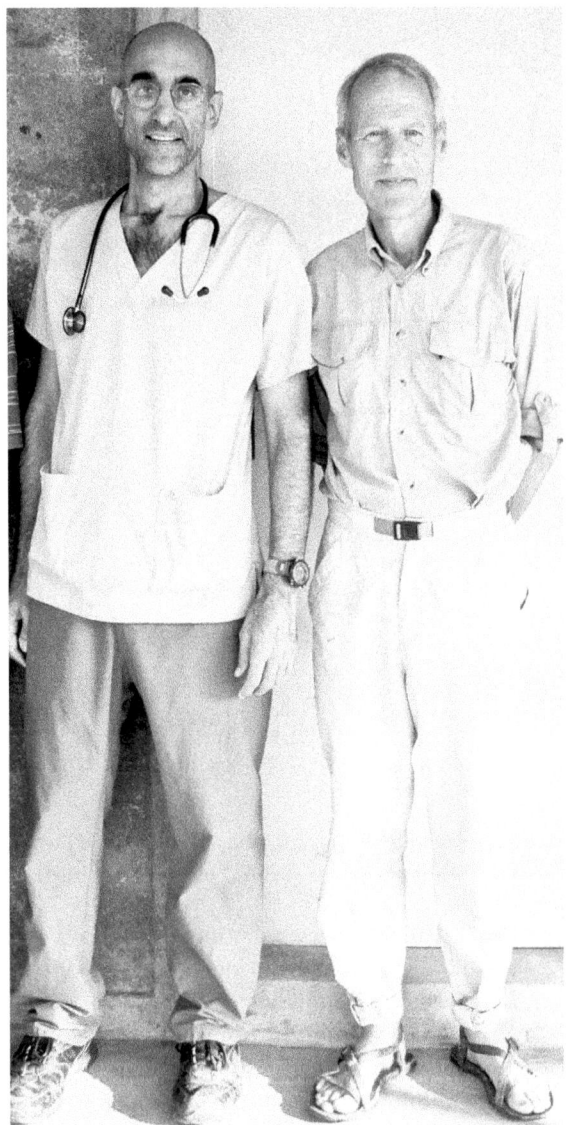

October 2011. Dr. Catena (left) and Dr. Perrinjaquet at the door of Dr. Catena's house (Dr. C. Louis Perrinjaquet).

Sister Mary Carmen from Mexico remembers going to meet an airplane [in Kauda last summer] and running from the airstrip and diving to the ground as bombs landed behind her; doing that back to back, three times, caring for another sister who was crying because she couldn't run as she was older with bad knees, lying on the ground praying, "God help us." They both dove to the ground as the bombs from the Antonov landed around them, got up and tried to run from the airship again, as the Antonov circled back three times. The memories are so terrifying she trembles when she hears the Antonovs.

Many children dying of malaria because of the lack of medicine in the tiny and extremely rudimentary clinics that dot the Nuba region. Added to that, al-Bashir had

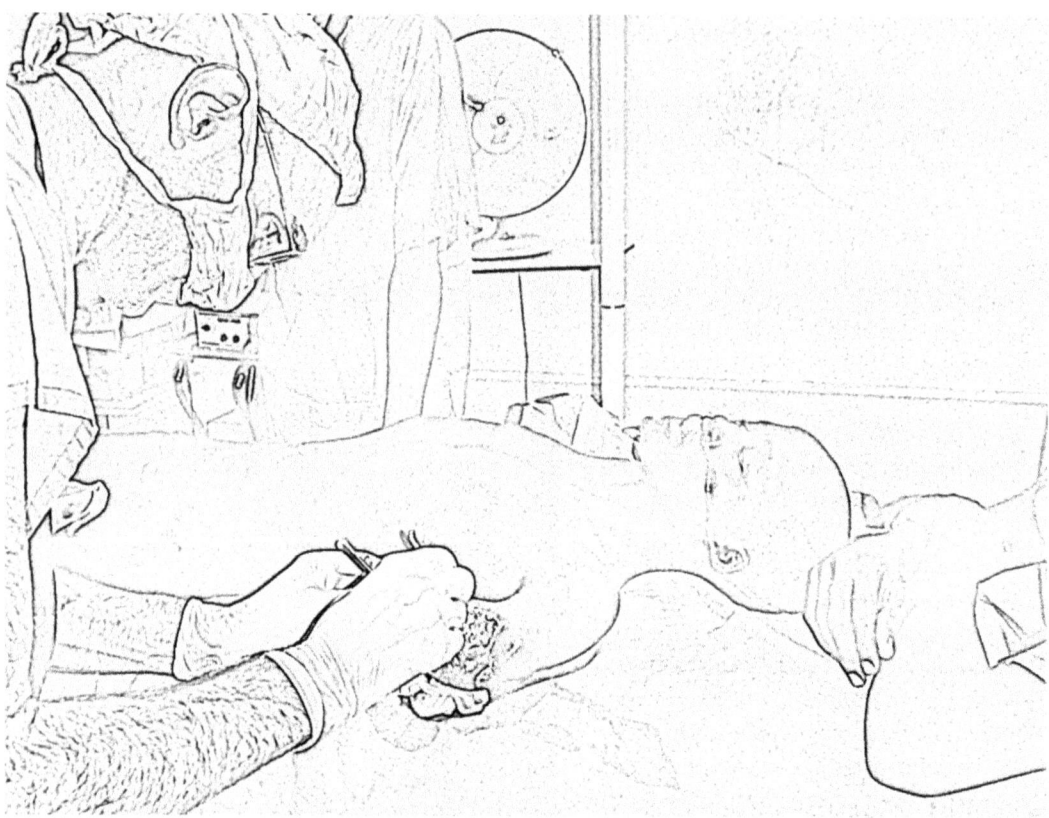

May 15, 2014. A "drawing" produced from a photograph of Dr. Tom Catena attending a young man whose arm was severed by a mortar shell (Dr. C. Louis Perrinjaquet).

banned all international humanitarian aid organizations (including the UN) from entering the region to deliver food and medicine to those in dire need—both a war tactic and a war crime.

Placed a traction pin through a young man's tibia for femur fracture when an Antonov bomb blew off his left buttock. Eight of us worked to construct a two-part mattress to allow access to dress the wound. The lower part of the bed supported his legs and the upper part supported his torso. What was left of his buttock hung open in the gap so it could heal without pressure being applied to the area. Now he has to lie on his back in traction and the nurses have to get underneath him to clean and dress the massive wound down to his pelvis, whole left buttock gone.

Oct. 17—Two children die during morning rounds today. Less than 1-year-old child in feeding program for the past week, fever, not doing well, gave few agonal breaths (agonal breaths of a person in agony are slow dying gasps) as we entered ward, his mother sobbing and holding scarf over her face as the father rocked the baby.

As soon as I left this part of the children's ward, a nurse summoned me to help adjust the dose of IV Quinine for a six-year-old boy who had been admitted in a coma the night before with cerebral malaria. He had a seizure as we approached his bed. There was little to do but wait and see if the medicine would work or not. Later that morning I knew he had died with I heard the wailing of a crowd of women gathered outside the main walls of the hospital and then noticed that the boy's bed was now empty.

Oct. 20—Togor (3½ hour drive north of Kauda) Am at the Save the Children clinic here. Fighting taking place in Dalami, just another hour north of here. People are fleeing to the south, seeking shelter in caves along the way.

Clinic Administrator, Abass: "No medicine. No gauze. Solar fridge needs battery, kerosene fridge not working, but there are no vaccines, so it doesn't really matter." Staff working free since May—13 staff including 2 guards and 2 cleaners.

Abass is monitoring children under five for starvation. Advising people from outside this area to travel to refuge camps in South Sudan—to Bentiu—many days or weeks walking.

50 yards away from the clinic I am shown bomb craters where shrapnel injured two sisters, one lost her right hand, a crude bandage covers the stump of her mid-forearm, the other has a flesh wound to her side.

12:30 Sabat (a small community we visited while driving south back towards Kauda from Togor). Am at a Nuba Community Clinic. Nice set of buildings, well maintained, but there are no patients because there's no medicine. Has not had supplies—except few packets of ORS (oral rehydration salts)—for months. Potential patients enter but leave empty-handed, so to speak. Many come seeking guidance on where they should go to obtain care, which everyone seems to already know is way too far away if one is badly injured or really sick.

Am spending the night in Lamba (just south of Sabat), at my guide's family's compound in which there were several tukuls made, of mud and grass, all in a circle and surrounded by a fence of thorn bushes to keep the goats inside and safe for the night.

We've heard Antonovs twice today. They were far off, but still people ran for the caves.

Jibril, from the village of Omhitan, relates the following to me: "I walked nine hours with two women and thirteen children here to Lamba. We heard the SAF [Sudanese Armed Forces] was planning to another attack on our village, which only has civilians, no SPLA. For many days Antonovs dropped six to seven bombs at a time. Two people were injured, everyone was frightened. Most fled, leaving behind all their crops, cows, goats, all their wealth to run with their families in hopes of finding a safer place. Those who chose to stay are hiding in the rocks, caves, forests."

As I spoke to Jibril, we looked up and saw an Antonov silently passing high overhead to the west heading south.

A second Antonov, this one louder, close enough to photograph with my little point and shoot jungle camera but not close enough to prod everyone to run for a hole. But we discuss where to go if and when the planes circle back if they are closer.

I am told that SAF soldiers could literally run from where they're located to where we are in two hours. The locals hope rumors that the SPLA are in the mountains will keep the SAF away from this area.

Oct. 22—Kauda. Met with the Media Coordinator of The Nuba Relief, Rehabilitation and Development Organization (NRRDO) Internet Manager and Media Coordinator. He tells me to "expect hunger." People have not been able to cultivate, especially those on the "far farms," due to the bombing and ground fighting. He said that whenever groups of civilians begin migrating south to get away from the fighting, the Antonovs seem to follow them in order to bomb them, sending the people fleeing up into the mountains and caves again. He also spoke about how the GoS has established a blockade of medicines and supplies from reaching the Nuba. The GoS won't even allow the UN into the Nuba for the purpose of providing medical supplies.

Now, at the end of the rainy season, lots of cases of malaria and no medicine in the tiny clinics that dot the region. Mother of Mercy was adequately stocked for those patients lucky enough to still be breathing upon reaching Gidel.

Already 30–50 families daily are arriving in Kauda in search of food. Immediately, they head to NRRDO (the Nuba Relief, Rehabilitation and Development Organization), which had none. There are large fields in central Nuba Mountains that normally grow enough for all Nuba area and even export to Khartoum, but that large area is not able to be cultivated now due to the constant bombings.

Oct. 23—Kurchi (midway between Kauda and the Yida Refugee Camp in South Sudan). Everyone is friendly, cheerful but also alert to sounds of Antonovs in the distance. As soon as we arrived the people inside the NRRDO compound here showed us where the holes we are to run to if we hear planes.

I am filled in by a local about what has transpired here over the past six months or so. "First attack in July. Fifteen killed, 56 injured here in Kurchi." Continuing, with sadness in his voice, he says, "My father died of hunger." This was the first time I had someone tell me a member of their family had perished from hunger [actually starvation]. Unfortunately, it was not the last time.

Oct. 24—Kurchi Clinic. Eight staff members, no medicine.

A nurse: "We may see 40–90 people per day, some of them walking up to three hours to reach here. Before the war it was only 45 minutes travel by car to Kadugli. Now it's totally cut off [the SAF controls Kadugli]. We have instruments to suture wounds and dressings. Psychological effects rarely draw patients here [the clinic], but obviously it has its effect. We've also seen more skin problems since the outbreak of war [June 2011] due to poor hygiene, running and living in caves, sleeping on the ground and dealing with ticks and scabies, among other things. We've had more first trimester miscarriages, too; and we're dealing with malnutrition in the IDP's [internally displaced persons]. It's said that there are about 40,000 IDP's in this [the Kurchi] area—some in camps, many dispersed up into the mountains and caves. We're seeing watery bloody diarrhea, mainly from poor water and sanitation and crowding. We've also had an increase in pneumonia and meningitis." The staff is committed to continuing to providing services even though they are not being paid. They said they would hang on as long as they possibly could. Malaria medicine, they told me, is a priority.

Telabon Clinic (about an hour's drive north from Kurchi). The staff here told me they are seeing up to 250 patients per day. They are seeing a lot of malaria cases, especially among the young children. The clinic, though, has no meds for malaria. One of the staff members told me that the prospective patients are "footing for three hours to get here and go back with zero." Staff is sacrificing to serve people, meaning they are not working for money.

Limon Clinic. After days of driving over dirt paths and across dry river beds, the terrain all looks the same to me. As we drive toward Kurchi from Talabon we stop at a clinic near the village of Limon. They are seeing about 75 patients per day. Most are suffering from malaria. The clinic only has enough quinine to last one or two more days.

Oct. 25—Back in Gidel [location of Mother of Mercy]. 8:00 a.m. Finished with rounds, then assisted Tom with a C-section to remove the rotten, decayed baby three weeks after its mother's uterus had ruptured during labor. Opened abdomen and was hit with a foul gas like opening a tomb. The baby's skull came out in pieces. The mother had lost a lot of blood and was septic (badly infected), but with the surgery, IV antibiotics and good nursing care, she survived.

I donate blood for a fifteen-year-old woman with a two-week old ankle injury, which had been "blown out from shrapnel off a bomb dropped by an Antonov." We'll amputate tomorrow.

Personnel from the tiny health clinics that dot the Nuba are coming here to Gidel in search of supplies. All are facing crises and potentially disastrous situations as a result of the warfare. Not a word of exaggeration there.

2:30 p.m. Wow—I just gave the stuttering nurse tooth puller named Monday all my dental instruments, some I've had for ten years. Monday said he agrees to stay and work at this hospital and use these tools at least 15 years—"until he retires."

4:45 p.m. Three pickup trucks with wounded SPLA soldiers just arrived. We'd just finished amputating a guy's right leg below the knee after giving him spinal anesthesia. He couldn't feel pain but was awake and talking about home over the sounds of our sawing through his tibia, which shook the whole table. We had earlier amputated a man's right arm above the elbow, as his forearm had been blown apart and packed with dirt and burnt flesh.

Initially we did an exploratory laparotomy because the shrapnel that had entered the SPLA soldier's abdomen had torn a hole in it the size of my thumb. Luckily, Tom only found small fragments and no bowel perforation.

Besides the shrapnel wounds to his abdomen, he had several rib fractures that resulted in an unstable section of chest wall called a flail chest. A flail chest flails in and out as the patient tries to breathe.

He also had an open wound that collapsed his lung, which allowed air to suck in and out of the wound with every breath. Tom inserted a plastic tube the size of his finger in between two upper ribs that were not broken and sewed the wound closed. He then attached the tube to a large jug of water on the floor next to the patient's bed that served as a one way valve bubbling air out of the man's chest when he exhaled but not allowing air to go back in the chest when he inhaled, slowly reinflating his collapsed lung.

The patient's still a high mortality risk from infection. Now we can just hope for the best.

Tom's pretty quiet, sick himself with a bad cold, hoping it isn't another attack of malaria.

Oct. 26—No bombs or bombers today. Donated blood again, something concrete I can do. I feel fine even giving a 2nd unit in eleven days.

Removed five fingers from four peoples hands today. Two patients had gun shot wounds, another patient was an old woman with leprosy, and the last a young woman with gangrene from traditional treatment of stuffing a wound with leaves.

As I was leaving for dinner with several sisters [nuns who serve as nurses at Mother of Mercy,] a SAF soldier from yesterday's battle was picked up on the battlefield and brought here by SPLA. He had a gunshot wound that entered and exited his thigh, shattering his femur. Not bleeding, though, and a good pulse. Does have a fever—probably from malaria, though, and not the wound. Tom plans to put in a traction pin tomorrow.

Lots of people in courtyard shouting about this enemy soldier, but SPLA who brought him asked he be treated well—not like the brutal SAF treatment of their prisoners or so I understand.

Oct. 29—Yesterday we amputated the right leg of the previously mentioned fifteen-year-old girl. We had to amputate it above the knee. Shrapnel from an Antonov's bomb had struck her ankle. The second unit of blood I donated the other day was running in her arm as I filed smooth the freshly sawed end of her thighbone. She felt no pain. The spinal anesthetic worked well for that, but she was wide awake and we made eye contact as I looked over the surgical drape to make sure she was OK. Experiencing both sorrow and relief.

After the rounded stump was cleanly wrapped and the surgical drape lowered she raised her head to see her future. Her lifeless leg was lying on the operating room floor. It took all I had not to project my sadness onto her own emotions.

I am overwhelmed by the injustice suffered by these innocent people, "The enemies of Omar al-Bashir" as Dr. Tom refers to his patients who have suffered such senseless violence.

October 2012: Yida Refugee Camp, The Republic of South Sudan

In October of 2012 I returned to the region during to work at Samaritan Purse's therapeutic feeding center at the refugee camp in Yida, which is just south of the border from the contested area of South Kordofan, Sudan. There are somewhere in the order of 65,000 refugees here [Yida], who have fled fighting and famine in the Nuba Mountains. The refugees are mostly women and children who walked for days to reach here, no telling what they had to eat, if anything. In certain cases, it may have been leaves, grasses and insects. Most of the men stayed behind to tend what few animals they have and/or to begin tending their crops as the rainy season subsides. (While in the region, I managed to take a short break and deliver a couple of boxes of my mother's chocolate chip cookies to Dr. Tom up in Gidel. Since the main focus of my trip was to work at the therapeutic feeding center in Yida, I returned there pretty quickly.)

Our initial system of screening for malnutrition is a simple measurement called the MUAC (the Mid-Upper Arm Circumference). MUAC is the circumference of the left upper arm, measured at the mid-point between the tip of the shoulder and the tip of the elbow. Especially in children ages 1–5, MUAC is useful for the assessment of nutritional status because this part of the body is less effected by accumulated fluids/edema that may accumulate in the abdomen, face or ankle from protein deficiency that often accompanies total calorie/energy deficiency.

We classify children as normal, mild, moderate, or severe malnutrition and treat accordingly with specialized formulas and protocols, with feedings every three hours. With severe malnutrition we treat with antibiotics because their bodies may be too weak to have a fever or show signs of infection the way a normally nourished person would.

Weight for age or height/weight rations were also helpful to classify and customize treatment plans and improve survival.

The last two weeks I was at Yida I took care of a single teenage mom, Najat. She and her 4-year-old son, Mohammed had walked for days to escape famine in the Nuba Mountains and both had severe acute malnutrition. Najat weighed 28 kilograms (61.6 pounds) and her son, Mohammed, weighed 10 Kg (22 pounds) when they arrived weak and despondent. Mohammed's face and ankles were swollen from his body's inability to produce the proteins needed to hold fluid in his blood vessels, so he needed to get stronger and actually lose this extra "water weight" before he could start gaining "lean body mass." His light colored brittle hair was evidence of chronic malnutrition for the months before he arrived in Yida.

Tia was my favorite little guy. He was two years old and weighed an unbelievable 9½ pounds when he arrived—less that a bag of sugar! Some babies weigh that much when they are born in the United States. He couldn't hold up his own head when, Caylin, one of the aid workers spotted him.

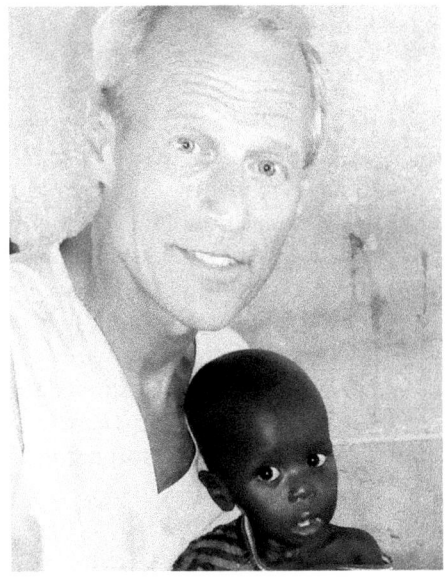

October 2012. Dr. Perrinjaquet working at a Therapeutic Feeding Center, Yida Refugee Camp, South Sudan, with his favorite patient, a two-year-old survivor of severe acute malnutrition (Dr. C. Louis Perrinjaquet).

He was hanging limp in his mother's arms as she stood in line at the food distribution and she brought him to the feeding center. It took a week of *attention to every detail of his care* before I was confident he would live. In seven days his weight increased to about twelve pounds. He could reach out to feed himself and smile and melt my heart.

Soon he'd be able to go "home"—at least leave the center with his mother to live with his extended family here in the camp and someday return to his real home in the Nuba Mountains.

Watching their recovery was dramatic. They came to life like putting water on wilted flowers. They became alert, interactive, and even playful. In two weeks, after the initial stabilization & resuscitation phases, Mohammed had increased his weight by 10 percent and his mother, Najat, had gained 6.2 kg (13.6 pounds) or 22 percent of her admission weight. That would be like me starting at 154 pounds and gaining 34 pounds in 14 days.

They were not yet at their target weights when they left the inpatient program to return to their extended family in the camp, but will return weekly for supplemental food rations of "Plumpy Nut"[1] until they have.

Most of the children who made it alive to our therapeutic feeding center survived. We didn't have the level of care in our center that was available at the MSF Hospital (also in Yida), so if we had a child who was not responding to treatment as expected we carried them to MSF.

Most mothers told stories of daughters and sons who did not live to adulthood, most dying under the age 5 of one of the "big three": diarrhea, pneumonia, or malaria. Lack of enough food, clean water and hygiene weakens a person's immune system, and thus they end up dying of something other than starvation—quite similar to a person with HIV/AIDS, who doesn't usually die directly from the virus, but dies from an overwhelming infection.

Some also told of the weaker members of their families, the very young or very old, who just collapsed and died during their journey to Yida.

Even if Khartoum stops bombing the Nuba Mountains, they are still guilty of preventing humanitarian aid organizations such as the United Nations and World Food Program access to the region. Contingent on how this all plays out, this could result in another case of what scholars have referred to as "genocide by attrition." (See Samuel Totten's book, *Genocide by Attrition: Nuba Mountains, Sudan*. Second Edition [New Brunswick, NJ: Transaction Publishers, 2015].)

This is the first time I've worked in a disaster area of this scale; that is, where large, well organized and well-funded organizations are needed in order to effectively address the situation, but are no where to be seen. As for Samaritan's Purse, it is Christian organization that has been working in the Nuba Mountains for decades.

November 14, 2012: Washington, D.C.

I'm on my way home after working for five weeks at a refugee camp in Yida, South Sudan. I'm writing from a friends yacht on the Potomac River within walking distance of the White House.

It's hard to reconcile the contrasts of starving women and children escaping war and famine in their homeland and the excesses of materialism with the obesity in my homeland. And by "starving," I don't mean the way the word is used in the developed world when dinner isn't ready on time. I mean the relentless gnawing stomach cramps that many Nuba women, children and men feel all day, every day that they try to calm by eating boiled grass and leaves or bugs that eventually leads to worsening degrees of nutritional deficiencies, inadequate protein, insufficient total calories/energy a body needs to function, loss of electrolytes, fluids, micronutrients, organ failure and death.

May 2, 2014: Mother of Mercy Hospital, Gidel, South Kordofan, Nuba Mountains, Sudan

Yesterday morning I had just been told, "Land Cruiser needs fixed again. No trip to the outreach clinic today." As I was walking back to the outpatient department at Mother of Mercy to help out, I suddenly heard a jet. Fearful, I glanced up. Within seconds it was on top of us. Chaos ensued: people screaming and running for at least some type of cover.

I remembered Dr. Tom's instructions—"Don't run! Just get down!" I dove to the ground and covered my head as a loud explosion came from the south, the area of TB/Leprosy Village. Huge gusts of wind, sand, dust exploded around us.

I took a quick glance about. People running in every direction, no longer screaming—or maybe I just couldn't hear yet.

I noticed the hospital's pharmacist running with purpose so I jumped up and started in her direction. She tripped over a wire fence she didn't seem to see, and tumbled into an overfull foxhole. I turned and saw Mother of Mercy's Director of Emergency Response

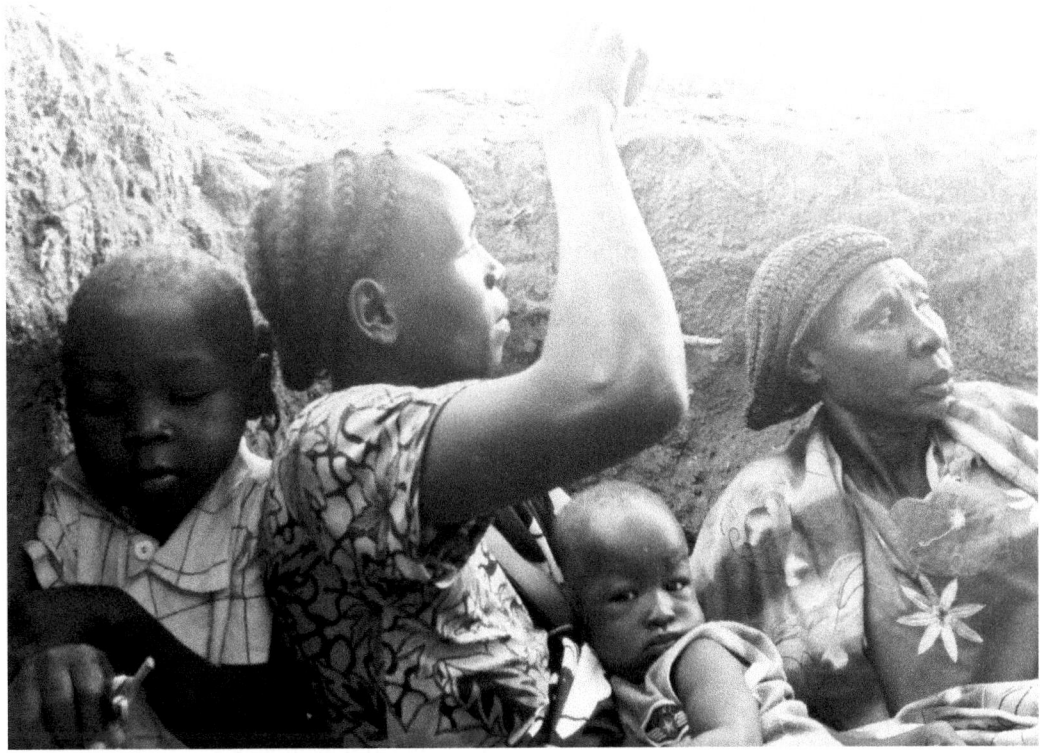

A family in a foxhole during an aerial attack by the Government of Sudan (Dr. C. Louis Perrinjaquet).

also moving with purpose. Thinking that she seemed to be the person to follow, I sprinted behind her a couple 100 yards through the gate to the doctors' compound and followed her into a foxhole—a hole 6 × 6 ft. square, 3 ft. deep.

And then we waited. Not long, though, as the jet, LOUD, flew by, fast right over us. Moments later, very near us, there was an even louder explosion.

Then, more waiting. Five minutes, ten minutes. Warily, we crawled out of the hole. Gotta head to the hospital to help with any casualties.

I saw Dr. Tom enter the children's ward. Then, NOT OVER! No time to even think. Jet upon us, just like that. I jumped into the nearest foxhole, body against body with women & children. One mass of quivering humanity.

Moments later another explosion, again close enough to shake the ground. Didn't hit the hospital though.

No one moves. Children are absolutely silent. Our collective hearts pounding, my head on the scarf of the woman behind me, my left elbow under the head of the woman in front of me, a custom fit puzzle of necessity.

We all knew the jet would be circling back. A few rapid breaths and an eternity later, here it comes. It's suddenly upon us and then closer and closer, roaring.

I would die in an instant if we were struck ... or survive. There was nothing more to do. I accepted that reality and felt a great calm. The noise was deafening ... then just as quickly it faded.

The rest of yesterday was spent inspecting the damage and cleaning up. The second missile struck 30 yards behind our small cinder block doctors' quarters. The ground was a thick mat of shredded leaves, which had been ripped off the now bare branches of the nearby tree. The back fence was destroyed. Where the fence had been was now a 6 foot across 1 foot deep crater. Metal shards of shrapnel had the force to sheer 8-inch limbs off trees. Incredibly, the only loss of life was one goat when the same jet attacked the next village. Not a single significant physical human injury. Psychologically however everyone to some degree or another is shaken. The rest of the day was quiet. Unless paralyzed or in traction, most patients left the hospital to head up the side of the mountain and seek the safety of the caves.

The roof in our quarters is damaged. Dr. Tom's room had a back door that was blown off its hinges. The inside of his room looked, well, "like a bomb had gone off."

Over a warm Russian beer, over dinner, while walking to and from the hospital, everyone was telling and retelling their own experience, encouraging each other that it would not happen again. And then it did.

During rounds on Men's ward around 10:00 a.m., we heard the low distant rumble of an Antonov high altitude bomber.

Tom casually said, "Too far away to worry right now."

But, in fact, it was getting closer.

"Move everyone out!" Tom shouted.

But then almost immediately, he yelled, "No time! Just lie down!!!"

Flat on my belly, eyes clenched shut, hands clasped behind my head, ears covered by my upper arms. BOOM BOOM!

The ground rumbled as dust seemed to spew up from everywhere.

A half minute later, we jump up and run outside. Debris is still falling from the sky near a dry riverbed a half mile away. I join mostly old men and a local nurse, Anna, who was crying and uttering she just wanted to go home to her baby.

We managed to get Anna into a foxhole knowing the plane would be circling back before she could make it home. I also helped lower into the hole a patient, who was on crutches, already having had one leg amputated due to the injuries he incurred from the shrapnel of a bomb an Antonov had dropped in his village.

We waited. And waited some more, keeping our heads low to the ground. And then there it was!

BOOM BOOM! The return pass missed us by about a ½ mile.

And then we began the wait all over again.

The plane circled back two more times, dropping four more bombs. Eight in total. Only one casualty.

This time a person was injured. A man who had sought shelter inside a hollow Baobab tree was struck in the foot by shrapnel that had penetrated the six inch outer trunk of the tree. He had a three-inch chunk of metal sticking out of the side of his right foot. Most of the bones of the foot were broken. With good wound care he may be able to keep his foot, but will likely limp in pain the rest of his life.

This second day of back-to-back bombings unequivocally resulted in psychological casualties. Everyone's asking, and if not asking, certainly thinking along the lines of: "Will they return this morning?" "Will they come at night?" "Is this going to be a regular occurrence now?"

There's enough work to focus on that these thoughts are not all consuming, but they do come and go. They are there. You can't shake them. And yet, personally, I am surprisingly calm. I am not proud or ashamed of the fact because I've not done anything to be calm. I just am—for now.

May 11, 2014

The young woman with open femur fracture is improving. Her hut was struck by a mortar shell when her village of Tongoli, in Delami County, was attacked the night of April 28 around 3:00 a.m. Her two nieces, who had been sleeping on a cot next to her, were killed. She arrived at the hospital the day before we were bombed. On May 1st when the first of five fighter jet missiles landed a few hundred meters from the hospital, everyone who could run for the caves did. She somehow threw herself out of bed and crawled to the hallway for help. Her leg was still attached to a bag of sand by a rope tied to a pin in her lower leg to provide the traction for her femur fracture.

Two weeks after she was first injured, after we finished changing her bandages, I held up my fingers to count and she had 8 wounds total. I give her a thumbs up for encouragement. She pointed to the sky and said, "Allah" with a peaceful smile, a smile she was able to maintain for the hour we took to do her daily wound care. Two wounds on her thigh were so deep I couldn't touch the bottom with my index finger which must have been excruciating.

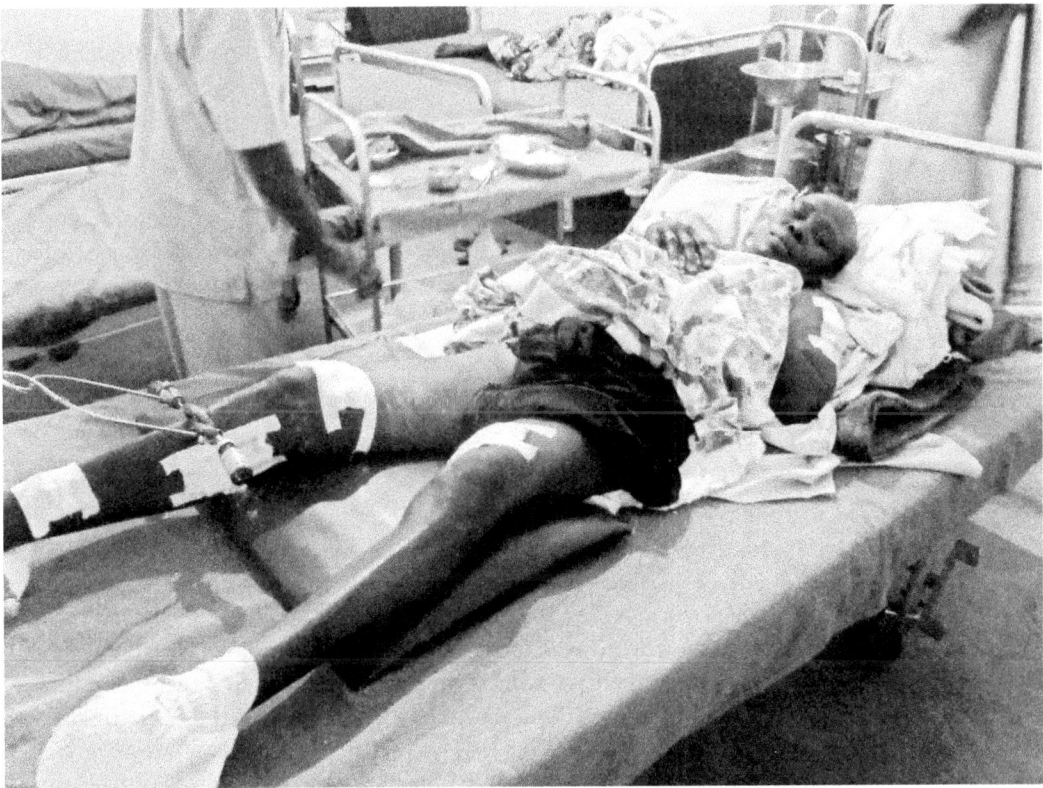

May 11, 2014. My inspiration. This woman was struck by a mortar shell in her home, and later threw herself from a traction bed (which she was in because of a femur fracture) when the hospital was attacked by an aerial bombardment (Dr. C. Louis Perrinjaquet).

I guess we all have to endure whatever may come to us, but she did so with such peace, strength and grace. I am humbled every time I think of her, which is often.

We continue to receive casualties from an area of fighting several hours' drive to the North. One was a seven month old boy who was hit by shrapnel while he was in his mother's arms as they hid in the rocks above their village near Kwalib. He will survive the gash on his forehead.

Tom says to me in frustration, "Seriously! What kind of person would do that? Indiscriminately shell innocent women and children hiding in caves?"

May 19, 2014

Casualties brought from Kadugli. I only saw the two worst. I first heard of their arrival when I walked into the clinical officers' tiny dining room for a piece of bread and coffee around 7 a.m. By the time I rushed to the operating room, Tom was already prepping the first guy to open his abdomen. None of his surgical staff had arrived yet, so he was glad to see me. Tom was making incisions as I was connecting suction, cautery, adjusting light, pulling a unit of O negative "universal donor" blood from the lab. When the lab determined his blood type was A+, the same as mine, I was sent to donate. His brother then volunteered his A+ blood and mine was saved for another day. The patient had been shot in the abdomen. He had a small entrance wound on the left, larger exit wound on the right, leaving three holes in the small intestine.

Tom removed the damaged areas, then as he continued to explore the abdomen he found that the large intestine was "blown apart" and that a hard mass of stool sat freely exposed in the abdomen. He removed about ½ of his large intestine and made an illeostomy hole in the abdominal wall to connect the small intestine to a bag on the outside. The abdomen was flushed with a couple liters of saline, and then several surgical drains were inserted. He was given a massive amount of antibiotics," IV Fluids, and blood transfusions—and now needs a lot of luck. He had been shot about 3 p.m. the day before, so to have eighteen hours of feces free in his abdomen, along with significant blood loss, carries a high risk of death.

The second casualty had been struck by shrapnel, which shattered his right knee. The shiny joint surface at the end of his femur was clearly visible from across the triage area. His lower leg was shattered so the only option was an above the knee amputation.

We had almost finished the operation when Tom noticed the patient's oxygen levels were going down. Then, suddenly, his heart stopped. Tom immediately started CPR, and directed his assistant to turn off the anesthesia. Slowly, the man's pulse and blood pressure returned and Tom finished the case. A few hours later he's come out of the anesthesia, sitting up in bed, "smoking and joking" as Tom would say. Maybe he had had a fat embolism (when bone marrow from an exposed fracture finds its way into a large vein and goes to the lung like a blood clot). Or maybe it had something to do with the anesthesia nurse not noticing that several hours worth of the anesthetic drug Ketamine that was in an IV for maintenance had run over by one hour by mistake. Whatever it was, that guy who Tom resuscitated had better odds than the abdomen full of feces guy. Hopefully they'll both survive, but it will take several months before either leaves the hospital if they do.

May 1, 2015

One year after the hospital is bombed.

I arrived at Mother of Mercy late this morning, went to the operating room to let Tom know I had arrived, then headed straight to the lab to donate a unit of blood. Tom lets me donate two units in three days because his patients often need transfusions, and living at high altitude my blood count is high so I can tolerate it well. Plus, I really like the idea of so literally giving of myself to help the Nuba.

I returned to the OR just as Tom was draining an abscess in a two-year-old's neck and hit an artery. Blood kept welling up in the incision and he couldn't find the bleeder to tie it off. He told me to check the child's chart for blood Type. He was A+! Tom is rarely rattled by anything, but this time he raised his voice and said, "Go get that unit of blood you just gave and we'll give it to this kid. Tell the lab guy to bring it right now and not to screw around!" Tom was swearing and sweating. He extended the incision and finally clamped the bleeder, but the boy had lost a lot of blood.

Apparently it's still very hard to get family members to donate blood, plus Type A+ is uncommon in the Nuba. Before my blood had cooled off it was running in this small patient's vein and he was waking up. I've never made a more dramatic gift.

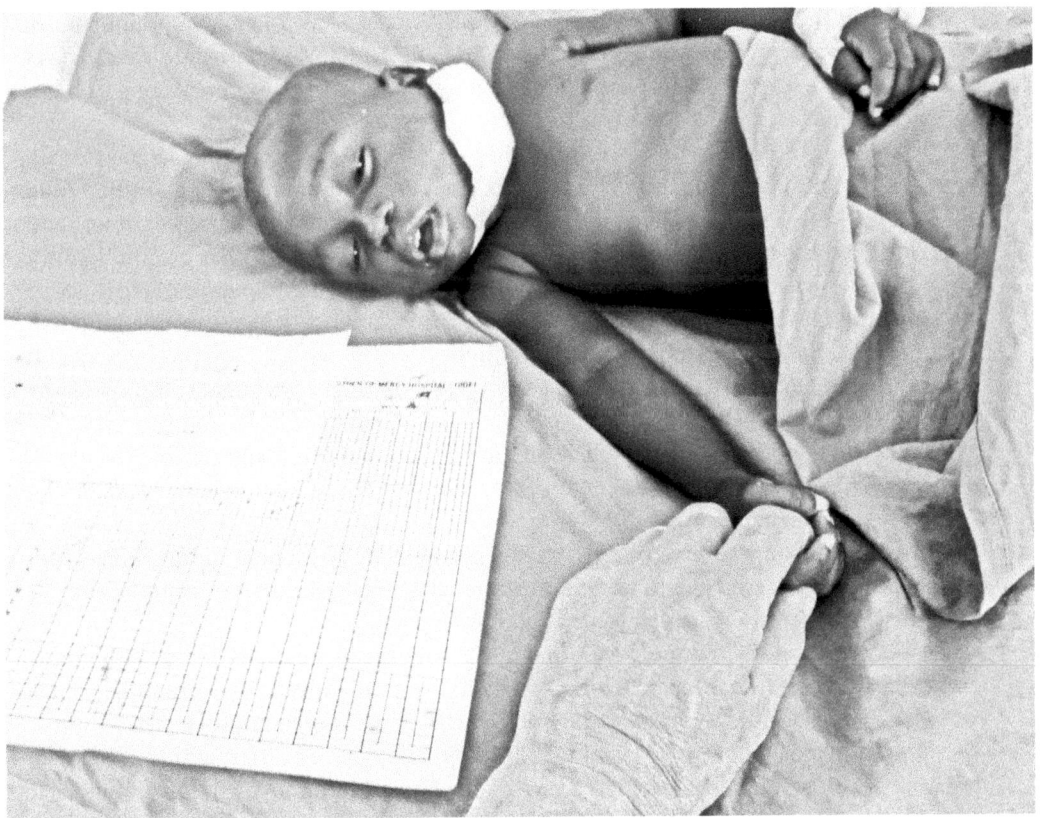

May 1, 2015. A+ Blood Brothers. The recipient of my still warm unit of blood recovering from blood loss after a neck abscess was drained.

Some Concluding Thoughts

The Nuba are by nature a joyful people. I have been fortunate enough to observe a rich culture of Nuba singing and dancing at every occasion. I also witnessed the heroic stoicism of patients smiling up from hospital beds despite missing limbs, lying for weeks in traction, having lost family members and all their possessions. Their spirit is strong and will eventually overcome the suffering that is being brought to them by an unjust government.

The government of Sudan continues to attack Nuba civilians at will—mostly via aerial attacks by Antonov but also, increasingly, by Sochki jets. Somewhere in the order of a million black African farmers have been displaced to IDP camps in the middle of nowhere, while others have fled to dusty, crowded refugee camps.

For those who may not know it, it is a fact that the International Criminal Court (ICC) has already issued an arrest warrant against Sudanese President Omar al-Bashir on five counts of crimes against humanity—murder, extermination, forcible transfer, torture and rape; two counts of war crimes—intentionally directing attacks against a civilian population as such or against individual civilians not taking part in hostilities and pillaging; and, three counts of genocide—by killing, by causing serious bodily or mental harm and by deliberately inflicting on each target group conditions of life calculated to bring about the group's physical destruction.

Framing this situation in a positive way, humankind has an amazing opportunity in this one small place to learn how to end war. The Nuba Mountains are roughly the size of Iowa. We, the 6 billion people on Earth, who are living on more than a dollar a day, can do this!

That is not to say that it will be easy. Indeed, it will likely be complicated. After all, the Nuba Mountains of Sudan is just north of the new boundary between South Sudan and Sudan where oil fuels both economies. It lies between the world's largest desert and the world's largest swamp where rock outcroppings and slightly higher ground allow a sparse population to subsist on goats and sorghum. Most of the population live in stone and grass huts. Even before the current conflict, women's death rate during childbirth and infant mortality rates were among the highest in the world. Malaria, leprosy and exotic diseases developed countries have eradicated decades ago are as common as the common cold.

But, be that as it may, it is, I believe, incumbent upon us, humanity across the globe, to figure out a way to protect innocent people who want the same things we all want: the freedom to pursue happiness.

If we do nothing, we can be sure we've been absolutely no help to the Nuba. And, in fact, at least as far as I see it, we will be guilty as a result of our very complacency. If we at least try, then there's a chance that good will grow.

When all is said and done, I think people across the globe are more alike than different. We all want to be free, love and be loved, live peacefully with our families, have enough eat, and be able to practice the religion that is most meaningful to us.

Finally, in closing, it is also a fact that different people need different things to make them happy. By volunteering in places such as the Nuba Mountains, I'm just doing what makes me happiest: helping those in greatest need. Interestingly, and perhaps tellingly, recent psychological research findings verify that people who *do* things are happier than people who *have* things.

I have this wild idea—kind of an experiment, really—of committing myself to trying to follow the advice of the major saints and scriptures of various religions which all say pretty much the same thing. "Be nice. Be generous. Take the risk to help people in need, and you will be happy." I know from my own experience, they are right.

NOTE

1. Plumpy'Nut is a peanut-based paste in a plastic wrapper for treatment of severe acute malnutrition. The ingredients in Plumpy'Nut include "peanut-based paste, with sugar, vegetable oil and skimmed milk powder, enriched with vitamins and minerals" referred to in scientific literature as a Ready-to-Use Therapeutic Food (RUTF).

Afterword

ISRAEL W. CHARNY

This is an absolutely exciting and captivating book—one of the truly gripping reads I've had in recent years.

I didn't expect it. I figured I was once again doing my duty and going to review another documentation of tragedy (what is happening in Nuba *is* a tragedy) written in correct academic prose. To my increasing amazement, in essay after essay by the contributors that Samuel Totten has gathered here, I found myself enthralled and, heaven forgive me, even enjoying deeply a "whodonit" and a "when, where, how and why the who done it" in the Nuba Mountains in Sudan. Presumably one should not "enjoy" reading about genocide but I did—without it reducing my protest and outrage.

But first I want to pay tribute to the untitled part of this book—especially for professional genocide scholars. I am referring to the work of Samuel Totten, a veteran and prolific genocide scholar. He has grown into being a Great Man because he is the rare academic in genocide studies who has gotten off his ivory seat and actually gone into the dangerous world of ongoing crimes against humanity (and a potential genocide). The overwhelming majority of us—genocide scholars—sit in comfortable critics' perches above the terrifying misery of genocide. As of this writing, Totten has now risked his life four times going directly to the killing fields of the Nuba. In the process, he has not only gone to study, record and analyze what is happening for our intellectual understanding, but has also carried with him tens of tons of food for the starving Nuba who are being cruelly attacked by the government of Sudan via aerial and ground attacks. I would add that much of the expense of these trips and supplies have been his, let alone that he has taken on collecting contributions from good people for his dedicated missions.

And now it turns out that the people whom Totten has successfully invited to contribute to this book are, one after the other, cut from the same cloth of wonderful human beings who have made profound spiritual commitments to devote much if not all of their lives to helping the persecuted Nuba, (see, for example, "Sojourns through Worlds of Suffering" by John Jefferson, or "Sowing Seeds of Peace: My Life at Mother of Mercy Hospital," by Margaret Camarca, who was raised in a devout Catholic family that "exemplifies the importance of family, service and forgiveness").

To me it is indisputably a fact that unless we go through a fundamental paradigm change in regard to how our world community is to respond to reports of mass killing, we will remain doomed forever to the ugly politics of competitive, combative and destructive countries, ethnicities, religions, and more. The current international political-legal system virtually guarantees that any and all attempts at intervention of small and large genocidal massacres and mass killing is maddeningly presaged by tedious and disputatious intellectual/political process that masks the truths of the self-centered, self-interested motives even of the more decent players in the international game. I remember, for example, the United Nations Human Rights Commission deliberating over two years whether a genocide was being executed in Cambodia during which time tens of thousands more died at the vicious hands of the Khmer Rouge.

For me the logic of intervention in situations of mass killing is ridiculously "simple." Just as in most societies a citizen can call the police and expect help to stop a killer, so I believe nations and other collective entities should be able to call on an international police force for immediate intervention. No political process should stand in the way of the "cops" arriving on the scene.

Over the years any number of scholars have proposed the creation of—you name it—an International Police Force, a Rapid Reaction Force, or in my own writing, an International Peace Army (IPA). In my proposal, the IPA would be composed of at least three major "armies" that would work closely together under a unified command:

- The IPA Military
- The IPA Medical and Humanitarian Army
- The IPA for the Rebuilding of Safe and Tolerant Communities

From the outset, the IPA would be charged not only with containing and destroying the killers, but with responding to immediate health and rehabilitation needs, and it would be dedicated to the wisest interventions, re-educational programs, and methods of community reorganization that have the promise of laying to rest age-old rivalries, animosities, and prejudices between different segments of our quite stupid killer humanity.

As noted, the contributors to this book are each exemplary persons who have dedicated much of their lives to helping and protecting a people under intense destructive fire, and this despite the fact that they themselves have to dive for the safety holes and caves when the attacking Sudanese appear in whatever forms, including Antonov bombers and fighter jets. Tomo Križnar, a journalist and documentary maker who has dedicated himself "to helping prevent the extermination of the Nuba people," movingly asserts: "We are at the beginning. We are looking for support and like-minded people. We need advice. We need support of all kind of professionals, anthropologists included."

There are several essays by deeply devoted physicians about the running of an unbelievable hospital—Mother of Mercy—right at the front lines in Sudan. It is striking how many of the humanitarians who contribute to this book describe their own backgrounds as being guided by a true devotion to medical helping and/or to deep religious convictions. (Thus, Sister Deirdre M. Byrne combines the two—"a general surgeon and religious sister.") I am reminded of a good number of studies of humanitarians in the past who saved lives by hiding potential victims of a genocide, such as those designated "Righteous Gentiles" by Yad Vashem (the main memorial and research center on the Holocaust in Israel) for saving Jews in the Holocaust. A good number of them also reported being guided by basic religious convictions. (One of my favorite stories is of the rescuer who, when interviewed after the war, explained that he really disliked Jews but he "simply" had no choice. It was the right thing to do.)

I wish to comment on several of the essays herein, though it should be understood that each and every one is inspiring reading.

Dr. Tom Catena stands out among the wonderful contributors to this book. He is a doctor who is spending his life in Sudan and devoting himself to 24-hour days, 7 days a week, doing surgery and caring for the wounded. It is utterly impossible not to be deeply moved by his accounts of the medical dramas in which he participates. (Incidentally, Catena comments on the cowardly *realpolitik* of any number of international organizations, such as the United Nations and not a few of its branches—that are devoted to humanitarian relief of the needy in the world but seemingly readily sideline their authority and expertise in order not to antagonize tyrannical governments such as Sudan.)

George Tutu provides an entirely different perspective than our wonderful Western professionals, for he himself is a son of the Nuba who grew up in the mountains without electricity or running water, and was, early on, under the attacks of Baggara Arabs who attacked their villages and farms with the complicity of the government of Sudan. Shades of a classic story of the immigrant boy who does well, he pulls himself up by the bootstraps, receives an education in the big city, even succeeds in moving to the United States with his family and gains American citizenship, but then responds to the call inside of him and returns to Nuba as a humanitarian helper.

In Tomo Križnar's essay I met up with the biggest surprise I had in this book. It is not necessarily the most important part of his story, but it absolutely blew my mind to have "Hitler appear in the Nuba Mountains." By that strange remark I mean that Tomo Križnar describes at length an unforgettable experience with no less than Leni Riefensthal, the legendary photographer, screen writer, film director, and producer of propaganda for the Nazis, and by all accounts a rare friend of Adolf Hitler. Riefensthal always insisted that she had no awareness of the Holocaust, but most people don't believe her—as we shall see with good reason.

Križnar brings to our attention that she is also famous for her professional photographs of the Nuba people in the early 1970s, with two books published in 1974 and 1976. Because of that he is interested in meeting her and succeeds in being invited to her home. Križnar begs Leni to go back to the Nuba Mountains and film their tragic suffering. He promises her that "history [will] remember you as a shining example to all humanitarians worldwide." In an unforgettable scene he is briefing her at great length about what is happening, and among other things, describes how Chevron, the American oil company, found oil in southern Sudan and how the grab for oil added another dimension to the war. Riefensthal replies excitedly, *"Nein! Nein! The Jews are to blame…. Die Juden! Die Juden!"* And then, according to Križnar, she adds, "I am interested solely in art and beauty … politics I do not care about." Intriguingly, Riefensthal does return to the Nuba Mountains, where the government of Sudan tries to profit from her return in order to create a propaganda picture of how well life is there is for the Nuba. (Križnar compares it to the Nazis' deception at Theresienstadt, their model concentration camp for the International Red Cross, where all seemed tranquil, but where thousands of the inmates were shipped periodically to Auschwitz.) Even Leni got the message that the government of Sudan was faking what they showed her.

To conclude, it is also touching and heart rending how many of the writers in this book refer to the Nuba as an unusually good people which then heightens the sense of tragedy. In this respect, John P. Sutter, M.D., one of the humanitarian volunteers who volunteered at Mother of Mercy Hospital, comments as follows:

> The Nuba are good people and it is odd how their plight for the most part is ignored, especially by the West.... The Nuba I met have values and traits that mirror what we strive for in the West—tolerance (Muslims and Christians living together without issue in Nuba), a fair rule of law, respect for women and children, an appreciation for education, and an emphasis on the preservation of the family unit. I am lucky to have been able to work with them and I am inspired.... It is a shame that no one has stepped up to stop the bombers from carrying out their daily bombing missions.

Another contributor, Dr. Corry Chapman (who started medical school at age 33 after having earned a college degree in history and worked at a bevy of jobs, in construction, retail, and clerical), has this to say: "Despite how harsh the environment is, the Nuba is stunningly beautiful and populated by people you'll meet nowhere else on earth. Seeing the Milky Way every night, living simply.... The Nubans are generous, kind, low-key and love to laugh."

Continuing, Chapman adds: "They are also very guarded, given the constant persecution in their history, and one's heart tears at the rupture of an almost idyllic picture." (We humans mess up life everywhere, don't we?)

One of the many aspects of this book that I greatly appreciate is that it gets away from the miserable intellectualization about genocidal events where scholars are so narcissistically busy with their "understanding" that they ignore and forget what was really happening to people. When masses of unarmed people are killed, it is obscene to spend hours arguing about whether or not it constituted genocide, crimes against humanity, ethnic cleansing, or what have you.

Personally I have come to the painful conclusion that mass killing is a way of nature—our natures as human beings as well as the larger picture of our universe that is constantly subject to entropy, instability and destruction. It is unbearably consistent with the nature of life that death comes prematurely to mass numbers of people.

Yet it seems to many of us that the most real and deepest challenge to our puny species, at the level of evolution that we represent, is to stand up to these challenges to life and seek to protect, extend, enhance, and enrich life for the largest number of human creatures possible. The challenge for mankind is to devote our magnificent intelligence to find new solutions to problems of overpopulation, climate change, rampant killer diseases, military belligerence, genocidal killing, and more.

This beautiful book is an inspiration and a call.

Israel W. Charny is a professor emeritus of psychology, Hebrew University (Jerusalem, Israel), the founder of the Institute on the Holocaust and Genocide (Jerusalem), a co-founder of the International Association of Genocide Scholars (IAGS), and the editor-in-chief of the Encyclopedia of Genocide.

Annotated Bibliography

Books and Reports

Africa Watch (1991). *Sudan: Destroying Ethnic Identity: The Secret War Against the Nuba.* New York: Africa Watch. 12 pp.

An early report that addresses the unremitting attacks by the Sudanese Government against the Nuba people, their culture, and their way of life.

African Rights (1995). *Facing Genocide: The Nuba of Sudan.* London: African Rights. 344 pp.

This highly informative book constitutes the first major and detailed report on the plight and fate of the Nuba Mountains people at the hands of the Government of Sudan under the dictatorial regime of Sudanese President Omar al-Bashir. It provides an overview of the history of the conflict, an in-depth commentary on the actors involved, the atrocities perpetrated, the actions and reactions of the victims, and how and why the Sudanese government's actions constituted "genocide by attrition." One of the coauthors of the report/book, Alex DeWaal, is a noted specialist on Sudan.

African Rights (1995). *Sudan's Invisible Citizens: The Policy of Abuse Against Displaced People in the North.* London: African Rights. 60 pp.

This report is comprised of the following chapters: "Internal Migration in Sudan"; "Forced Acculturation and the Moslem Brother's Project for Transforming Sudan"; "Demolition, Forced Removal and Removal and Population Transfer"; "Discrimination and Abuse: The Daily Struggles of the Displaced"; and "Response and Resistance."

African Rights (1997). *A Desolate Peace: Human Rights in the Nuba Mountains, Sudan.* London: African Rights. 27 pp.

A discussion of the horrific situation the Nuba faced at the hands of the Government of Sudan.

African Rights (1997). *Justice in the Nuba Mountains of Sudan: Challenges and Prospects.* London: African Rights. 43 pp.

Subtitled "A Report on African Rights' Involvement with Access to Justice in the Nuba Mountains, 1995–1997," this is an examination of the difficulties that continued to plague the Nuba Mountains well into the late 1990s, as well as the challenges and potential for gaining some sort of justice for the Nuba Mountains people.

Amnesty International (1993). *Sudan: The Ravages of War: Political Killings and Humanitarian Disaster.* London: Amnesty International. 29 pp.

In part, this report presents information on major human rights violations (including "ethnic cleansing") perpetrated by GoS troops and their militia cohorts against the Nuba people.

Burr, Millard (1993). *A Working Document: Quantifying Genocide in Southern Sudan and the Nuba Mountains, 1983–1993.* Washington, D.C.: American Council for Nationalities Service. 66 pp.

In this report, the author, based on his experience as director of logistics operations for the U.S. Agency for International Development (USAID) in Sudan, estimates that 1.3 million people had died in southern Sudan due to war and war-related causes. That death total was nearly twice as large as earlier estimates. The conclusions of the study were generally accepted and used by policy makers, international media, humanitarian and human rights workers, and many Sudanese themselves.

Burr, Millard (1998). *Working Document II: Quantifying Genocide in Southern Sudan and the Nuba Mountains, 1983–1998*. Washington, D.C.: U.S. Committee for Refugees. 84 pp.

This report updates and expands on the first study (see above) by Burr. Burr suggests that approximately six hundred thousand additional people perished in southern and central Sudan since 1993, raising the toll to 1.9 million deaths. This updated report expands the scope of research to include the Nuba Mountains area of central Sudan.

Burr states that this report was "based on a review of thousands of articles and studies. Rather than simply quantifying incidents both by province and by year, three new elements were added to the study. The first dealt with the purposeful Government aerial bombardment of civilian populations. The second new element, a chapter titled 'The Nuba Genocide,' describes the degradation and massacre of Nuba Mountains tribes by Government forces. The third new element in the updated study was a section titled 'Genocide in Bahr al-Ghazal.' It discusses the activity of Government forces and the Government's Arab militia (Murahaleen) to depopulate the Kiir River region of northern Bahr al-Ghazal."

De Waal, Alex (2006). "Averting Genocide in the Nuba Mountains, Sudan." 12 pp. Available at: http://howgenocidesend.ssrc.org/de_Waal2/.

In this update of "Facing Genocide: The Nuba of Sudan," de Waal discusses the status of the Nuba ten years after his initial report.

Human Rights Watch (1994). *Sudan: "In the Name of God"—Repression Continues in Northern Sudan. Human Rights Watch Report 6, No. 9*, November. New York: Author.

The authors state, "This report highlights excerpts from the diary kept by a resident of Kordofan from late 1992 to April 1993 that describes the large-scale displacement of Nubans, their forcible relocation under intolerable conditions, the abduction of children, the forced recruitment of boys as young as thirteen into military service, the destruction of churches, the abuse of women in displaced persons' camps, and the manipulation of relief for Islamic proselytization purposes, among other abuses.

"This diary reinforces the findings on the situation in the Nuba Mountains presented in the February 1994 report of the U.N. Special Rapporteur on Human Rights in Sudan."

This report also "covers the plight of displaced persons and squatters in urban areas of northern Sudan, including Nubans and southerners displaced by the war. In 1992 hundreds of thousands of the displaced and urban squatters were summarily evicted from their homes in urban areas. Their property was destroyed under a purported urban renewal campaign which targeted the large non–Arab and non–Muslim population of the capital. This campaign continued in 1993, and in 1994 an estimated 160,000 more people were similarly displaced from Khartoum and moved to unprepared sites far from water, work, or education."

Human Rights Watch (1999). *Famine in Sudan, 1998: The Human Rights Causes*. New York: Human Rights Watch. n.p.

One section of this report is entitled "Nuba Mountains: Under Siege by the Government." In part, it discusses the GoS's strategy to starve the Nuba people into submission.

Jok, Madut (2001). *War and Slavery in Sudan*. Philadelphia: University of Pennsylvania Press. 211 pp.

This study of war and slavery in Sudan examines the contemporary practice of slavery in Sudan through the lens of the long history of the conflicts between those residing in the north (Arabs with power) and those in the south ("the black African peoples," many of whom are disenfranchised and comprised of both Christians and Muslims).

It addresses, in part, the issue of slavery in the Nuba Mountains, and, more specifically, how the Nuba people have been historically viewed as slaves by the powers that be in Sudan.

This book is comprised of the following parts and chapters. "Introduction: Slavery in Sudan: Definitions and Outlines": Part I, The New Slavery (1) "The Revival of Slavery During the Civil War: Facts and Testimonies"; (2) "Slavery in the Shadow of the Civil War: Problems in the Study of Sudanese Slavery"; (3) "The Suffering of the South in the North-South Conflict"); and Part II: Underlying Causes of the Revival of Slavery in Sudan (4) "The Legacy of Race"; (5) "The South-North Population Displacement"; (6) "The Political-Economic Conflict"); and "Conclusion: Has No One Heard Us Call for Help? Sudanese Slavery and International Opinion."

Manger, Lief (1993). *From the Mountains to the Plains: The Integration of the Lafofa Nuba into the Sudanese Society*. Uppsala: Nordiska Afrikainstituet. 173 pp.

In this study of the Lafofa Nuba, Manger examines the interaction between Nuba and Arab groups, illuminating the impact of Arabization and Islamization.

Nazer, Mende, and Damien Lewis (2003). *Slave: My True Story*. New York: Public Affairs. 350 pp.

This book relates the story of Mende Nazer, who was kidnapped in 1993 by Arab raiders and sold into slavery. It relates her years as a "black slave," as she was called by her wealthy Arab owners, and relates the physical, sexual, and mental abuse to which she was subjected up until she regained her freedom.

Rahhal, Suleiman (Ed.) (2001). *The Right to Be Nuba: The Story of a Sudanese People's Struggle for Survival*. Trenton, NJ: Red Sea Press. 136 pp.

This highly informative book delineates the plight faced by the Nuba people and their struggle for survival as the Sudanese government continued to perpetrate major human rights abuses against them. It is comprised of pieces by prominent Nuba scholars, Nuba activists, and Nuba leaders, as well as others.

The book is comprised of the following chapters: "The Right to Be Nuba" by Alex de Waal; "The Nuba" by Ahmed Rahman Saeed; "The Nuba of South Kordofan" by George Rodger; "Things Were No Longer the Same" by Yousif Kuwa Mekki; "Focus on Crisis in the Nuba Mountains" by Suleiman Musa Rahhal; "The State of Sudan Today" by Peter Woodward; "Voices from the Nuba Mountains"; "The Survival of the Nuba" by David Stewart-Smith; "The Nuba Relief, Rehabilitation and Development Organization" by Neroun Phillip Kuku; "Nuba Agriculture: Poverty or Plenty?" by Ian Mackie; "Democracy under Fire in the Nuba Mountains" by Julie Flint; "Unity in Diversity: Is it Possible in Sudan" by Ahmed Ibrahim Diraige; "What Peace for the Nuba?" by Suleiman Musa Rahhal. Note: Select chapters are annotated separately in this annotated bibliography.

Rottenburg, Richard, Guma Kunda Komey, and Enrico Ille (2011). *The Genesis of Recurring Wars in Sudan: Rethinking the Violent Conflicts in the Nuba Mountains/South Kordofan*. Halle, Germany: University of Halle. 31 pp.

An outstanding and extremely detailed report about the latest crisis in the Nuba Mountains. It is comprised of the following sections: Background. Part One, "What Can Be Known? The Structure of Evidence"; Part Two, "Which Kind of Violence Takes Place? The Military Situation" (The Escalation of Violence in June 2011; Processes of Militarization Before 2011); Part Three, "Why Does Violence Take Place? The Political Situation" (The Election as a Process and Its Disputed Results; and the CPA and Its Failure); Part Four, "Where Does the Violence Come From? The Economic and Cultural Situation" (Patterns of Economic Marginalization and Exploitation; Patterns of Suppression of Ethnic and Cultural Identity); "Conclusion: The Genesis of Recurring Wars in Sudan."

Small Arms Survey (2008). "Insecurity and Militarization in the Nuba Mountains." *Sudan Issue Brief*, No. 12, August. Geneva: Small Arms Survey. 22 pp.

A highly informative report on an outbreak of fighting between Government of Sudan troops and the SPLA of the South.

Special Rapporteur of the Commission on Human Rights (1993). *Interim Report on the Situation of Human Rights in the Sudan*. A/RES/48/147. 85th Plenary Meeting, December 20.

This UN report decries the grave human rights abuses by the GoS against its people residing in various parts of Sudan. It includes a line that reads: "…it is essential to put an end to the serious deterioration of the human rights situation in the Sudan, including that in the Nuba Mountains."

Sullivan, D., and S. Orcutt (2012). "Sudan's Man-Made Catastrophe: A War on Civilians in South Kordofan and Blue Nile." Washington, D.C.: United to End Genocide. 13 pp.

A short report that says, in part: As the rainy season reaches its peak, the people of South Kordofan and Blue Nile are being forced to make an impossible choice between continued attacks and starvation in their homeland or disease and malnutrition en route to flooded camps across the border.

Totten, Samuel (2015). *Genocide by Attrition, Nuba Mountains, Sudan*. Second Edition. New Brunswick, NJ: Transaction Publishers.

This book is largely comprised of detailed interviews by survivors of the genocide by attrition they suffered through in the Nuba Mountains in the late 1980s and throughout the 1990s. It also includes a detailed historical overview of the genocide by attrition, and a useful Afterword that brings the reader up to the current crisis (war between the Government of Sudan and the Sudan People's Liberation Army–North) in the Nuba today (June 2011–present).

254   Annotated Bibliography

Totten, Samuel, and Amanda Grzyb (Eds.) (2015). *Conflict in the Nuba Mountains: From Genocide by Attrition to the Contemporary Crisis in Sudan*. New York: Routledge. 314 pp.

This edited volume is comprised of the following parts and chapters. Part One, The Nuba People and The Nuba Mountains: "The Nuba Plight: An Account of People Facing Perpetual Violence and Institutionalized Insecurity" by Guma Kunda Komey; "The Dilemma of the Nuba" by Mudawi Ibrahim Adam; and "Sudan: The Islamist Project" by Gillian Lusk. Part Two, The Nuba Mountains: Mid 1980s–1990s: "Nuba Mountains, Sudan" by Alex de Waal; "Quantifying Genocide in Southern Sudan and the Nuba Mountains, 1983–1998" by J. Millard Burr; and "The Problem of Impunity: A Signal That Crimes Against Humanity and/or Genocide Are Forgivable?" by Samuel Totten. Part Three, The Outbreak of New Violence in the Nuba Mountains in 2011: "Sudan's Comprehensive Peace Agreement and How the Nuba Mountains Was Left Out" by Jok Madut Jok; "South Kordofan State Elections, May 2011" by John Young; "The Nuba Mountains Crisis: Facts and Factors" by Siddig Kafi; "Perspectives on the Blue Nile" by Wendy James; "Who Will Remember the Nubans? The International Community's Response to the Nuba Mountains Crisis, 2005–present" by Rebecca Tinsley). And "Eyewitness": Interview with Dr. Tom Catena, Physician/Surgeon at Mother of Mercy Hospital in Gidel, South Kordofan (Nuba Mountains), Sudan. Conducted by Samuel Totten.

Chapters in Books/Booklets/Reports

African Rights and Justice Africa (2001). "Voices from the Nuba Mountains," pp. 59–84. In Suleiman Rahhal (Ed.) *The Right to Be Nuba: The Story of a Sudanese People's Struggle for Survival*. Trenton, NJ: Red Sea Press.

This chapter contains four first-person testimonies, each of which addresses a different issue faced by the Nuba people: abduction and rape, the beginning of the war in the Nuba Mountains, extrajudicial executions, and the burning of a mosque. It also contains a section entitled "Stories from an Offensive" in which different individuals relate their personal experiences ("softening up," full-scale assault, scorched earth policies and actions, shelling, land mines, abduction to garrisons and peace camps, killings, hunger, and displacement).

De Waal, Alex (2012). "The Nuba Mountains," pp. 421–445. In Samuel Totten and William S. Parsons (Eds.) *Centuries of Genocide: Critical Essays and Eyewitness Accounts*. 4th Edition. New York: Routledge.

An analytical essay about the GoS's attack on the Nuba Mountains in the late 1980s and early 1990s by an expert on the Sudan. It is accompanied by a small selection of first-person accounts taken from interviews conducted by Samuel Totten in the Nuba Mountains.

Mohamed, Mona A., and Margaret Fisher (2002). "The Nuba of Sudan," pp. 115–128. In Robert K. Hitchcock and Alan J. Osborn (Eds.) *Endangered Peoples of Africa and the Middle East: Struggles to Survive and Thrive*. Westport, CT: Greenwood Press.

In addition to providing a "cultural overview" of the Nuba (The People, The Setting, Traditional Subsistence Strategies, Social and Political Organization, Religion and Worldview), this chapter also discusses "the threats to survival" faced by the Nuba (including the attacks carried out against them by the Government of Sudan). In a subsection entitled "Response: Struggles to Survive Culturally," the authors assert that "From the Perspective of the Nuba, the most pressing issues they are facing are survival, resistance to genocidal policies, sovereignty, the right to make their own political decisions, and the right to practice their own cultural traditions and speak their own languages" (p. 123).

Rahhal, Suleiman (2001). "Focus on Crisis in the Nuba Mountains," pp. 36–55. In Suleiman Rahhal (Ed.) *The Right to Be Nuba: The Story of a Sudanese People's Struggle for Survival*. Trenton, NJ: Red Sea Press.

This chapter is a must-read for those who wish to begin to understand the origins and evolution of the crisis facing the Nuba people. Among the issues covered herein are: a succinct overview of events leading up to the conflict, the roots of the conflict (the religious factor, the racial factor, issues over power-sharing, the lack of economic development, land sequestration, and human rights violations), that which ignited the conflict, the jihad against the Nuba, extrajudicial killings, food as a weapon of war, and the international response.

Saeed, Ahmed Abdel Rahman (2001). "The Nuba," pp. 6–20. In Suleiman Musa Rahaal (Ed.) *The Story of a Sudanese People's Struggle for Survival*. Trenton, NJ: Red Sea Press.

This chapter provides a succinct but informative overview of who the Nuba are, early Nuba history, Nuba customs and traditions, the traditional religion of the Nuba, status of women in the Nuba community, and the impact of Islam in the Nuba Mountains.

Suliman, Mohamed (1999). "The Nuba Mountains of Sudan: Resource Access, Violent Conflict, and Identity." In Daniel Buckles (Ed.) *Cultivating Peace: Conflict and Collaboration in Natural Resource Management*. Washington, D.C.: ICRC/World Bank.

This chapter "attempts to explain the complex web of cooperation and conflict that binds the Nuba and the Baggara [the Arab group used by government as a militia to fight the Nuba]. It also documents three peace agreements reached between the two warring groups."

Winter, Roger (1999). "The Nuba People: Confronting Cultural Liquidation," n.p. In Jay Spaulding and Stephanie Beswick (Eds.) *White Nile Black Blood: War, Leadership, and Ethnicity from Khartoum to Kampala*. Lawrenceville, NJ: The Red Sea Press.

Roger Winter, the former director of U.S. Committee for Refugees and a former administrator at USAID, provides a highly readable and engaging overview of the plight of the Nuba people as it stood in the late 1990s. In doing so, he provides key facts, addresses major issues, and interweaves the latter with personal stories and observations based on his visits to Sudan and the Nuba Mountains.

Refereed Journal Articles

Bradbury, Mark (1998). "Sudan: International Responses to War in the Nuba Mountains." *Review of African Political Economy* 77 (September 25): 463–74.

Bradbury examines the effectiveness of the international response to the Government of Sudan's all out attack against the Nuba and finds that it was minimal, at best.

Gettleman, Jeffrey (2012). "The War Against the Nuba." *The New York Review of Books*. August 16, 59(13): n.p.

A overview of the Nuba crisis by a *New York Times* journalist: causes, key actors, the plight of the civilians in the region, etc.

Reeves, Eric (2014). "Failure to Prevent Genocide in Sudan and the Consequences of Impunity: Darfur as Precedent for Abyei, South Kordofan, and Blue Nile." *Genocide Studies International*, 8(1): 58–74.

The abstract of this article states, "The responsibility to protect, adopted with such enthusiastic fanfare at the September 2005 UN World Summit, has proved an abject failure in defining international policy in Sudan. On the contrary, impunity continues to be afforded to even the most egregious atrocity crimes committed by Khartoum's National Islamic Front/National Congress Party regime, which has been waging a genocidal counterinsurgency campaign in Darfur since early 2003. This impunity extends to the worlds' refusal to respond meaningfully to the regime's military seizure of the contested Abyei region—displacing more than 100,000 of the indigenous Dinka Ngok—and the subsequent genocidal campaign against the people of South Kordofan and Blue Nile. Sudan loomed as a test case for the responsibility to protect doctrine as defined by paragraph 138 and 139 of the World Summit's Outcome Document. In the assessment of this essay, its failure has been complete."

Salih, Mohamed A. (1995). "Resistance and Response: Ethnocide and Genocide in the Nuba Mountains, Sudan." *GeoJournal* 36(1): 71–8.

This article delineates the origins of Sudan's abuse and oppression against the Nuba and spells out how the government's policies and actions constitute both ethnocide and genocide.

Salih, Mohamed A. (1999). "Land Alienation and Genocide in the Nuba Mountains, Sudan." *Cultural Survival* 22(4): 36–8.

The author argues that "the current situation of indigenous peoples in the Sudan is the result of the independent state's [in other words, Sudan's] adoption of land and other policies identical to those introduced by colonialists more than a century ago. The Sudanese state has unwittingly maintained some colonial coercive institutions and brutally deployed them against its indigenous peoples."

Tinsley, Rebecca (2014). "The Nuba People: Out of Sight, Out of Mind." *Genocide Studies International* 8(1): 75–85.

In Tinsley's précis of her article, she says, "Despite the improved international architecture for the prediction, prevention, and punishment of mass atrocities since the Rwandan Genocide 20 years ago, the fate of Sudan's Nuba people has been overlooked. Since May 2011, the Nuba have been under attack by the Sudanese regime, which has been using the same tactics it employed to devastating effect during the 1990s.... The international community's attention to continuing human rights abuse in the Nuba Mountains has been inconsistent and easily deflected onto low-level hostilities between South Sudan and Sudan. Meanwhile, Sudan has rallied regional leaders, defying the International Criminal Court's indictment of President al-Bashir. The United States and the United Kingdom, guarantors of the 2005 Comprehensive Peace Agreement (CPA), have declined to press Khartoum to fulfill its obligations under the CPA, to enact constitutional reform, or to cease bombing the Nuba for fear that a Sudanese Arab Spring might bring unknown actors to power in Khartoum."

Totten, Samuel (2014). "Paying Lip Service to R2P and Genocide Prevention: The Muted Reponses of the US Atrocities Prevention Board and the USHMM'S Committee on Conscience to the Crisis in the Nuba Mountains." *Genocide Studies International* 9(1) (Spring): 23–57.

A stinging critique and rebuke of the lack of attention (and ostensible concern) by the United States Atrocities Prevention Board and the United States Holocaust Memorial Museum's Committee on Conscience to the current crisis (June 2011–present) in the Nuba Mountains.

Totten, Samuel (2016). "The Forgotten War in the Nuba Mountains." *Social Education* 80(1) (January/February): 52–57.

A short overview of the author's effort to deliver food to those in most desperate need during the current war between the Government of Sudan and the Sudan People's Liberation Army–North.

Totten, Samuel (2016). "Humanitarian Missions to the Nuba Mountains, Sudan: Delivery of Food to Those in Critical Need." *Genocide Studies International* 9(2): 248–268.

The following reports delineate the most recent experiences and insights gleaned by Samuel Totten, a scholar of genocide studies based in the United States, as he traveled up into the war-torn Nuba Mountains in Sudan during December 2014 and April–May 2015. During the course of both trips, accompanied by an interpreter and a driver, both from the Nuba Mountains, he served as a witness to the ongoing aerial attacks by the government of Sudan against Nuba civilians (in their villages, on their farms, in open marketplaces, in their schools, and in places of worship) and delivered food (sorghum, lentils, dried beans, salt, sugar, and cooking oil) to those Nuba in the most dire need. An untold number of Nuba have been forced out of their villages and off their farms due to the aerial bombings, and without access to their farms and stores of food, many, particularly those residing in the remotest regions, are experiencing everything from malnutrition to severe malnutrition to starvation.

Articles

Africa Watch (1991). "Sudan: Destroying Ethnic Identity: The Secret War Against the Nuba." *News from Africa Watch* 3(15) (December 10): 9.

A short piece that provides insight into the Government of Sudan's attempted destruction of the ethnic identity of the Nuba.

Pilchinski, Dorothy (2011). "Terror in Sudan: Nuba Mountains Genocide." Available at: www.redruby slippers.org/2012/04/terror-in-sudan-nuba-mountains-genocide.html.

A short but fascinating article on the efforts of Adidan Hartley and Daniel Bogado's to film "extensive documentary footage from the war zone [in the Nuba Mountains], and to film the heroic doctors who are saving children in a largely hidden war being perpetrated on civilians by one of the world's most brutal dictatorships."

Speeches

Suliman, Mohamed (1997). "Ethnicity from Perception to Cause of Violent Conflicts: The Case of the Fur and Nuba Conflicts in Western Sudan." Talk at the CONTICI International Workshop. Bern, Switzerland, July 8–11. Available at: http://www.ifaanet.org/ifaapr/ethnicity_inversion.htm

In speaking of the Government of Sudan's attacks against the Fur and Nuba in western Sudan, the author argues that "Most violent conflicts are over material resources, whether these resources are actual or perceived. With the passage of time, however, ethnic, cultural and religious affiliations seem to undergo transformation from abstract ideological categories into concrete social forces. In a wider sense, they themselves become contestable material social resources and hence possible objects of group strife and violent conflict."

The section on the Nuba ("The Armed Conflict in the Nuba Mountains") is comprised of the following sections: The People, The History of the Nuba People, The Baggara Enter the Mountains, The Post-Independence Period, The Conflict, The Response of the Jellaba Government, The Causes, Resource Depletion, Against Mechanized Farming in the Nuba Mountains, Climate Variations, and Conflict Resolution.

Letters/Calls for Action

Africa Watch (1992). "Sudan: Eradicating the Nuba: Africa Watch Calls for the United Nations to Investigate Killings, Destruction of Villages and Forced Removals." *News from Africa Watch* 4(10) (September 9).
A clarion call for action.

International Women's Committee in Support of Nuba Women and Children (1997). "Nuba Mountains Letter." *Africa Policy E-Journal*, n.p.
A letter of protest over the ongoing onslaught against the Nuba people. It includes information from various sources vis-à-vis the "genocidal human rights abuses" by the GoS in the Nuba Mountains region.

Films

Eyes of Nuba (Available on-line at www.aljazeera.com/programmes/witness/2014/01/eyes-nuba-2014 12214233201165.html).
Filmmakers John Dickie and Will Sherman relate the story of a remarkable group of citizen journalists formed in the Nuba Mountains in 2011 under the guidance and leadership of American Ryan Boyette. The film follows one of the citizen journalists with *Nuba Reports*, Ahmed Khatir, as he travels throughout the Nuba Mountains reporting on the daily bombings by Antonovs and the destruction, injury and death they had wrought.

Nuba Conversations (52 minutes; produced in 2001 Nuba Survival, PO Box 486 Hayes, Middlesex, UB3 3WZ, United Kingdom, e-mail: nubasurvival@googlemail.com).
Described by *The New York Village Voice* as "A film that works both as searing journalism and a passionate first-person account of the unaccountable, a document of what has to many Western eyes remained an invisible cataclysm."

Nuba: Pure People (Distribution: Bela Film, Beljaska 32, 1000 Ljubljana; Fax: (00 386 1) 515 00 25; and Nuba Survival, PO Box 486 Hayes, Middlesex, UB3 3WZ, United Kingdom; e-mail: nuba survival@googlemail.com).
"Award-winning documentary about the illegal journey of the Slovene writer Tomo Križnar to the Nuba Mountains in Sudan [in order to capture] the story of the unknown genocide perpetrated for fifteen years against the Nuba people."

The Right to Be Nuba (35 minutes; produced in 1993 Distributed by Filmmakers Library).
The struggles of the Nuba people are presented herein as they are caught in the middle of a civil war between the Government of Sudan and the SPLA.

About the Contributors

Ryan Boyette is a Christian and human rights activist based in the Nuba Mountains in Sudan, where he has lived for the past fourteen years. He initially worked with Samaritan's Purse in the region, overseeing the construction of churches and schools for the Nuba as well as waterholes and hand-pumping systems for the local people. After the outbreak of war in June 2011, he founded a citizens journalist group, which is now known as Nuba Reports. In 2014, he received the Human Rights First Award.

Sister/Dr. Deirdre M. Byrne is a POSC Religious Sister with the Congregation Little Workers of the Sacred Hearts, medical director of the D.C. Catholic Charities Medical Clinic and general surgeon for the impoverished in Washington, D.C. In the Nuba Mountains, she was a volunteer general surgeon who provided care at Mother of Mercy Hospital. She served as a volunteer in the Nuba during 2010, 2011, and 2013. She has also worked in the Kakuma Refugee Camp in Kenya.

Margaret Camarca, RN, M.P.H., is a nurse and senior study director at Westat in Rockville, Maryland. In November 2013 she joined the Catholic Medical Mission Board to serve as a fulltime medical volunteer at the Mother of Mercy Hospital in the South Kordofan state of the Sudan. She resides in Gaithersburg, Maryland.

Dr. Tom Catena is the only surgeon at the only fully functioning hospital in the Nuba Mountains. He is a U.S. citizen with a medical degree from Duke University and has what is aptly described as legendary status in the Nuba Mountains, and he cares for anyone who shows up at Mother of Mercy Hospital in Gidel. Prior to arriving in Sudan in 2008, he was a military doctor and then a physician who attended the poor and sick in the slums of Nairobi, Kenya.

Matt Chancey is a founding director of the Persecution Project Foundation (PPF), a Christian organization providing physical relief and spiritual hope to the victims of genocide and religious persecution. Since 2005, he has traveled extensively through South Sudan and the contested border areas of the Republic of Sudan. On July 4, 2011, he made the first of many trips to the Nuba Mountains to document war crimes committed by the Sudan government. His work with the PPF helps to provide safe water, medical, educational, and crisis relief programs in the Nuba Mountains.

Corry Chapman, M.D., is a physician with Neighborhood Health in Alexandria, Virginia. He has made three separate visits over the period 2008–2014 to the Nuba Mountains in order to work with Dr. Tom Catena at Mother of Mercy Hospital. While there, he provided general medical care, and saw firsthand the killing of civilians by Sudanese government bombs in 2014. He has also gone on medical missions to Haiti and Ecuador.

John C. Jefferson is one of the co-founders of ENG (End Nuba Genocide) Project, and the founder of the Greater Nuba Action Coalition. He has undertaken humanitarian relief and compassionate ministry activities in the Nuba Mountains and refugee camps in the surrounding region since shortly after the outbreak of hostilities in 2011. Traveling by foot, tractor, and truck to access the embattled region, he has worked to form coalitions responsible for getting tons of food, medicines and supplies to some of the most desperate and isolated people in the world.

About the Contributors

Tomo Križnar is a journalist, author, documentary filmmaker, and peace activist. In 2006, he entered the Darfur region with the help of Darfur rebels during the ongoing conflict there. Ultimately, he was arrested and imprisoned by Government of Sudan authorities and was only released upon diplomatic efforts by Slovenian officials. In 2011, he delivered video cameras in Southern Kordofan to the local ethnic Nuba civilians in order to help them collect the evidence of North Sudan military's war crimes against them.

C. Louis Perrinjaquet, M.D., M.P.H., known universally as "Doc PJ," earned his medical degree at the University of Iowa and completed his family practice residency at the University of Iowa Hospitals and Clinics. He earned his Masters in Public Health (M.P.H.) from Harvard University. He is a founding diplomat of the American Board of Holistic Medicine, and has a certificate of added qualification in sports medicine, and a diploma in tropical medicine and hygiene from the University of London.

John P. Sutter, M.D., has an interest in global health and tropical medicine, and has volunteered for medical missions in remote areas of Africa and Southeast Asia. He is most grateful to Bishop Macram Gassis of the Diocese of El Obeid through whom he was able to volunteer at Mother of Mercy Hospital in Gidel, Nuba Mountains. He lives in the Washington, D.C., area and works at a health center for homeless veterans.

Samuel Totten is professor emeritus at the University of Arkansas, Fayetteville (1987–2012). His areas of research include the Darfur genocide and the genocide by attrition in the Nuba Mountains, Sudan. In 2004, he served as one of the 24 investigators with the U.S. State Department's Atrocities Documentation Project (ADP), collecting data on whether genocide had been perpetrated in Darfur by the Government of Sudan (GoS). For the past twelve years he has conducted field-based research in the refugee camps in eastern Chad and in the Nuba Mountains of Sudan.

George Tutu was born in the Nuba Mountains, but now resides in Denver, Colorado. A longtime activist, he has returned time and again to the war-torn Nuba Mountains in order to provide food and medical supplies to his people. He is a founding member of ENG (End the Nuba Genocide), and has been a major advisor to the group and the leader of many of its missions into the Nuba Mountains. He is also the founder of the Nuba Christian Family Mission, Inc.

Index

aerial bombings 5, 11, 13, 14, 39, 45, 47, 48, 67, 90, 94, 113, 124, 132, 136, 142, 154, 157, 173, 190, 196, 200, 215, 216, 217, 218, 234, 240, 256, 257
African Rights 12, 19, 251, 254
Amnesty International 18, 124, 251
amputations 49, 62, 74, 198, 206, 208, 209, 242
Andudu, Right Reverend 86, 88, 129
Animists 14, 22, 81, 105, 164, 175
Antonovs 2, 3, 4, 7, 8, 14, 28, 35, 45, 49, 51, 53, 55, 57, 58, 59, 60, 71, 89, 90, 94, 109, 110, 111, 116, 130, 131, 132, 134, 137, 138, 141, 142, 143, 144, 145, 146, 147, 148, 150, 151, 153, 156, 157, 177, 192, 195, 196, 197, 198, 200, 201, 202, 203, 213, 215, 216, 231, 232, 233, 234, 235, 236, 240, 244, 247, 257
Arabization 2, 105, 253
Arabs 4, 24, 25, 27, 29, 42, 45, 52, 75, 77, 78, 81, 83, 95, 96, 110, 120, 121, 133, 248, 252
Aziz, Abdel el Hilu 13, 30, 32, 50, 52, 86, 90, 106

Baggara 77, 78, 81, 82, 93, 175, 248, 255, 257
Bashir, Omar al 1, 2, 3, 6, 7, 9, 12, 13, 14, 16, 17, 21, 23, 25, 30, 31, 32, 35, 42, 47, 48, 52, 62, 80, 82, 83, 84, 85, 87, 89, 104, 105, 106, 108, 109, 110, 111, 112, 123, 124, 125, 133, 152, 177, 211, 217, 230, 231, 236, 251, 256
Black Africans of Darfur 21, 31, 83, 116, 117, 119, 120, 121, 124, 125, 227, 229
Blue Nile State 13, 18, 31, 32, 33, 34, 35, 42, 44, 45, 47, 52, 80, 82, 83, 87, 161, 162, 164, 168, 253, 254, 255
Boyette, Ryan 3, 4, 17, 32, 38–48, 90, 100, 110, 124, 134, 136, 146, 159, 257, 259
Byrne, Deirdre 4, 18, 50, 64–74, 189, 205, 247
bystanders 7, 16, 17, 127, 259

Camarca, Margaret 9, 210–224, 246, 259
Catena, Tom 4, 8, 9, 10, 17, 49–63, 64, 66, 67, 68, 69, 71, 73, 90, 98, 107, 108, 132, 133, 140, 149, 150, 154, 155, 156, 190, 193, 194, 195, 196, 197, 198, 200, 201, 202, 203, 204, 205, 206, 207, 208, 209, 212, 222, 230, 231, 232, 235, 236, 238, 239, 240, 242, 243, 248, 254, 259
Catholicism 4, 15, 18, 50, 54, 65, 66, 77, 78, 85, 98, 189, 201, 205, 210, 211, 246, 259
caves 2, 3, 15, 48, 55, 90, 92, 94, 108, 109, 132, 136, 138, 144, 159, 233, 234, 240, 241, 242, 247
Chancey, Matt 5, 101–113, 259
Charny, Israel W. 126, 246–249
children, Nuba 2, 6, 9, 10, 11, 12, 26, 29, 35, 46, 47, 49, 51, 52, 53, 57, 60, 61, 62, 66, 69, 71, 72, 78, 81, 90, 94, 95, 96, 107, 108, 109, 110, 111, 112, 113, 122, 125, 133, 140, 147, 153, 154, 155, 159, 164, 171, 172, 175, 177, 178, 181, 182, 187, 190, 194, 195, 197, 200, 206, 207, 216, 217, 220, 222, 231, 232, 233, 236, 237, 238, 239, 242, 252, 256
Christians 1, 3, 4, 5, 6, 7, 8, 12, 14, 15, 16, 27, 38, 32, 45, 64, 73, 74, 76, 77, 78, 81, 82, 84, 85, 86, 87, 88, 93, 94, 101, 103, 105, 106, 107, 112, 122, 124, 127, 136, 138, 161, 164, 168, 171, 175, 182, 188, 203, 209, 210, 211, 212, 224, 230, 238, 249, 252
citizen journalists 4, 32, 257
civilians, Nuba 2, 3, 4, 9, 11, 13, 14, 15, 18, 28, 29, 30, 34, 34, 40, 45, 46, 49, 71, 90, 124, 125, 129, 130, 134, 137, 141, 145, 146, 147, 152, 164, 167, 173, 175, 177, 179, 201, 216, 217, 227, 228, 231, 233, 244, 253, 255, 256
cluster bombs 28, 111, 113, 147
Comboni missionaries 29, 55, 78, 201, 213, 214, 224
Comprehensive Peace Agreement (CPA) 1, 6, 13, 14, 32, 123, 164, 253, 254, 256

Conflict in the Nuba Mountains: From Genocide by Attrition to the Contemporary Crisis 15, 19, 254
The Congressional Record 126
Cox, Baroness Caroline 1–10

Darfur 9, 13, 18, 21, 31, 32, 33, 34, 35, 41, 42. 44, 45, 47, 52, 83, 87, 104, 105, 111, 112, 116, 117, 118, 119, 120, 121, 122, 124, 125, 227, 228, 229, 255
"Dar Fur: For Water" (documentary) 21
deaths from aerial attacks 5, 11, 13, 14, 39, 45, 47, 48, 67, 90, 94, 113, 124, 132, 136, 142, 154, 157, 173, 190, 196, 200, 215, 216, 217, 218, 234, 240, 256, 257
Doctors Without Borders 13, 18, 109, 182, 198, 221, 222, 237; *see also* Médecins Sans Frontières or MSF
drones 35, 36, 73, 131, 132, 157, 215
"Drones Over Roots of Humanity" (documentary) 36

election: Governor of South Kordofan 13, 14, 32, 52
El Obeid Diocese 55, 71, 260
End Nuba Genocide (ENG) 7, 91–93, 93–96, 96–98, 99, 127, 128–132, 134, 136, 166, 168, 169, 174, 177, 179, 183, 184, 185, 187, 259, 260
Episcopal churches 77, 78, 79, 81, 82, 84, 85, 86, 87, 93, 128, 184
Eyes and Ears of God (organization) 32, 33, 100, 257
"Eyes and Ears of God—Video Surveillance of Sudan" (documentary) 33

Facing Genocide: The Nuba of Sudan 19, 23, 251, 252
Flint, Julie 23, 25, 31, 32, 253
food insecurity 18, 151, 152, 153, 157
foxholes 14, 57, 59, 60, 89, 129,

261

262 Index

138, 174, 196, 197, 201, 207, 216, 217, 234, 247
Friends of Nuba (organization) 31

Gabush, Father 78, 79, 80, 81
Garang, John 31, 80, 99
Gassis, Bishop Macram 50, 68, 69, 71, 72, 73, 191, 202, 211, 260
genocide by attrition 2, 3, 7, 12, 14, 15, 19, 121–124, 127, 251 253, 254
Genocide by Attrition: Nuba Mountains, Sudan 15, 238, 253
Genocide in Sudan: Investigating Atrocities in the Sudan 117
German Doctors Hospital 27, 30, 155, 156
Golden Rule 16
Government of Sudan (GoS) 1, 2, 3, 5, 6, 7, 13, 14, 15, 18, 23, 26, 30, 31, 35, 45, 48, 49, 72, 79, 83, 84, 85, 86, 89, 92, 93, 94, 96, 99, 105, 106, 107, 109, 111, 116, 117, 119, 120, 121, 122, 123, 124, 125, 128, 134, 136, 137, 138, 141, 142, 143, 146, 147, 150, 151, 152, 153, 154, 156, 157, 158, 162, 163, 164, 165, 166, 168, 169, 173, 175, 176, 177, 178, 211, 215, 218, 219, 227, 234, 251, 252, 253, 254, 257, 260
Graham, Franklin 38, 220
Greater Nuba Action Coalition (GNAC) 7, 98, 183–188, 259

Haroun, Ahmed 13, 14, 32, 52, 123, 124
Heiban 4, 32, 53, 82, 109, 138, 142, 146, 147, 148, 156, 159, 196, 218
holes (foxholes) 14, 57, 59, 60, 89, 129, 138, 174, 196, 197, 201, 207, 216, 217, 234, 247
Holy Cross Primary School (Nuba Mountains) 9
Human Rights Watch 18, 124, 159, 251, 252
humanitarian aid 75–100, 101–113, 114–159, 160–188

injuries from GoS aerial attacks 2, 3, 4, 7, 8, 14, 28, 35, 45, 49, 51, 53, 55, 57, 58, 59, 60, 71, 89, 90, 94, 109, 110, 111, 116, 130, 131, 132, 134, 137, 138, 141, 142, 143, 144, 145, 146, 147, 148, 150, 151, 153, 156, 157, 177, 192, 195, 196, 197, 198, 200, 201, 202, 203, 213, 215, 216, 231, 232, 233, 234, 235, 236, 240, 244, 247, 257
Internally Displaced Persons (IDPs) 123, 125, 137, 147, 148, 150, 153, 154, 155, 173, 187
International Criminal Court (ICC) 13, 105, 124, 244, 256
International Media 4, 42, 112, 124, 125, 126, 166, 188, 251, 255
Islam 12, 16, 105, 106, 150, 164, 212, 227
Islamists 1, 2, 23, 25, 34, 83, 105, 106, 107

Islamization 1, 5, 25, 105, 164, 175, 253

Janjaweed 34, 83, 105, 116, 117, 119, 227, 228
Jefferson, John 7, 91, 95, 98, 127, 134, 160–188, 246, 259
Jesus Christ 4, 8, 53, 54, 64, 73, 74, 76, 77, 94, 136, 182, 188, 209, 210, 211, 224
Jihad 1, 5, 6, 83, 111, 254

Kadugli 6, 14, 25, 32, 52, 79, 82, 86, 106–107, 123, 125, 134, 137, 138, 153, 234, 242
"The Kafi Story" (documentary) 23
Kao Nyaro 7, 34, 93–96, 96–98, 99, 134, 151, 153, 174, 176–179, 181, 183, 185, 187, 188
Kauda 9, 13, 14, 32, 50, 52, 53, 54, 55, 57, 60, 62, 67, 106, 107, 110, 122, 123, 124, 128, 129, 131, 132, 137, 138, 141, 142, 146, 147, 150, 151, 152, 153, 156, 157, 192, 196, 207, 217, 219, 222, 230, 231, 233, 234
Kelley, Alan 161, 162, 163, 166, 179, 187
Kodok 33, 34, 93, 96, 97, 98, 99, 176 179–184, 185, 187, 188
Kristof, Nicholas 42, 124. 125, 126, 166, 167, 188
Kriznar, Tomo 3, 18, 21–37, 247, 248, 257, 260
Kuwa, Yusef 6, 25, 30, 79, 80, 81, 103, 105, 253
Kurchee 32, 129, 130, 137, 157, 158, 234
Kwalib 137, 138, 139, 141, 146, 147, 151, 153, 156, 157, 159, 242

landmines 90, 162
The Last of the Nuba 3, 22, 37
Little Workers of the Sacred Hearts 4, 5, 65, 66, 259

Mahdi, Sadiq al 78, 80, 82
Malakal 79, 93, 96, 98, 134, 174, 179
malnutrition 4, 6, 11, 12, 15, 39, 71, 72, 91, 122, 129, 132, 133, 140, 144, 148, 151, 153, 154, 155, 159, 161, 163, 177, 178, 181, 182, 190, 194, 231, 234, 236, 237, 245, 253, 256
MASH Unit 8, 53, 206
Médecins Sans Frontières (MSF) 13, 18, 109, 182, 198, 221, 222, 237
medical care 4, 5, 8, 9, 10, 18, 49–63, 65–74, 108, 110, 189–203, 204–209, 210–224, 225–245, 238–245, 259
medical missionaries 49–63, 65–74, 189–210, 204–209, 210–224, 225–245
Mother of Mercy Hospital 4, 5, 8, 9, 18, 49–63, 65–74, 90, 108, 110, 189–203, 204–209, 210–224, 230–236, 238–245

Mother Teresa 9, 65, 224
The Muslim Brotherhood 81, 95
Muslims 1, 4, 8, 12, 14, 22, 42, 45, 73, 81, 105, 106, 124, 164, 203, 249, 252

National Congress Party 255
National Intelligence and Security Service 83
National Islamic Front (NIF) 1, 5, 6, 103, 104, 255
Neroun, Phillip 5, 103, 253
"New Sudan" 13
Nile River 33, 93, 96, 98, 134, 136, 179, 180, 181, 187, 255
Nimeiri, Gaafar el 29, 79, 80, 81, 82
No-Fly Zone 2, 68, 128, 157
"No Go Zones" 6, 104
Nuba Christian Family Mission (NCFM) 5, 85, 86, 87, 168
Nuba Mountain Political Association 78, 79
Nuba Relief, Rehabilitation, and Development Organization (NRRDO) 2, 5, 24, 28, 32, 85, 87, 90, 93, 103, 128, 129, 130, 153, 156, 169, 174, 176, 177, 188, 233, 234
Nuba Reports 4, 23, 41, 43, 90, 100, 110, 113, 137, 145, 257, 259
Nuba Revolutionary Movement 78, 79
Nuba Survival (an organization) 23, 257
"Nuba, the Pure People" (documentary) 24, 25, 29, 31, 257
Nuba Water Project 230

Oil and Conflict in Sudan 27
Operation Lifeline Sudan (OLS) 30, 103, 104, 161, 162

"peace camps" 26, 254
The People of Kau 3, 22, 34, 37
Persecution Project 5, 6, 103, 104, 105, 106, 109, 110, 112, 143, 159, 259
Perrinjaquet, C. Louis 9, 87, 90, 225–245, 260
Phillips, Brad 5, 102, 103, 104, 105, 106, 107, 108, 109, 143, 145, 159

Rahal, Suleiman 23, 31
rainy season 5, 27, 46, 91, 94, 118, 127, 133, 136, 143, 159, 170, 171, 175, 185, 194, 205, 218, 220, 221, 234, 253
referendum 13, 31, 32, 52, 63, 123
The Republic of South Sudan 1, 13, 15, 17, 236
Riefenstahl, Leni 3, 21–26, 29, 34, 36, 37, 248
Russia 28, 72, 83, 192

Samaritan's Purse 3, 38, 39, 41, 137, 151, 154, 158, 162, 220, 238
Satellite Sentinel Project 43
Second Sudanese Civil War (1983–

2005) 13, 23, 27, 63, 81, 123, 133, 162, 164, 212, 215, 217
Sharia law 14, 31, 79, 80, 81, 82, 124
starvation 2–4, 6–7, 12, 14, 15, 19, 39, 46, 91, 121–124, 127, 134, 153, 161, 164, 171, 178, 206, 233, 234, 237, 251 253, 254, 256
Sudan fatigue 47
Sudan Islamic Medical Association (SIMA) 227, 228
Sudan People's Liberation Army (SPLA) 24, 30, 31, 32, 50, 51, 53, 79, 80, 81, 82, 83, 84, 86, 99, 158, 161, 163, 168, 169, 171, 188, 253, 257
Sudan People's Liberation Army—North 3, 8, 13, 14, 33, 34, 39, 45, 52, 87, 88, 89, 90, 91, 92, 93, 95, 98, 112, 128, 133, 139, 140, 146, 152, 153, 154, 156, 157, 158, 180, 188, 198, 200, 211, 219, 233, 235, 236
Sudanese Armed Forces (SAF) 15, 53, 57, 90, 125, 147, 178, 192, 193, 196, 200, 230, 233, 234, 235, 236

"Sudan's Secret War" (a documentary) 23
Sukhoi fighter jets 2, 3, 53, 55, 57, 59, 60, 62, 111, 137, 146, 147, 148, 153, 159
Sutter, John 8, 189–203, 248, 260

Television Slovenia 25, 29, 33
terror 3, 6, 44, 51, 105, 108, 132–133, 173, 209, 231, 256
Theresienstadt 26, 37, 248
Tomo Križnar Foundation 3, 35
Totten, Samuel 1, 6, 7, 11–19, 91, 114–159, 167, 168, 169, 174, 184, 238, 246, 253, 254, 256, 260
Tuto, George 5, 17, 75–100, 134, 168, 169, 175, 177, 185, 187, 248, 260

Umduran 157
UNICEF 27
United Nations 4, 5, 13, 15, 16, 18, 27, 34, 257; Declaration on Human Rights 11, 19; High Commissioner for Refugees 34; Human Rights Council 43; Peacekeeping Force (Nuba Mountains, 2011) 14; Security Council 34
United States Holocaust Memorial Museum's Committee of Conscience 126, 256
United States State Department's Atrocities Documentation Project 115–117

Waal, Alex de 23, 27, 31, 251, 252, 253, 254
"War on Terror" 6, 111
Werni 93, 95, 96
White, Billy 7, 127
World Food Program (WFP) 136, 229

Yida Refugee Camp 54, 68, 69, 87, 88, 90, 91, 92, 93, 128, 130, 131, 132, 134, 136, 137, 138, 142, 143, 145, 146, 147, 150, 151, 155, 156, 157, 158, 159, 170, 171, 173, 176, 181, 190, 191, 192, 193, 201, 202, 207, 208, 219, 220, 221, 234, 236, 237, 238

www.ingramcontent.com/pod-product-compliance
Ingram Content Group UK Ltd.
Pitfield, Milton Keynes, MK11 3LW, UK
UKHW050539150426
5217IPUK00026B/2000